Praise for *Reset Your Child's Brain*

"This practical and easy-to-read guide is a much-needed wake-up call for this digital age. Buy *Reset Your Child's Brain* for your family, your school, and your local library."

— **Kerry Crofton, PhD**, cofounder and executive director of Doctors for Safer Schools and author of *A Wellness Guide for the Digital Age*

"One of the problems worldwide that relates to this book is sleep deprivation. This has many consequences and — to put it bluntly — makes the sleep-deprived person fat, lazy, stupid, and depressed! The more that books like this expose the problem, the sooner we will be moving to a higher and more secure state of well-being!"

— **John J. Ratey, MD**, clinical associate professor of psychiatry, Harvard Medical School, and author of *Spark*

"This book looks at how electronic media use can affect the central nervous system long after the offending device has actually been used — an effect similar to that of drug addiction. It presents new studies that show how, as with drug use, functioning may not be impaired immediately, and in some cases it may even improve initially but then becomes worse. Finally, Dr. Dunckley outlines issues in diagnosis, in assessment, and most important, in treatment for battling and resetting the brain to overcome the rapidly emergent condition of Electronic Screen Syndrome."

— **Dr. Kimberly S. Young**, founder and director of the Center for Internet Addiction and www.NetAddiction.com

"Victoria Dunckley makes a convincing case that parents should be very concerned about their children's constant exposure to electronic screen–based entertainment. Citing medical research as well as her work with hundreds of patients, Dr. Dunckley explains how electronic media overwhelm children's nervous systems and impair their physical and mental functioning. Families who follow her practical approach to discontinuing electronic screen-time will see dramatic improvement in their children's health and behavior."

— **Jessica Solodar**, award-winning medical journalist and former medical writer for Massachusetts General Hospital Department of Psychiatry and the Child & Adolescent Bipolar Foundation

RESET YOUR CHILD'S BRAIN

RESET YOUR CHILD'S BRAIN

A Four-Week Plan to
End Meltdowns, Raise Grades,
and Boost Social Skills by
Reversing the Effects
of Electronic Screen-Time

Victoria L. Dunckley, MD

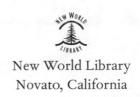

New World Library
Novato, California

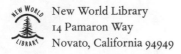

New World Library
14 Pamaron Way
Novato, California 94949

Text design by Tona Pearce-Myers

Library of Congress Cataloging-in-Publication Data
Dunckley, Victoria L., date.
Reset your child's brain : a four-week plan to end meltdowns, raise grades, and boost
social skills by reversing the effects of electronic screen-time / Victoria L. Dunckley.
       pages   cm
Includes bibliographical references and index.
ISBN 978-1-60868-284-3 (paperback) — ISBN 978-1-60868-285-0 (ebook)
  1. Video games and children—Health aspects. 2. Behavior disorders in children—Prevention. 3. Problem children—Behavior modification. 4. Internet and children. 5. Electronics—Social aspects. 6. Parenting. I. Title.
HQ784.V53D86 2015
004.67'8083—dc23   2014046885

First printing, August 2015
ISBN 978-1-60868-284-3
Printed in Canada on 100% postconsumer-waste recycled paper

New World Library is proud to be a Gold Certified Environmentally Responsible Publisher. Publisher certification awarded by Green Press Initiative.
www.greenpressinitiative.org

10   9   8   7

To all the parents, kids, and young adults I've worked with who took the road less traveled by going screen-free. Your efforts, candid feedback, and creative ideas have helped many others already, and will hopefully help many more through this book. I salute you all.

CONTENTS

Part Two — The Reset Solution:
A Four-Week Plan to Reset Your Child's Brain

Part Three — Beyond the Reset:
Action Plans for Home, School, and Community

SOMETHING WICKED
THIS WAY COMES

Several months ago, a colleague I barely knew pulled me aside as I passed by her in the hallway at work. "Can I talk to you?" she whispered urgently. Without waiting for an answer, she launched into the litany of problems she was having with her eight-year-old son, Ryan. Over the past year, Ryan had become increasingly depressed, irritable, and isolated. Meltdowns and tears over seemingly minor incidents had become a daily occurrence. He was spending less time with his friends, preferring to remain alone in his room for hours, playing games on his cell phone. He was failing nearly every subject in school, and his teachers felt frustrated with his distractibility and lack of organization.

Ryan had been evaluated and treated by two child psychiatrists and three therapists over a six-month period. He was first given a diagnosis of attention deficit disorder, then high-functioning autism, and finally bipolar disorder. He was on his fourth medication trial, but his mother felt each regimen only made him worse.

"I don't know what to do at this point," she said, frowning. "I feel like something's being missed. I wanted your opinion about all this medication."

Sidestepping the medication question, I explained to her that I see children with Ryan's "problem" every day, and I gave her some background on how electronic screen devices irritate the brain and overstimulate the nervous system, especially in children. And I advised her to try a seemingly radical — yet simple — plan before considering any more changes: to remove all video games, handheld electronic devices, computers, and cell phones from Ryan's possession for three weeks — in essence, to put Ryan on an "electronic fast."

As we talked further, the explanation began to make sense to her, especially when it occurred to her that Ryan had received his first cell phone — a "smart" one at that — the year before, shortly before the onset of his troubles. Desperate for some improvement, my colleague immediately took action and stuck to the plan I outlined.

Four weeks later, she sought me out and excitedly reported that Ryan was doing "much, MUCH better." Her face, body, and even her speech seemed more relaxed. She was inspired enough to continue the "electronic abstinence," and six months later, Ryan would be weaned off all medication. His grades had improved, and he was playing outside with his friends again.

"He's back to himself," she told me proudly.

Why had Ryan been so significantly misdiagnosed, even by well-respected professionals — two of whom were faculty at a major academic institution in Los Angeles? And why had he been placed on so many medications, none of which seemed to help? Unfortunately, Ryan's experience with receiving ineffective mental health treatment is hardly unique. But before we get to the underlying reasons, consider some emerging trends in childhood mental health disorders. In a mere ten-year span from 1994 to 2003, the diagnosis of bipolar disorder in children increased forty-fold.[1] Childhood psychiatric disorders such as ADHD (attention deficit hyperactivity disorder), autism spectrum disorders, and tic disorders are on the rise.[2] Between 2002 and 2005, ADHD medication prescriptions rose by 40 percent.[3] Mental illness is now the number one reason for disability filings for children, representing half of all claims filed in 2012, compared to just 5 to 6 percent of claims twenty years prior.[4]

Now consider that this rise in childhood psychosocial and neurodevelopmental issues has increased in lockstep with the insidious growth of electronic-screen exposure in daily life. Not only are children exposed to ever-increasing amounts of screen-time at home and in school, but exposure is beginning at ever-younger ages. Children aged two to six now spend two to four hours a day screen-bound — during a period in their lives when sufficient healthy play is critical to normal development.[5] Computer training in early-years education — including in *preschool* — has become commonplace, despite lack of long-term data on learning and development.[6] And according to a large-scale survey conducted by the Kaiser Family Foundation in 2010, children ages eight to eighteen now spend an average of nearly *seven and a half hours a day* in front of a screen — a 20 percent increase from just five years earlier.[7]

Handheld and mobile devices account for most of the more recent growth. These devices compound toxicity due to the fact that they are held closer to the eyes and body, are used more frequently throughout the day, and tend to be used during activities that previously facilitated conversation (such as riding in the car and eating out). From 2005 to 2009, cell phone ownership among children nearly doubled; about one-third of ten-year-olds now have their own mobile phone.[8] Two-thirds of American teens now own cell phones, and 70 percent own an iPad, tablet, or similar device with Internet capability.[9] And according to a 2010 Nielsen report, US teens text over four thousand times a month, or about 130 times a day.[10]

No doubt, modern-day life presents unique challenges to children's brains, minds, and social development for parents and clinicians alike that have never been encountered before. The explosion of Internet use, video gaming, cell phone use, and texting is a relatively new phenomenon, and the full implications of such excessive technology exposure have yet to be played out. As I write this, the iPad and other tablets have taken us by storm in just a few short years. Meanwhile, despite a growing body of evidence that suggests electronic screen media exposure inherently causes harm — beyond simply wasting time or being sedentary — much of the research on this development remains disparate, highly technical, or overly focused on limited concerns, such as violent games or Internet addiction. Review of the research on "typical" use is difficult to evaluate, in part because what is typical is constantly evolving, and in part because relevant studies are being conducted in a variety of fields, ranging from sociology to quantum physics, making findings difficult to assimilate.

Adding to the confusion is the unfortunate fact that the public receives conflicting messages about electronic media's effects on the brain from the press on a nearly daily basis. People have no way of easily determining whether a particular study is considered methodologically sound, whether any of the researchers had financial conflicts of interest, whether the media sensationalized the findings, or whether they're hearing about a study so prominently because of a heavily funded and carefully orchestrated press release. As such, it's difficult to get a sense of what the balance of unbiased research shows. Parents are given vague advice to "moderate" usage and are often led to believe that limiting screen-time only applies to video game play. They're told to avoid violent games, but that educational games might give a child an "edge" over peers or even enhance his or her intelligence. They've heard of Internet and gaming addiction, but they are encouraged to feel safe if their child does not meet strict addiction criteria.

Nevertheless, many parents sense intuitively that electronic screen activity has unwanted effects on their children's behavior and mood, but they are unsure what to do about it. They feel helpless because of the sheer prevalence of electronic devices, at home and at school. At the same time, parents are *acutely* aware that it has become increasingly common for families to have at least one "problem child" who is suffering from enough dysfunction that a parent or teacher seeks help. Since the child's struggles frequently include meltdowns, falling grades, or loss of friendships, parents feel increasingly desperate to find answers *now*.

So, what's really happening to our children? Like Ryan, many youngsters exhibit ill-defined but disruptive symptoms that baffle clinicians, teachers, and parents alike, leading to premature or wrong diagnoses in a misguided attempt to name the problem and take action. In a word, these children are *dysregulated* — that is, they have trouble modulating their emotional responses and arousal levels when stressed. In fact, in 2013, a controversial new diagnosis — Disruptive Mood Dysregulation Disorder, or DMDD — debuted in the long-awaited fifth edition of the *Diagnostic and Statistical Manual of Mental Disorders* (*DSM-5*). The presentation of a child with chronic irritability, poor focus, rages, meltdowns, and truly disruptive oppositional-defiant behavior has become disturbingly commonplace, and there is legitimate concern that these children are being misdiagnosed with bipolar disorder or other conditions and being prescribed antipsychotic medication.[11] In the face of an increase in such diagnoses, psychiatrists felt it was necessary to define a new disorder that more accurately matches these children's symptoms, despite a lack of definitive proof that these symptoms indeed represent a true, organic mental health disorder.

But what if this "disorder" characterized by dysregulation is not some mysterious new plague, but environmentally related? If we ask ourselves, "What has been the biggest change in our children's environment compared to only one generation ago?" the answer is not gluten, pesticides, plastics, or food dye,* but the advent of the Internet, cell phones, and wireless communication. Might DMDD really be merely a by-product of constant bombardment from electronic screen devices, causing the brain to short-circuit?

And what if systematic removal of such screen devices provided much-needed relief, almost immediately?

A Doctor's Journey

I first became aware of the negative effects of screen-time in the early 2000s while working with particularly sensitive patients. These were children with psychiatric disorders complicated by psychological trauma. Some of these kids lived in group homes, others were in foster care, and still others had been adopted into a new family. Regardless of their current situation, they all shared a number of symptoms due to universal changes the brain and body make when presented with repeated trauma — namely, a "hair trigger" response to perceived stress that put their little bodies into a nearly constant state of fight-or-flight. This state was marked by emotional reactivity, trouble following direction, meltdowns over small frustrations, and high physiological arousal (getting "revved up" easily).

Through regular observation of these sensitive children over months and years, I discovered that even *small* amounts of video game play triggered this fight-or-flight response — the same response we were trying to assuage with therapy and blunt with medication. I started advising parents and group home staff to avoid letting these children have any video game play altogether. These kids had enough strikes against them — why add fuel to the fire? Although my advice was often met with resistance, when the intervention was followed, many of the more egregious symptoms abated quite rapidly.

---

* Admittedly, these are all offenders of mental health, but they do not constitute the biggest change in one generation.

One especially striking intervention occurred in a residential treatment facility where I worked with the children (and their staff) on site. Every week when the treatment team met, I'd be barraged with all the unfortunate events that had taken place over the previous week and pressured to make changes in medication to alter the children's behavior. Each "house" at this center had video game consoles that were used as incentives for good behavior, and every week I'd hear things like, "Jacob hit Robert over the head while they were playing a video game together on Saturday." Or "Joaquin was the only kid in the house who had good behavior on Wednesday, so we rewarded him with some video game play, but he wound up becoming really agitated and threw a chair."

I'd often get exasperated and ask things like, "Why do we even *have* video games in the house in the first place?" Most of the time my complaints fell on deaf ears, but one day some of the staff from one house approached me after the weekly meeting and said they also suspected that the games were a problem. The house leaders had held a meeting and decided they wanted to try removing the games to see if it helped keep the whole house calmer. Sure enough, one month later, the number of "special incident reports" (which were reserved for severe behaviors like overt aggressive acts) for that house dropped by one-third. Interestingly, staff also noticed that the children stopped asking about the games fairly quickly and turned naturally to healthier activities. Years later, one of the male staff who had initiated the removal of the games contacted me to ask if I was still working on increasing awareness about using this intervention and offered to write a testimonial. The dramatic difference it had made in the behavior of the children in his house stayed with him.

Another group of patients I discovered early on to be sensitive to video game play were those with tics or Tourette syndrome.* In these children, overactive areas of the brain were causing involuntary motor activity. The exacerbation of symptoms caused by video games in this group was even more obvious. With some of these children, gaming increased their overall tic frequency and severity, and with others the tics would ratchet up whenever the child actually played the game or used the computer. As with the trauma patients, removal of the video games often produced significant relief and sometimes helped us avoid medication altogether.

---

* Tourette syndrome is characterized by two or more motor and one or more vocal tics.

For all of these children, there was something about playing video games that seemed to exacerbate both neurological and psychological symptoms by putting the brain and body into overdrive. Although my initial observations and efforts focused specifically on video games, over time it became apparent that fight-or-flight reactions occurred with other interactive screen devices as well, such as laptops and smartphones. Eventually, I found these effects were noticeable not just in children with major psychiatric disturbances, but also in children with "plain-old" ADHD symptoms. Ultimately, I realized even "typical" children (without any diagnoses) could experience less extreme but nonetheless disruptive symptoms — which meant it wasn't just highly sensitive children or those with psychiatric disorders who were vulnerable to adverse effects, but potentially *any* child.

Feeling certain I was on to a significant connection, I began prescribing video game restriction more widely and more strictly — with startling results. While perhaps only a minority of children are truly "addicted" to video games, I observed how the vast majority of children exhibited certain symptoms surrounding game play — symptoms strikingly similar to amphetamine exposure — that resolved within days or weeks of complete abstention. I watched what happened before and after the intervention, which I came to call an *electronic fast*, tracked objective measures (like grades or homework completion), and observed what happened when parents inevitably "reintroduced" screens. I paid attention to what it took to convince parents that the fast was worthwhile, what anxieties they had about how to do it, and what impact my delivery had. I learned by watching the children over long periods what worked and what didn't, and I noticed how their development would grow by leaps and bounds when screens were most restricted. I also saw how screen-time had a sneaky way of reinserting itself into families' lives, and that — much like management of diet or finances — screen-time management was an ongoing process.

Importantly, I realized that the more information the parents had and the better they understood the underlying mechanisms connecting screen-time and symptoms, the better they were at regulating exposure, and the more quickly they could get a handle on problems before they spun out of control. When I set up an online course based on my experience (dubbed "Save Your Child's Brain"), I received dozens of emails from mothers around the world, and I learned from those examples, too. Many of the mothers said they intuitively thought screens might be the cause of their child's symptoms but that their concerns had been ignored by their child's doctor or therapist. Hearing about the experiences of other parents helped them to stick to their guns and lose the screens, and I was encouraged that my message was resonating and having such a positive effect.

Perhaps serendipitously, even as I was continuing to counsel parents about reducing their children's exposure to electronic screens, I began experiencing pronounced electronic screen sensitivity myself! If I spent several hours writing, and especially if I was on the Internet for extended periods poring over studies, I'd wind up feeling spacey, forgetting things, lashing out at my husband, and sleeping poorly. I'd even experience a rash on my face around my eyes if I used my laptop for an extended period of time. By necessity, I was forced to find ways to make my brain and body tolerate the time I needed to work at my computer; fortunately, I devised numerous helpful strategies, which I'll discuss in chapter 10.

Finally, about five years ago I began expanding my studies into the fascinating world of integrative medicine. Integrative practitioners learn to look at patients in a holistic manner, and they systematically uncover environmental influences — such as diet, lack of exercise, or exposure to toxins — that may be triggering and maintaining a patient's symptoms. Modifying these factors not only reduces aggravation, it frees up the body to self-heal. In general, for most chronic conditions, integrative clinicians favor natural methods over pharmaceuticals; they do prescribe medications, but they seek to use them sparingly. This is because, aside from nasty side effects we can see, we are now discovering that many medications (including psychotropics) deplete various nutrients or cause some other metabolic imbalance in the brain or body. In psychiatry, it's often the case that medication solves one problem but produces another. For example, medications that help with attention often cause sleep problems, and medications that address mood often cause lethargy or weight gain. Thus, the importance of avoiding *unnecessary* medication in children — whose brains and bodies are more sensitive — cannot be overstated. This is not to say psychiatric medications are never appropriate for children; indeed, they serve an important role. But they should be used conservatively, always with risks and benefits in mind, and always in conjunction with other interventions that minimize the need for them. And they certainly shouldn't be used merely to counteract overstimulation arising from environmental influences that are within our control.

It is astonishing how much chronic disease is caused by lifestyle choices. But while it takes more energy, both on the physician's and the patient's part, to heal in a natural, integrated fashion rather than just getting a quick fix with a prescription, it is equally astonishing how much can be reversed.

How to Use This Book

This book is intended to expose and explain how interactive screen-time creates and exacerbates psychiatric symptoms, and it provides parents with a practical, proven solution to reverse such changes. Part 1 introduces the phenomenon I call *Electronic Screen Syndrome* (ESS) — a constellation of symptoms from exposure to electronic screen media characterized by a state of hyperarousal (fight-or-flight) and mood dysregulation — and it examines case studies ranging from the severely emotionally disturbed child to the high-functioning child with isolated behavior or social issues. We'll explore how screen devices interface with a child's physiological systems, altering brain chemistry, arousal level, hormones, and sleep, ultimately interfering with thinking, mood, behavior, and social skills. We'll see how these changes can eventually masquerade as full-blown psychiatric disorders, whether the child has any underlying disorders or not, and create growing dysfunction across multiple dimensions, as well as how a "screen-liberated" brain improves over the weeks, months, and years to come.

Part 2 provides the detailed, step-by-step plan I've used with hundreds of children and parents to minimize and reverse the harmful effects of ESS. This proven four-week program consists of a week-long preparation phase and a three-week electronic fast, and it can effectively "reset" a child's brain. Much of the plan is dependent on proper planning and structure, and you'll receive plenty of practical instruction on how to set yourself up for success, as well as how to handle any pitfalls you may encounter, such as handling resistance from others. You'll also learn how to navigate screen-time *after* the Reset, both in the immediate aftermath and over the long haul. Part 3 addresses concerns parents inevitably bring up as they embark on the program — what to do about school-related screen-time, how to protect children if complete lack of screen exposure isn't possible, and how to build community awareness. There are also three appendices: one outlines screen-time's various physiological effects in table format; one describes the potential health effects of electronic-related radiation; and one answers the most frequently asked questions I hear from parents.

Although you may be tempted to jump right to the Reset itself (part 2), to get the most out of the book and maximize the program's effectiveness, I suggest you read part 1 first. The more you understand about the nature of ESS, the more conviction and motivation you'll have to follow through. If you are eager to get right to it, though, you could read part 1 during the first week of the fast. My hope is that this book empowers you to take action and inspires you to implement a treatment strategy that's effective, broad-reaching, 100 percent safe, and essentially free.

So what you can you expect from the Reset? Based on utilizing a strict electronic fast in over five hundred children, teens, and young adults, and observing the changes during and following the fast, I have found that in children with diagnosed psychiatric disorders, about 80 percent will show marked improvement (symptom reduction of at least 50 percent) *across all psychiatric symptom and diagnostic categories*. In children without an underlying disorder, the percentage may be even higher, and of those who respond positively, about half will show a complete *resolution* of symptoms (that is, cessation of tantrums, chronic irritability, poor focus, and so on), and the other half will show marked improvement. You can expect to see a happier child with better focus and organization, improved compliance, and more mature social interactions. Beyond relief from the worst aspects of ESS, my goal for your child is not just symptom relief, but optimization of brain, mind, and social development.

PART ONE

IS YOUR CHILD'S BRAIN AT RISK?

The Inconvenient Truth about Electronic Screen Media

CHAPTER 1

ELECTRONIC SCREEN SYNDROME

An Unrecognized Disorder

In diagnosis, think of the easy first.
— Martin H. Fischer

Consider the following questions:

- Does your child seem revved up a lot of the time?
- Does your child have meltdowns over minor frustrations?
- Does your child have full-blown rages?
- Has your child become increasingly oppositional, defiant, or disor-ganized?
- Does your child become irritable when told it's time to stop playing video games or to get off the computer?
- Do you ever notice your child's pupils are dilated after using elec-tronics?
- Does your child have a hard time making eye contact after screen-time or in general?
- Would you describe your child as being attracted to screens "like a moth to a flame"?
- Do you ever feel your child is not as happy as he or she should be, or that your child is not enjoying activities like he or she used to?

- Does your child have trouble making or keeping friends because of immature behavior?
- Do you worry your child's interests have narrowed recently, or that these interests mostly revolve around screens? Do you feel his or her thirst for knowledge and natural curiosity has been dampened?
- Are your child's grades falling, or is he or she not performing academically up to his or her potential — and no one is certain why?
- Have teachers, pediatricians, or therapists suggested your child might have bipolar disorder, depression, ADHD, an anxiety disorder, or even psychosis, and there's no family history of the disorder?
- Have multiple practitioners given your child differing or conflicting diagnoses? Have you been told your child needs medication, but this doesn't feel right to you?
- Does your child have a preexisting condition, like autism or ADHD, whose symptoms seem to be getting worse?
- Does your child seem "wired and tired," like they're exhausted but can't sleep, or they sleep but don't feel rested?
- Does your child seem lazy or unmotivated and have poor attention to detail?
- Would you describe your child as being stressed, despite few or no stressors you can clearly point to?
- Is your child receiving services in school that don't seem to be helping?

If these questions strike a familiar chord, like many other parents you may be confronted with difficulties all too common in today's electronically saturated world. These days, parenting a child who is struggling with behavior, mood, or cognitive issues is fraught with confusion and frustration: What's causing the problem? Where do we focus our resources? Does my child need formal testing? Should we get a second opinion, and from whom — a neurologist? A psychiatrist? A psychologist or educational specialist? And so on. Many parents feel lost; they are unsure of what's going on and often receive conflicting advice, leading them to feel pulled in different directions. They seek multiple opinions, scour the Internet for information, ask other parents what's worked for them, and agonize over whether to try medication. Parents often report that the process winds up feeling like they're simply going in circles. This paralysis of analysis is costly — in terms of time, money, resources, and a child's self-esteem.

You might notice that the quiz questions above cover a wide variety of dysfunction, but they all represent scenarios — related to symptoms, functioning, or treatment effectiveness — that can occur when a child starts operating from a more primitive part of the brain. During this state, two things tend to happen: 1) symptoms and functioning worsen, and 2) interventions don't work very well. Thus, the goal is to find out what's causing this state. Regardless of what your child's particular issues are, if they're not being managed adequately, it's safe to assume that *something is being missed*. Wouldn't it be nice if that *some*thing could be the *same* thing for each and all of these issues? If addressing one thing improved functioning across the board, whether your child carried multiple diagnoses or none at all?

To see how this might be possible, consider the following three cases:

Diagnosed with autism, six-year-old Michael was receiving in-home behavioral services. When he suddenly developed severe obsessive-compulsive symptoms, his treatment team called me for a consult. Upon learning he was earning video game time daily as a reward, I convinced the family and treatment team to try the Reset Program before initiating any medication. Four weeks later his obsessive-compulsive symptoms had diminished substantially, and as an added bonus he made better eye contact and displayed a brighter mood.

Calla was a high school junior who struggled with severe mood swings and insomnia. Calla's treatment providers suspected she was bipolar, and her defiant attitude and dramatic displays of emotion had recently landed her in a class reserved for kids with emotional problems, which only made things worse. Frustrated after a particular medication trial caused a rapid weight gain, Calla and her mother wound up in my office. After much discussion, they agreed to try the electronic fast as part of an overall treatment plan. Six weeks later, the sweet girl underneath all that turmoil resurfaced. Within six months, Calla was sleeping soundly, following the rules at home and school, and had lost ten pounds. By the end of the school year, she was back in mainstream classes.

Eight-year-old Sam was a typical kid with no formal diagnosis who had always enjoyed learning. But in third grade, Sam's math and reading achievement scores dropped inexplicably, and he began to dread going to school. He was nearly constantly in trouble for being disruptive, and both his teacher and the school psychologist suggested to his mother that Sam might have ADHD. Yet within two months of completing the Reset Program, Sam was turning in more assignments, getting glowing reports from his teacher about his "attitude change," and making steady progress in math and reading.

Though their individual presentations varied, each child was essentially in a state of *dysregulation* — that is, they lacked the ability to modulate mood, attention, and/or level of arousal in a manner appropriate to the given environment or stimulus. Something was irritating these kids' nervous systems, making it difficult to handle everyday life. All three kids felt miserable and out of control, their families felt taken hostage by whatever had taken hold of their child, and their support teams struggled to identify what was being missed. Yet all three children responded to the same simple intervention. The fact that each child's nervous system renormalized with an electronic fast suggests that screen-time played a role in the development of each child's decline.

The Dawn of a New Disorder

Like many other aspects of our fast-paced but often sedentary lifestyle, screen-time is introducing new variables into the health equation. Screen-time affects our brains and bodies at multiple levels, manifesting in various mental health symptoms related to mood, anxiety, cognition, and behavior. Because the effects of screen-time are complicated and diverse, I've found it helpful to conceptualize the constellation of common phenomena as a syndrome — what I call *Electronic Screen Syndrome* (ESS). Importantly, ESS can occur in the absence of a psychiatric disorder and yet mimic one, or it can occur in the face of an underlying disorder and exacerbate it.

ESS is essentially a disorder of dysregulation. Because it's so stimulating, interactive screen-time shifts the nervous system into fight-or-flight mode, which leads to dysregulation and disorganization of various biological systems. Sometimes this stress response is immediate and obvious, such as while playing a video game. At other times the stress response is more subtle, taking place gradually from repetitive screen interaction, such as frequent texting or social media use. Or it may be delayed, brewing under the surface but managed well enough, then erupting once years of screen-time have accumulated. Regardless, over time, repeated fight-or-flight and overstimulation of the nervous system from electronics will often eventually culminate in a dysregulated child. The sidebar "Characteristics of Electronic Screen Syndrome in Children" (page 17) provides a good idea of what ESS looks like.

One way to think about the syndrome is to view electronics as a stimulant (in essence, not unlike caffeine, amphetamines, or cocaine): electronic screen device use puts the body into a state of high arousal and hyperfocus, followed by a "crash." This overstimulation of the nervous system is capable of causing a variety of chemical, hormonal, and sleep disturbances in the same way other stimulants can. And just as drug use can affect a user long after all traces of the drug are out of the body, electronic media use can affect the central nervous system long after the offending device is actually used. Furthermore, also like drug use, functioning may not be impaired immediately, and in some cases it may even *improve* initially, but then become worse. In fact, abuse and addiction of stimulant drugs such as cocaine and methamphetamine have a very similar presentation to that of ESS, including mood swings, concentration problems, and restricted interests outside of the substance or activity of choice.

Characteristics of
Electronic Screen Syndrome in Children

1. The child exhibits symptoms related to mood, anxiety, cognition, behavior, or social interaction due to *hyperarousal* (an overly aroused nervous system) that cause significant dysfunction in school, at home, or with peers. Typical signs and symptoms mimic chronic stress or sleep deprivation and can include irritable, depressed, or rapidly changing moods, excessive or age-inappropriate tantrums, low frustration tolerance, poor self-regulation, disorganized behavior, oppositional-defiant behaviors, poor sportsmanship, social immaturity, poor eye contact, insomnia/non-restorative sleep, learning difficulties, and poor short-term memory. Tics, stuttering, hallucinations, and subtle or overt seizure activity may also occur. Irritability and poor executive functioning* occur in most cases and are hallmarks of the disorder.

---

* Executive functions include reasoning, judgment, task completion, planning, problem solving, and critical thinking; they take place primarily in the brain's *frontal lobe*.

2. The symptoms of ESS may occur in the absence or the presence of other psychiatric, neurological, behavioral, or learning disorders, and they can mimic or exacerbate virtually any mental health–related disorder.

3. A child with ESS is often described by parents and teachers as "stressed out," "revved up," "wired," or "out of it." Family members often remark that they "have to walk on eggshells" around the child.

4. Symptoms markedly improve or resolve with an electronic fast; that is, the strict removal of interactive electronic screen media for several weeks. To have a lasting impact, a three-week fast is typically necessary, but it may not be sufficient in some cases.

5. Symptoms often recur with the reintroduction of electronic media following a fast, particularly if screen-time exposure returns to previous levels. After a fast, some children can tolerate small amounts of screen-time with strict moderation, while others seem to relapse immediately if reexposed.

6. Frequently, the child will be intensely drawn to screen devices and will have difficulty pulling away from them.

7. Certain factors increase risk for ESS. These include male gender; younger age; preexisting psychiatric, neurodevelopmental, learning, or behavior disorders; concurrent or past psychosocial stressors; addiction tendencies or family history of addiction; younger age when first exposed to screen-time; and higher amounts of total lifetime exposure. Possible risk factors include environmentally sensitive medical conditions like asthma, food or chemical sensitivities, and sensory dysfunction. Generally speaking, boys with ADHD and/or autism spectrum disorders are at particularly high risk.

It's the Medium, Not the Message

Now that ESS has been broadly defined, let me clarify some terms and address some questions readers may have at this point.

For instance, if mental health issues arise because of screen-time, the first question is often: Is it because of the sheer *amount* of screen-time, because of the *type of activity*, or because of the *nature* of what's seen? The truth is, research suggests that *all* screen activities provide unnatural simulation to the nervous system and can cause adverse effects. But contrary to popular belief, content isn't as important as amount, and interactive screen-time causes more dysfunction than passive.

Strictly speaking, the term *screen-time* refers to any and all time spent in front of any device with an electronic screen, such as computers, televisions, video games, smartphones, iPads, tablets, laptops, digital cameras, e-readers, and so on. It includes any screen-related activity, whether for work, school, or pleasure. This includes time spent texting, video chatting, surfing the Internet, gaming, emailing, engaging in social media, using apps, shopping online, writing and word processing, reading from a device, and even scrolling through pictures on a phone.* It includes activities like playing electronic Scrabble or solitaire, "educational" electronic games or apps, and reading from a Kindle.

Interactive vs. Passive Screen-Time

In terms of impact, perhaps the most important distinction is between interactive and passive screen-time. *Interactive screen-time* refers to screen activities in which the user regularly interfaces with a device, be it a touch screen, keyboard, console, motion sensor, and so on. *Passive screen-time* refers to watching movies or television programs on a TV set from across the room. Nowadays parents often let their children watch TV shows or movies on an iPad, laptop, or handheld device, but because viewing media this way is more stimulating and dysregulating (for reasons I'll get into later), I consider this to be interactive screen-time.

Generally speaking, both interactive and passive screen-time are associated with health issues. Research indicates both types are involved in obesity,

---

* I note this particular activity because many of my adolescent female patients spend substantial time scrolling through pictures or filming short segments of things around them, and then view them throughout the day; using a phone or camera for this purpose represents a source of screen-time that may be overlooked.

attention problems, slower reading development, depression, sleep problems, diminished creativity, and irritability, to name a few.[1] What is somewhat counterintuitive with ESS, however, is that interactive screen-time is much worse than passive. Many families I work with already limit passive screen-time (such as television) but not interactive. This is because we associate passive viewing with inactivity, apathy, and laziness. In fact, parents are often encouraged to provide interactive screen-time (particularly in favor of passive screen-time), with the rationale that surely this type of activity engages the child's brain. Children are forced to think and puzzle rather than just watch, so it must be better, right? But interaction is in and of itself one of the major factors that contributes to hyperarousal,[2] so sooner or later, any potential benefit of interactivity is overridden by stress-related reactions. Furthermore, interactivity is what keeps the user engaged by providing a sense of control, choices, and immediate gratification, but unfortunately these attributes are the same ones that activate reward circuits and lead to prolonged, compulsive, and even addictive use.[3]

Burgeoning research comparing the two supports this theory that interactive screen-time is more dysregulating to the nervous system than passive. A 2012 study surveying the habits of over two thousand kindergarten, elementary, and junior high school children found that the minimum amount of screen-time associated with sleep disturbance was just thirty minutes for interactive (computer or video game use) compared to two hours for passive (television use).[4] A 2007 study demonstrated that sleep and memory were significantly impaired following a single session of excessive computer game playing, while a single session of excessive television viewing produced only mild sleep impairment and had no effect on memory.[5] And a large 2011 survey of American adolescents and adults demonstrated that interactive device use before bedtime was strongly associated with trouble falling asleep and staying asleep while passive media use was not.[6] Notably, this study also revealed that adolescents and young adults under thirty were the age group most likely to use interactive devices before bedtime, and they also reported the most sleep disturbance. Moreover, of those experiencing sleep problems, 94 percent also reported an impact on at least one area of functioning: mood (85 percent), school/work (83 percent), home/family life (72 percent), and social life/relationships (68 percent). Not coincidentally, these are the very areas of functioning the Reset Program addresses! And finally, we know that actual *brain damage* occurs from excessive Internet and video game use that looks remarkably similar to that from drug and alcohol abuse,[7] so something about the interactive nature either directly (through hyperarousal) or indirectly (through addiction processes) makes interactive screen-time more potent as well as distinct.

When implementing the electronic fast in the Reset Program, I typically allow small amounts of television or movies under certain conditions (as discussed in chapter 5). If these conditions are met, the fast is still highly effective. On the other hand, allowing even small amounts of gaming or computer play often renders the Reset useless. Thus, for the Reset Program, we are primarily concerned with eliminating *interactive* screen-time. Additionally, most parents become overwhelmed at the thought of taking away all electronics, so allowing a small amount of passive viewing of appropriate, calm content provides parents with a bit of a respite. That said, I do not take television's effects lightly, especially on the very young,* and I applaud anyone who removes *all* passive screen-time in addition to the other requirements of the fast. Regarding computer use for school purposes, I typically allow it during the Reset, but certain exceptions and rules apply (as discussed in chapters 5 and 10).

Common Misconceptions about Problematic Screen-Time

Misconceptions abound when it comes to screen-time, even among mental health professionals. For starters, it's not just violent video games that can cause dysregulation, but *any* video game — including educational or seemingly benign games, like puzzles or building games. Another myth is that it's only children who are "addicted" to gaming, Internet use, or social media who experience issues, or that screen-time only becomes a problem when parents don't restrict it. In fact, many children display symptoms from screen-time without being addicted per se, and some children become overstimulated and dysregulated with only minimal amounts of screen exposure. I see many families in which the parents limit usage to levels at or below what

---

* The American Academy of Pediatrics recommends that children under the age of three be screen-free (of both passive and interactive screen activities).

the American Academy of Pediatrics recommends (no more than one to two hours total screen-time daily),[8] but if some or most of that time is interactive, it can easily create a problem.

The truth is, every child is affected differently. Comparing your child's screen-time to his or her peers isn't helpful either, as it doesn't necessarily provide protection if it's less than others'. The average child is exposed to several fold–higher levels of electronic screen media compared to just one generation ago — not to mention the constant bombardment of wireless communication that often accompanies it.

This fact bears emphasizing: "moderate use" today amounts to exposing your child to levels of electronics use never before seen in history.

This is why I caution parents against trying to distinguish between "good" and "bad" screen-time or between "too much" and "only a little." Though understandable, this mind-set is risky. The purpose of the Reset is to provide the brain with a clean break and adequate rest to return to its natural state. The reality is that there are likely many variables — too many to sort out — between various screen activities and each individual child's makeup and vulnerabilities. But even if we could distinguish them all, these differences would likely be meaningless in the larger picture. Among all the various kinds of problematic screen-time, research is uncovering more similarities than differences. Thus, when approaching a Reset, the easiest and most productive thing to do is to lump all interactive screen-time together.

Kindle, Cartoons, and Cognitive Load

So why is it that reading a book before bed is soothing, while viewing an e-reader can be just the opposite? In either case, we are reading the same content, whether that be an adventure story or an historical account. It's that the medium itself affects the amount of energy needed to process and synthesize information, a factor researchers call *cognitive load*. Parents often ask if e-readers like the Kindle or Nook "count" as interactive devices. After all, these particular devices do not emit light, they use electronic "ink," and they are supposed to read like a regular paper book. Only they don't. Studies show that reading is slower and that recall and comprehension is impaired when using an e-reader, suggesting that the brain doesn't process the information as easily.[9] Conversely, research suggests that the sensory feedback of a real book helps us incorporate information: the weight, texture, and pressure felt from holding a book; the cracking of its spine and flipping of its pages; the buildup of turned pages that provides a sense of how far along you are in the story — all reduce the cognitive load needed to absorb the information. Finally, while e-ink displays are less visually fatiguing than LCD screens, they are still hard to visually and cognitively process because they are pixelated, display a "flash" when refreshing between pages, and don't provide 3-D input.

High cognitive load is also the reason I eliminate fast-paced cartoons for the Reset. If some TV is allowed, what's watched should be, above all, slow-paced. Cartoons of all kinds are typically much more rapidly paced today. Scene changes, movement within scenes, and plot points unfold very quickly, and all of this the brain must digest. A recent study demonstrated that just nine minutes of viewing a fast-paced cartoon impaired memory, the ability to follow direction, and the ability to delay gratification in toddlers compared to viewing a slower-paced cartoon.[10] It's not just pace, either. Intense color, fantastical events, and sudden or loud noises also contribute to sensory and cognitive overload.

The Controversy Over Electromagnetic Fields and Health

Do manmade electromagnetic fields (EMFs) play a role in ESS or other health conditions? No one denies that manmade EMFs — which arise from electronic devices themselves as well as from wireless communication (such as WiFi or mobile phone frequencies) — have biological effects. It is a basic tenet of physics that nearby electromagnetic fields influence one another. The question is whether those biological effects are meaningful. In other words, do higher levels of everyday EMF exposure translate into health issues the average person wouldn't have experienced otherwise?

At present, research on the kinds of fields produced by wireless communication is still relatively "young," and the findings are not always consistent. However, there is a growing body of objective, non-industry-funded research — that includes studies from highly respected institutions such as Columbia, Yale, and Harvard — that suggests these fields may be harmful.[11] Some of the research is highly technical and difficult to grasp; for example, some evidence suggests that extremely weak fields may be more harmful than stronger ones. Interestingly, some of the findings are strikingly similar to those found in screen-time studies, so there may be synergistic mechanisms occurring, particularly for individuals with sensitive constitutions. Personally, I feel there's fairly strong evidence that, at a minimum, manmade EMFs cause inflammation. I also think appreciating how they can interact with the nervous system (which is, after all, electrical, and thus produces an electromagnetic field itself) adds to our understanding of how electronics impact us. My best guess is that EMFs are a portion of the stress from electronics, and that proportion varies widely depending on the individual's chemical and electrical makeup.

Regardless, the *precautionary principle* dictates that when the science regarding the risks of a new technology is not yet fully conclusive — and in this case it won't be for decades — that we should proceed with caution and minimize exposure wherever possible, particularly when it comes to children. At the same time, when one fully understands the EMF science and believes there is even possible risk to the developing child, it opens a whole new can of worms — especially considering the explosive growth of wireless communications in public places, like schools.

Because this is such a complicated and emotionally charged topic, the bulk of relevant EMF information is presented in appendix B, "Electromagnetic Fields (EMFs) and Health: A 'Charged' Issue." Additionally, since it's not totally necessary to appreciate or accept the role of EMFs to address Electronic Screen Syndrome, "carving it out" reduces the amount of information you'll need to process in order to take action. You can think of the EMF appendix as an additional layer to digest whenever you're ready.

An Inconvenient Truth

Let's face it. Hearing that video games, texting, and the iPad might need to be banned from your child's life does not fill one with glorious joy. Rather, for many, it creates an immediate urge to find a way either to discredit the information or to work around it. Sometimes when I tell parents what they need to do in order to turn things around, I sense that I am losing them... their eyes shift away, they squirm, and they look like they're in the hot seat. This is not what they want to hear. It's as though I'm telling them they need to live without electricity — that is how ingrained screens are in our lives. The inconvenience of what I'm proposing can seem overwhelming. Aside from dreading the inconvenience, though, discussing ESS and the Reset often produces other negative feelings. Some folks feel as though their parenting skills are being judged, or that their efforts or level of exhaustion are under-appreciated. Other parents feel guilty or irresponsible for not setting healthier screen-time limits to begin with, or they become acutely aware that their own screen-time use is out of balance.

Let's dig a little deeper into some other negative reactions parents experience upon hearing about the effects of electronics or the fast itself. These are feelings that are sometimes pushed outside of everyday awareness, and these same feelings, when left unacknowledged, can undermine your success. Conversely, getting in touch with where any resistance is coming from will help you work through it, and it will help you understand others' resistance, too. These challenges are discussed throughout the book, but because these concerns can be preoccupying, I'd like to acknowledge them here. Below are some of the reactions parents commonly experience:

- Parents feel overwhelmed by the sheer pervasiveness of screens and are convinced that removing them all will be "way too hard."
- Parents fear the child's reaction and worry that a fast will be met with rage, despair, and tantrums.
- Parents feel guilty about taking away a pleasurable activity, and/or they are concerned the child will no longer fit in with peers.
- Parents worry about, and even resent, losing their "electronic babysitter," and they wonder how they will get household tasks done without it.
- Parents doubt that electronics are the problem, or they don't believe removing them will solve their child's problems.
- Parents worry about what others (in their family or community) will think. Will others undermine their efforts to limit screens, or view them as extremist or alarmist — and therefore not take their concerns seriously?
- Parents are annoyed by the inconvenience of removing or restricting laptops, iPads, and mobile devices they themselves use.

Of all the reactions, perhaps the hardest to deal with is guilt. No parent wants to feel they have unwittingly contributed to their child's difficulties. And many parents already harbor guilt regarding the use of electronics.

Whatever rules they have set or usage they allow, they often already feel that they are allowing "too much" and that their own use does not set the good example they'd like it to. Nor do any parents want to do something they know will put their child into a genuine state of despair; for some parents, even the *thought* of removing electronics causes them to feel tortured.

Guilt is an exquisitely uncomfortable emotion, and, as such, it is human nature to avoid feeling it. When it comes to electronics, one way parents assuage guilt is to rationalize its use: "Screen-time is the only time my kids are quiet." "Electronics allow me to get things done." "Screen-time is the only motivator that works." "It's what all the kids do, and anyway my child uses it a lot less than others." "I only let her play educational games." And so on. If you find yourself rationalizing use, simply cut yourself some slack and keep reading. I don't want you to dwell on what's already happened; I only wish to show you *there's a way out*. On the other hand, if you think you might be rationalizing use to avoid guilty feelings over taking electronics away, then just acknowledge this fact, and know that these feelings will diminish as you take action and start to see positive changes.

Aside from guilt, parents also experience anxiety about the potential impact of an electronic fast on their child: they worry about how the child will react, about what his or her peers will think (particularly if the child already has social problems), and about whether screen restrictions will breed resentment and put additional strain on an already tense parent-child relationship. Even when parents agree that screen-time is a problem, many fear that the Reset will only produce *more* stress — more headaches, more tears, more *work*. Yet while many parents feel overwhelmed initially, most report that the Reset is far easier than they imagined. This is in part because the child "gets over it" a lot faster than the parents expect, and in part because as the relief and pleasure grow from seeing their child become happier, better behaved, and more focused, the restrictions become easier for everyone to follow.

Lastly, some parents question the concept of Electronic Screen Syndrome itself. They want *scientific proof* behind the claims I make. After all, how could something so pervasive have been overlooked as a problem until now, and don't "positive" studies regarding interactive screen-time come out on a regular basis? I have two answers to this question. The first is to emphasize that despite seemingly conflicting studies presented by the popular press, there is a solid consensus in the medical community that screen-time is associated with multiple adverse outcomes — including academic, emotional, sleep-related, behavioral, and physical health issues — and that these effects may be long-lasting.[12] Indeed, this now rather large body of research is cited throughout this book, and there has been a push by the American Academy of Pediatrics to encourage physicians to discuss screen-time health risks with parents.[13] And positive studies? Even I admit there may be special cases where video games might be helpful, such as rehabilitating a limb after a serious injury. But those instances are the exception, not the norm. The vast majority of positive findings don't transfer to real-life functioning or are conclusions from studies that aren't considered methodologically sound. There will never be 100 percent consensus among researchers in any field, but with screen-related research, studies are often funded by powerful corporations or organizations with vested financial and political interests. These studies' findings are suspect to begin with, and they are also "spun" in terms of significance.

For instance, regarding the use of technology in education, it may *appear* that there is a division of scientific opinion regarding risks versus benefits. However, despite much hype and many promises, there is as yet no solid evidence that educational software enhances learning or brain development, while there is increasingly clear evidence that computer use may hamper both. Meanwhile, virtually all the "positive" research studies are industry funded.[14] Educational policy makers are often misled by such research, whose decisions trickle down to school administrators, who then buy software and licensing agreements, and so it goes.

In contrast, whether their focus is medical, psychological, or educational, serious researchers who don't have skin in the game also don't have huge public relations departments — which is why you don't always hear about their work. There is nothing inherently radical about linking screen-time usage with behavioral problems. Perhaps the most radical thing I've done is to gather a wide range of diverse symptoms under a single name and created an effective program to address it.

Which leads to my second answer to this question. Whatever specific studies show, whatever you believe about screen-time usage, the Reset Program works. That it works is the best evidence that screen-time usage, in itself, can cause behavioral, mood, and cognitive problems. Even if parents are unsure, the risks of trying an electronic fast are virtually nonexistent. The

Reset Program involves no real expenses, no medicine, and has no side effects. It's safe, widely applicable, and is shown to be highly effective across multiple domains. Yes, there are inconveniences, but what are they next to the difficulties your child is experiencing? Which, ultimately, is more inconvenient, losing the screen-time status quo or having a child who rages, who can't focus enough to learn, or who drives others away because of behaviors? What about the inconvenience of not sleeping at night because you're worried, of endlessly driving to fruitless appointments, or of spending money on treatments because you don't know what else to do? Acting on the information presented here requires mental energy and a leap of faith — but the payoff can be enormous.

Throughout the book, I present the stories and case studies of real children. Many of these stories are based on my formal work with my own patients and on my informal experience with children of friends and family, and some are from reports I've received from parents, grandparents, teachers, and therapists who've completed the website course, read my articles, or heard me speak. To protect identities, I've changed descriptive details and occasionally created composites, but the effects of screen-time and of the Reset Program are accurate to what actually happened. That said, even though I took pains not to exaggerate results, I realize that some stories sound a little too good to be true. Is it possible that something as simple as an electronic fast could resolve so many issues and situations so neatly? In fact, yes. Done properly, the Reset Program is that effective, and its benefits are that widespread. Further, these benefits can be maintained as long as the appropriate screen-time restrictions are maintained. That doesn't mean it's always easy, but for many parents, the most convincing proof that Electronic Screen Syndrome is real is seeing how the Reset Program improves the life of their own child.

Chapter 1 Take-Home Points

- When traditional mental health or educational resources are ineffective or insufficient for treating children with psychosocial issues, an environmental cause might be screen-time usage, manifesting as Electronic Screen Syndrome (ESS).

- The introduction and ubiquitous use of interactive screen devices represents a widespread new source of environmental toxicity, and it's capabilities to produce nervous system dysregulation are largely underestimated.

- Symptoms and issues associated with ESS are not due solely to screen addiction or violent content; even "moderate" screen-time can trigger fight-or-flight reactions.

- The concept of ESS was developed to capture the unifying features that explain the variety of symptoms and dysfunction that screen-time can induce.

- ESS is characterized by overstimulation and hyperarousal and defined by the presence of mood, cognitive, and/or behavioral symptoms that are relieved with strict removal of electronic devices (the Reset Program).

- Interactive screen-time is more likely to create hyperarousal and dysregulation compared with passive screen-time, and it is more likely to disrupt sleep and be associated with mood, cognitive, and social problems.

- Electronic devices create electromagnetic fields (EMFs), but whether and how EMFs negatively impact the brain is controversial and complicated; for more, see appendix B, "Electromagnetic Fields (EMFs) and Health: A 'Charged' Issue."

- Uncertainty about ESS and reluctance or resistance to trying an "electronic fast" are normal. The Reset Program requires changes in everyone's daily life in terms of screen-time usage. Anticipating these changes, and acknowledging and accounting for resistance, is essential for success.

ALL REVVED UP AND NOWHERE TO GO

How Electronic Screen Media Affects Your Child's Brain and Body

It is not stress that kills us, it is our reaction to it.

— Hans Selye

On the eve of his big sister Liz's high school graduation, nine-year-old Aiden sits with his parents and relatives at a celebration dinner, bored by their "adult" conversation and irritated at all the attention showered upon Liz.* He can't wait to get back to his video game! Before dinner, Mom had (annoyingly) called him away to join the family, and then she got mad when he spent a few minutes getting to the next level and saving his game. So many people in the house make him restless; he squirms uncomfortably and drums his fingers on the table, waiting to be excused.

Finally, he is allowed to escape the dinner table, and he settles into a corner of the living room couch to play his Nintendo DS. For the next hour or so, he is completely oblivious to the company in the house. Although he's already played much longer than his mother likes, she lets him continue, knowing these family situations are a little overwhelming for him. And besides, the game keeps him occupied. *What's the harm?* she thinks. *It's just for today.*

---

* This story is a dramatization based on true events.

However, in the meantime, a perfect storm is brewing. As the play continues, Aiden's brain and psyche become overstimulated and excited — on fire! His nervous system shifts into high gear and settles there while he attempts to master different situations, strategizing, surviving, accumulating weapons, and defending his turf. His heart rate increases from 80 to nearly 100 beats per minute, and his blood pressure rises from a normal 90/60 to 140/90 — he's ready to do battle, except that he's just sitting on the couch, not moving much more than his eyes and thumbs. The DS screen virtually locks his eyes into position and sends signal after signal: "It's bright daylight out, nowhere near time for bed!" Levels of the feel-good chemical dopamine rise in his brain, sustaining his interest, keeping him focused on the task at hand, and elevating his mood. The intense visual stimulation and activity flood his brain, which adapts to the heightened level of stimulation by shutting off other parts it considers nonessential.

The visual-motor areas of his brain light up. Blood flows away from his gut, kidneys, liver, and bladder and toward his limbs and heart — he's ready to fight or escape! The reward pathways in his brain also light up and are reinforced by the flood of dopamine. He is so absorbed in the game, he doesn't notice when his little sister, Arianna, comes over until she puts her chubby hand on the screen, trying to get his attention.

"DooOOON'T!!" he shouts and roughly shoves her out of the way. Arianna falls backward, bursts into tears, and runs to their mother, who silently curses herself for letting Aiden play this long.

"All right, that's it. Time to start getting ready for bed. Get your pajamas on and you can have a snack before you go to bed," she says, pulling the DS out of Aiden's hands and turning it off in one fell swoop.

Aiden looks at his mother with rage. How dare she ruin his game because of his stupid sister!

"Fine!" he shouts, runs up the stairs, and slams his bedroom door. His primitive brain is fully engaged now, turning him into an enraged animal ready to fight off all challengers. He rips all the sheets off his bed and then throws his lamp on the floor, providing a satisfactory crash and shatter. Thinking about how wronged he's been and filled with visions of revenge, he kicks the wall a few times and then pounds on his bedroom door, putting a big hole in it.

Downstairs, his relatives sit in quiet shock and murmur to each other how they've never seen him act like this. Dad runs up the stairs to contain his son. Calmly, his dad holds him in a bear hug from behind, waiting for the rage to subside.

As the dopamine in his brain and the adrenaline in his body begin to ebb, his rage loses its focus. Now, the pent-up energy takes on a disorganized, amorphous form. Aiden feels like he can't think straight or get himself together. While he spaces out, his dad helps him put his pajamas on and they go back downstairs. Stress hormones remain high, however, making it difficult for him to relax or think clearly. He seems a little confused, actually. His relatives look at him with a mixture of concern and love, but they also wonder why his parents let him "get away with" this kind of behavior. His mother intuitively knows that direct eye contact will overstimulate him again, so she approaches him slowly from the side, and rubs his back gently.

When his favorite aunt looks him in the face sympathetically, he immediately distrusts her intentions. Eye-to-eye interaction is interpreted by his primitive-mode brain as a challenge, and he starts getting revved up again. His mother intervenes, and takes him up to his room. She lowers the light, settles him into bed, and starts to read him a soothing story. His nervous system attempts to regulate itself back to normal, but it seems to still be held hostage by his hyped-up emotions. That night, after he does finally fall to sleep, Aiden awakens repeatedly with panic attacks — his heart races and blood pounds in his ears. He's scared of the dark, and worried that his angry outburst has upset and alienated his parents. His mother, meanwhile, confiscates the DS and decides to take it with her to work on Monday. (She really wants to throw it in the trash, but it was expensive!)

The following morning, the fight in Aiden has subsided, but the aftermath leaves him in a fog, listless, weepy, and exhausted. He experiences an increased craving for sweets while cortisol, the stress hormone, drives his blood sugar up and down erratically. It will take weeks before his body, brain, and mind return to some sense of balance.

Meanwhile, his mother reaffirms her commitment "to get rid of those damn video games."

Perceived Threat and the Fight-or-Flight Response

Does Aiden's story sound familiar? Why would a seemingly normal, loving child become so enraged and difficult after playing video games? Though his response may seem extreme, there's actually a completely natural explanation for Aiden's behavior.

Playing video games mimics the kinds of sensory assaults humans are programmed to associate with danger. When the brain senses danger, primitive survival mechanisms swiftly kick in to provide protection from harm. This response is instantaneous; it is hardwired in our genes and necessary for survival. Keep in mind that the threat does not have to be *real* — it only needs to be a *perceived* danger for the brain and body to react. Think of how you feel when watching a truly scary movie. Your heart rate increases, your stomach twists into knots, and your limbs tense, poised to react. Even though you know "it's only a movie," the graphic and threatening images produce an intense, undeniable physiological response. When this instinct gets triggered, our nervous system and hormones influence our state of arousal, jumping instantly to a state of *hyperarousal* — the fight-or-flight response. These feelings can be hard to shake off even after the movie is over, which is why even adults sometimes have nightmares afterward — usually of being attacked (fight) or of trying to run away from danger (flight).

While in medical school, we often heard this state referred to as "running from the tiger," since during ancient times humans protected themselves from predators by literally fighting or fleeing. Today, we still need this rapid stress response for emergency situations, and on a day-to-day basis mild stress reactions help us get things done. But for the most part, repeatedly enduring fight-or-flight responses when survival is not an issue does more harm than good. When the fight-or-flight state occurs too often, or too intensely, the brain and body have trouble regulating themselves back to a calm state, leading to an experience of *chronic stress*. Chronic stress is also produced when there is a "mismatch" between fight-or-flight reactions and energy expenditure, as occurs with screen-time; the physical energy needs to be discharged for the system to re-regulate. Once chronic stress sets in, brain function suffers. With children, whose nervous systems are still developing, this sequence of events occurs much faster than it does for adults, and the chronically stressed child soon starts to struggle. If your child is experiencing behavior issues, falling grades, mood swings, problems socializing, or other chronic difficulties, it is fairly safe to assume that his or her nervous system is being subjected to stress on a repeated basis.

As parents (and as clinicians), when we see children who are revved up all the time, we instinctively do all we can to make them feel safe and calm. We don't show them scary movies, take them bungee jumping, or let them hang out with rougher children. But in today's environment, our children are under nearly constant assault from electronic screen devices, and they react in the same way as they might to any other danger, resulting eventually in distressing symptoms and dysfunction — Electronic Screen Syndrome. When a child is experiencing ESS, it only makes sense to use the same strategy we use in other stressful situations: minimize stress where you can — electronic or otherwise — and minimize overstimulation. Whether or not other stressors are present, electronic screen media heightens stress states, and therefore all mental, neurological, and physical symptoms worsen in tandem. Conversely, many times when electronic stress is removed, other stressors become more manageable or are no longer experienced as stressors. Figure 1 depicts the cycle of stress and dysfunction, compounded by additional stress from interactive screen-time.

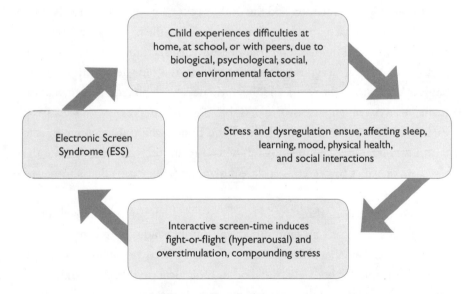

Figure 1. Electronic screen stress and stress reactions influence each other in a vicious cycle

Sensitive and Vulnerable: Eyes, Brain, and Body

Exactly *how* do electronic screen devices cause stress? To understand what factors may be affecting your child's nervous system, we need to take a closer look at the workings of the brain when confronted with the many electronic stimuli present in today's environment. Although in Aiden's case it was video game play that disrupted his behavior, it's essential to realize that *any* electronic screen interaction, regardless of content, can irritate the nervous system — "it's the medium, not the message." Why? Because the interface between the screen and your child's nervous system allows natural processes to be disturbed. The three main points of access for development of ESS are your child's eyes, brain, and body, including the body's natural energy fields. Understanding the various pathways by which electronic screens affect your child helps you appreciate why any kind of interactive screen-time can wreak havoc.

The Eyes

The eyes provide a particularly potent route for electronic screen toxicity, regardless of content being processed. How does this communication between unnatural screen stimulation and the brain occur? The eyes are directly connected to the central nervous system, which allows the physical environment to have a powerful influence on brain activity. In fact, the eyes are the only part of the central nervous system exposed to the outside world. Directly behind each eye are the retina and the optic nerve, which receive information from the environment in the form of light. The optic nerves extend back from each eye and then cross at the base of the brain, where they communicate with the small but vital pineal gland, whose main job is to help regulate the sleep-wake cycles by secreting a sleep hormone (melatonin) that's triggered by darkness.

There are at least three eye-related "routes" that can be accessed. First, because electronic screens emit unnaturally bright light, they convey information to the brain that's inconsistent with what's occurring in the real world, desynchronizing the body clock and other biological rhythms.[1] Second, interacting with a 2D screen alters normal eye muscle movements, including those used for changes in depth. This influences visual and vestibular (relating to sense of balance and body position) development, cognition, and mood regulation. Third, electronic media provides intense, unnatural, "arresting" visual stimulation that affects sensory and attention processes.[2] This is true no matter what the specific content is. Thus, screen devices affect your child through his or her eyes by light, muscle movement signals, and visual stimulation.

The eye itself may suffer as well. Aside from eye strain or "computer vision syndrome," which causes blurred vision, headaches, and dry, irritated eyes,[3] the LED light emitted from screens has been implicated in retinal damage in various laboratory and animal studies.[4] Both blue light and intense light have been implicated. Screen-time has also been linked incrementally to a narrowing of retinal blood vessels — a marker for cardiovascular disease.[5]

The Brain

The second point of access for screen activities is the brain itself. The brain is evolutionarily designed to respond to stimulating visual input — brightness, color, contrast, and movement — called the *orienting response*. Back in the day when we had to hunt, gather, or fish for our food, this kind of sensory input suggested the presence of prey or predators, and a rapid response to such input increased our odds of survival. In other words, the orienting response helps us assess a threat before we determine whether to fight or flee. When these stimuli are artificially created, however, the brain's orienting response gets hijacked, creating chemical, electrical, and mechanical shifts that raise arousal levels. When this happens repeatedly, the brain remains on heightened alert.

Screen devices access the brain on a psychological level as well; video games, for example, are purposely designed to exploit psychological needs and thus activate natural reward pathways, releasing feel-good chemicals in the brain. The brain is attracted to interactive screen-time for other psychological reasons, too, including our need for immediate gratification and responsiveness, aspects that gaming, social media, Internet use, and even texting can provide.

The Body

In addition to effects of electronic screens on the eyes and the brain are the effects on your child's body. With electronic screen interaction, blood flows away from organs like the gut and reproductive organs and toward the limbs and heart. Heart rate and blood pressure increase and stress hormones are released, preparing the body for fight-or-flight. This reaction might not be surprising when one considers how a child playing an action-oriented video game might respond, but in fact research tells us that all forms of screen-time create subtle changes in the cardiovascular system that can cause damage over time.[6] In addition, sitting for lengthy periods of time can cause unhealthy bodily changes within as little as thirty minutes, and the majority of screen-time is spent in a sedentary fashion.

The fact that screen-time is associated with *metabolic syndrome* is telling. Metabolic syndrome is a combination of high blood pressure, midsection weight gain ("spare tire"), abnormal cholesterol levels, and high fasting blood sugar. It's a serious condition that can lead to diabetes, heart disease, and stroke. Up until recently, it was rarely seen in children; now it's become common. It's unclear why it develops in some but not others, but it's thought to be related to chronic stress and poor sleep. Even more telling is the fact that the link between metabolic syndrome and screen-time holds true regardless of activity level — a finding that suggests that screen-time produces unhealthy physiological changes that are above and beyond changes seen in those with low activity levels.[7]

The Biofield

The matrix of biological electromagnetic fields present in the human body represents yet another potential interface between electronics and your child, but this will be discussed in more detail in appendix B on EMFs.

All Revved Up: Fight-or-Flight Mechanisms Related to Screen-Time

Thus, through the eyes, brain, and body, use of electronic screen media sends unnatural and overstimulating messages to the nervous system. Via these pathways, numerous mechanisms promote and maintain the fight-or-flight response, leading to the chronic hyperarousal associated with ESS. It doesn't take much screen-time exposure for some children to get all revved up because so many mechanisms can occur at once and then feed off one another. Each of these mechanisms is capable of self-perpetuating the stress cycle, while simultaneously lowering a child's resistance to future stress. Figure 2 depicts the array of screen-related factors that can elicit fight-or-flight reactions. Let's look at each of these factors in turn.

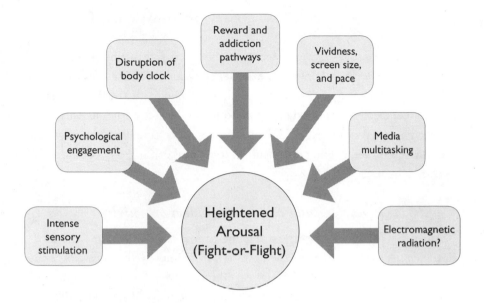

Figure 2. Screen-related factors contributing to hyperarousal or fight-or-flight

Intense Sensory Stimulation

Screen brightness, quick movements, and supersaturated colors all contribute to visual sensory overload.[8] Intense stimulation heightens attention and arousal, feeding into fight-or-flight.[9] Furthermore, excessive stimulation can overwhelm the sensory system, causing other parts of the brain to shut down in order to compensate. Afterward, the brain experiences a relative sensory deprivation, which can feel uncomfortable and lead to irritability. Some individuals may even suffer light- or screen-associated seizures, tics, and migraines when intense visual stimulation produces electrical excitability, or the overfiring of brain networks.[10] In Japan in 1997, over seven hundred people, mainly children, experienced seizures and vomiting after watching a particular Pokémon cartoon episode that utilized flashing colored lights in a scene depicting two characters in battle.[11] The vast majority of victims had never had a seizure before. While extreme, this example shows how intimate the relationship is between the eyes and the brain. We should view the visual effects from electronic screen interaction as a spectrum, with seizures, tics, and migraines representing the more severe or tangible manifestations on one end, and everyday "irritation" and general nervous system dysfunction on the other.

Another sensory-related reaction to extended screen-time is the *game transfer phenomenon*, where users experience visual hallucinations of game-related objects, like an imprint, after prolonged play.[12] Lastly, from a development perspective, repeated exposure to intense sensory stimuli leads to an overactive visual system; the child will attempt to pay attention to everything around him or her, making it difficult to focus and causing other sensory integration issues.[13]

Psychologically Engaging Content or Activity

Though not all screen activities are games, those that are add another layer to the fight-or-flight story. As the need to win or improve is repeatedly reinforced in some way during play (by earning rewards, escaping from threats, being promoted to the next level, and so on), the player becomes more and more hyperaroused. Meanwhile, the feel-good brain chemical dopamine is continually being released, causing the player to want to continue playing — often for longer than planned. The more engaging a game is, the more it increases dopamine-related attention and arousal, which reinforces itself over time and makes it harder to stop playing. Game designers are absolute *geniuses* at creating the timing and intensity of in-game rewards.[14]

In terms of content — for both video game and Internet use — violent, competitive, sexual, vivid, interesting, challenging, and bizarre images and situations all increase arousal or fight-or-flight reactions.[15] In terms of game type, role-playing games, such as multimember online role-playing games (MMORPGs), are known to be particularly addicting.[16] In part, they may be compelling because they play off of adolescent developmental needs, such as identity formation.[17] With younger children, the game Minecraft, which consists of building structures, items, and weapons out of various materials in the form of blocks — activities that seem relatively benign on the surface — is frequently described as "mesmerizing" by parents as their children become "obsessed" with it.[18]

Disruption of the Body Clock

Both natural and artificial light relay information to the brain and impact the body's biorhythms, including the sleep-wake cycle, a "circadian rhythm," and hormone cycles, which have daily, monthly, and seasonal variations.[19] As mentioned, when the brain is exposed to the unnaturally bright light of electronic screens, the sleep signal hormone melatonin is suppressed, and natural biorhythms are disrupted.[20] Additionally, light from screens tends to be rich in blue tones, which is particularly disruptive because blue light mimics daylight. Low melatonin is linked to depression and inflammatory states — such as cancer and autism — as well as alterations in hormone function, including reproductive hormones.[21] Aside from melatonin suppression, light-at-night is associated with other hormonal abnormalities, such as low growth hormone.[22] These changes in biorhythms and melatonin production result in poor sleep quality because the body does not enter the deeper phases of the sleep cycle as often or as long as is healthy. Studies also show that screen exposure delays the onset of sleep, suppresses REM sleep (which we need to "clean house" and solidify learning), and prevents the body temperature from dropping to levels supportive of deep sleep.[23]

Without restorative sleep, the brain does not function properly. Muscles become tense, and you feel tired the next day — even if the total sleep time was adequate. To compensate, the body releases more stress hormones to keep you awake, perpetuating a vicious cycle. Even short exposures to electronic screens (such as fifteen minutes) near bedtime can produce these changes. While a screen's blue tones are much more potent in terms of melatonin suppression, it's been shown that red light and dimmer displays during evening hours are still quite disruptive.[24] Interestingly, a study showed electromagnetic radiation from cell phone towers produced a similar degree of suppression in melatonin,[25] suggesting that exposure to a screen device plus EMFs may deliver a "double whammy" of sleep disturbance.

Light-at-Night: Effects on Sleep, Mood, and Cognition

In general, non-restorative sleep is associated with poor memory, irritability, and impaired school or work performance.[26] A 2010 sleep study conducted at the JFK Medical Center showed that over half of the children who used electronic media at night not only suffered sleep problems but mood and cognitive problems during daytime.[27] Other studies have linked light-at-night from electronics to depression and suicidality,[28] and some speculate that disrupted circadian rhythms lead to low serotonin levels — the brain chemical of well-being.[29]

There is no "safe dose" of after-lights-out texting that does not cause sleep disturbance and daytime sleepiness.[30] Teens are notorious for texting at night; some even sleep with their phones. Unfortunately, both children and teens also use the computer in the late afternoons and evenings for schoolwork, making screen-related sleep disturbance a ubiquitous problem.

Reward and Addiction Pathways

There is much discussion today about whether intense video game play or Internet use can be considered an addiction. The relationship between interactive screen-time, addiction, and stress is complex, but a number of key studies shed light on the issue. There is actually an abundance of evidence supporting the concept of screen or tech addiction, but perhaps most convincing are imaging studies. Brain scan research indicates that when heavy gamers — or even individuals who merely crave gaming — are shown computer game cues, their brains "light up" in exactly the same areas as the brain of someone addicted to drugs.[31] One study showed that in college students who reported cravings for online gaming, just six weeks of heavy Internet video game playing produced changes in those students' prefrontal cortex (part of the frontal lobe, the brain's executive center) similar to those seen in the early stages of addiction.[32] Internet and video game addiction studies in adolescent and young adults have found strong physical evidence that brain damage occurs with heavy use.[33] Other brain-scan studies have demonstrated that playing video games releases large amounts of dopamine,[34] the primary brain chemical associated with reward pathways activated in addiction.

How is all this occurring when there is no toxic "substance"? Compulsive video game and Internet use can be considered an *arousal addiction*

— that is, the user becomes addicted to high levels of stimulation and arousal and then needs more stimulation to achieve or sustain that feeling. Tolerance occurs because reward pathways — the exact same reward pathways in the brain that are involved in chemical addictions — become overactivated. In other words, the pathways become desensitized from overuse. Meanwhile, in addition to the "rush" of stress hormones released during use, the screen-addicted person experiences stress reactions at other times: when he or she is not able to play; when craving or negotiating for play; when experiencing physical or psychological withdrawal from play; and when play is cut short. Thus, the stress reactions related to the addiction process compound the stress of screen-time itself.

While true screen addiction is less common than ESS, it is possible that ESS may set the stage for tech and *other* addictions in children and adolescents. The cycle of craving play, playing, and then withdrawing not only creates stress but also causes the brain to be more *sensitive* to stress, resulting in a "hair-trigger response" to even mild stressors — a pattern known to develop in individuals with substance abuse.[35] The inability to deal with stress leads to the need to escape, and the user uses more. In fact, "escapism" — using screen-time to avoid reality — has been found to be a predictor of video game addiction.[36] Thus, repeated arousal and activation of reward pathways induced by electronics' use may "prime" the brain not just for tech addiction but for other addictions as well.[37]

Vividness, Screen Size, and Pace

Whatever the subject matter, the style or manner in which content is delivered has its own impact. Research indicates that movement, zooms, pans, cuts, and vividness (how "lifelike" images are) all trigger the orienting response and contribute to repeated fight-or-flight reactions.[38] Screen size affects arousal levels as well, with larger screens producing higher levels of arousal. It's worth noting that in today's market, whether the device is a handheld device, laptop, desktop monitor, or television set, the trend is "the bigger the better."[39] Regarding Internet activity, the speed and frequency of downloading and use of video all contribute to alertness and arousal, in addition to that contributed by the actual content.[40] As technology improves, so does its ability to engage and arouse.[41]

Media Multitasking

Multitasking could be more accurately called "task switching." Juggling more than one task at a time places increased cognitive demands on the brain, which increases arousal levels and stress. (And just because your child may be considered "good at it" does not mean multitasking is good for him or her!) Kids now chat while playing online games, Skype and text while doing homework, and email and surf the web on a smartphone while watching TV. Studies show that high multitasking is associated with physiological stress, impaired cognition, and negative mood due to frequent attentional switching, the experience and inefficiency of being frequently interrupted, and sensory overload.[42]

Radiation from Electromagnetic Fields (EMFs)

EMFs represent another possible source of hyperarousal and other stress reactions, at least for some people. Like other aspects of electronics, EMFs may induce stress directly, or immediately upon exposure, and indirectly, by affecting sleep quality. Several studies have demonstrated immediate effects on particular stress markers, and other research suggests sleep patterns and biorhythms may be affected. Stress reactions have been found to occur at the level of the cell as well. See the EMF appendix for a more detailed discussion of this research.

Chronic Stress, Hyperarousal, and Your Child

Chronic stress and hyperarousal generally lead to some form of *dysregulation* — the loss of the ability to modulate responses in a manner appropriate to the current environment. This can occur in anyone no matter what the source of stress, and as we've seen, it occurs in children from screen-time, leading to ESS.

As I describe in the introduction, working closely with children who'd experienced serious trauma from abuse and neglect helped me recognize that screen-time could induce symptoms that mimicked those seen in children who were perpetually in "survival mode." In this section, I look more closely at how chronic stress and hyperarousal affect children in terms of physiology and behavior, using Aiden's story to illustrate certain points. Because ESS is essentially a stress syndrome, examining how stress manifests in children can illuminate why ESS causes so many problems so easily. Figure 3 outlines the myriad of biological, psychological, and social dysfunctions produced by stress; all of these impacts are likewise seen with Electronic Screen Syndrome.

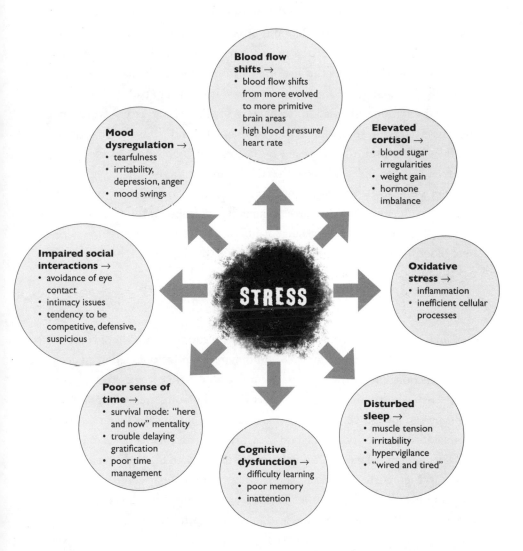

Figure 3. Effects of chronic stress and hyperarousal*

---

*   This graphic does not include all stress reactions, and some of these factors are interrelated.

Blood Flow Shifts

This mechanism has potential long-term implications for brain development. When under stress, blood flow in the brain is repeatedly shunted away from areas of higher thinking (the cortex, or "new" brain, at the outermost layer) and toward more primitive areas (the limbic, or "old" brain, seated deep within). In other words, blood is directed to the areas involved in survival. Similarly, when addiction of any kind occurs during adolescence, it tends to stunt development of the brain's frontal lobe, which is responsible for decision making, organization, attention, impulse control, task completion, and emotional regulation (to name a few!). If interactive screen-time induces a stress response *and* activates reward and addiction pathways, might it affect brain development by decreasing blood flow to the cortex and frontal lobe? Indeed, it very well might. Interestingly, when I've treated patients with the Reset Program and they continue to be screen-free afterward, they seem to mature developmentally in leaps and bounds — in a matter of months. This suggests that liberation from screens redirects robust blood flow back to the frontal lobe, thereby supporting healthy brain development.

Elevated Cortisol

Research suggests electronic screen activity is associated with altered cortisol regulation.[43] While adrenaline is the dominant hormone released in an *acute* stress reaction, the hormone typically associated with *chronic* stress is cortisol. Cortisol actually serves to protect the body from stress reactions, but high cortisol levels over time cause harm. In fact, chronically high cortisol is correlated with obesity, high blood pressure, diabetes, metabolic syndrome, and hormone imbalance.[44] During times of stress, when the body needs ready access to fuel, cortisol "loosens the reins" of blood sugar control by counteracting insulin. In the short term, this translates into unstable blood sugar levels, but in the long term it can lead to weight gain concentrated in the abdominal area and problems with insulin regulation. Recall how Aiden craves sweets after his episode; children under stress often crave sweets or other carbohydrates because of blood sugar fluctuations. As mentioned, research shows screen-time is a risk factor for metabolic syndrome regardless of activity level, and it is likely that high cortisol is one of the reasons why.

Additionally, elevated cortisol throws off the production of other hormones, such as thyroid and reproductive hormones, and over time excess cortisol damages the brain.[45] Chronically elevated cortisol wreaks havoc on the nervous, cardiovascular, metabolic, and hormonal systems.

Oxidative Stress

Chronic stress — electronic or otherwise — puts stress on the very system that fights stress! At a molecular level, all cellular reactions in the body produce free radicals, which are unstable, unpaired electrons that must quickly grab another electron in order to stabilize. When a cell is healthy, *free radicals* are "scavenged" by adequate amounts of antioxidants — which are both ingested as nutrients and produced by the cell itself — and balance is maintained. But when the cell's defenses are overwhelmed by too many stressors, antioxidants become depleted, and oxidative stress (excessive free radicals) ensues. As free radicals build unchecked, the unstable molecules containing them are forced to "grab" electrons from our own tissue. Nearby fats, proteins, and DNA are typically the elements vulnerable to being attacked. Eventually, this process creates inflammation, tissue damage, and inefficiency, further compromising the cell's ability to contend with acute and ongoing stress.

Unfortunately, the brain is highly susceptible to oxidative stress for several reasons. First, oxidative stress can cause disruption of the blood-brain barrier, making it more vulnerable to toxins it should be protected from. Second, it's also relatively hard to get antioxidant nutrients *into* the brain that could potentially provide the brain protection, so there's never much of a buffer. And third, oxidative stress tends to attack the fatty sheaths that insulate brain cells, which can cause aberrant firing of networks. Meanwhile, a developing brain — because it is highly dynamic with increased energy needs — is more vulnerable to oxidative stress than a fully formed adult brain. This means that a child's brain — especially if it is already compromised by a mental disorder — will develop damage from oxidative stress relatively quickly. The eyes are also vulnerable to oxidative stress; the retinal damage studies mentioned above also found markers associated with oxidative stress.[46]

Disturbed Sleep

The far-reaching effects of poor quality sleep have already been mentioned, and they can occur in children after just one night of not getting enough rest.

Poor sleep goes hand in hand with both acute and chronic stress. In Aiden's case, video game playing (and subsequent fight-or-flight rage) results in non-restorative sleep, which doesn't allow his brain adequate recovery. After a night of poor sleep, the body produces adrenaline to get through the day, which can then cause difficulty falling or staying asleep the following night. Non-restorative sleep compounds hyperarousal and leaves a child feeling "wired and tired."

Sleep hygiene is a set of practices sleep experts recommend to obtain quality rest on a daily basis. Recommendations include low levels of stimulation in the evening, exercise and exposure to lots of natural light during the day, banning electronics from the bedroom, and sticking to a regular sleep-wake schedule. Children and teens who are stressed tend to have poor sleep hygiene if left to their own devices.

Cognitive Dysfunction

If you've ever described your child as seemingly "out of it," you may be witnessing the cognitive dysfunction that occurs when the brain has just been exposed to something it considers stressful. When Aiden tries to get ready for bed after his episode, he can't quite get himself together and has trouble following sequential steps. After a poor night's sleep, he continues to struggle with focus, long after the game has been turned off. Stress affects the ability to assimilate new facts, retain new information, and execute tasks. Short-term memory suffers. Cognitive dysfunction then translates into forgetting to complete or turn in homework assignments, falling grades, and a tendency to lose things. Chronic or repeated stress causes even more alarming effects, including loss of neurons, or brain cells, particularly in the hippocampus — an area important for forming and storing memories.[47]

Poor Sense of Time

Both *sense of time* and *time management* can be affected by stress. If we were to ask Aiden in the moment how long he has been playing his game, in all likelihood he will underestimate the time spent — even if he is being honest and not trying to minimize in order to avoid getting into trouble. In fact, video gaming has been found to cause *time distortion* in players, nearly universally.[48] Both video games and Internet use cause problems with *managing* time as well: being late, underestimating how much time a task will take, procrastinating, forgetting appointments and activities, and so on. Interestingly, children with extensive traumatic histories have great difficulty with time perception. They appear to be forever stuck in the moment, unable to look forward or backward — an advantage if you're trying to survive. Focusing on the "here and now" serves self-preservation in extreme situations. But in everyday life, it translates into impulsive actions, repeating mistakes by failing to reflect on their consequences, and an inability to focus on future goals.

Impaired Social Interactions

The very essence of survival mode centers around defensiveness. While in this state, being open and intimate creates vulnerability and therefore poses a threat. During Aiden's episode, direct eye contact with his aunt provokes him. This is a primitive reaction, and it is why we don't stare unfamiliar dogs directly in the eye — they'll see it as a challenge. Try making sustained eye contact with your child after video game play — he or she will likely become uncomfortable and look away.

Chronically hyperaroused children get defensive easily when playing games and are often "sore losers." They may feel wronged when something happens by chance, and they may be more prone to cheating. These behaviors can happen online and in other settings, like the playground. As this defensiveness rises, the child's relationships can become affected. Interestingly, while both children and adults claim that social media helps them feel connected to others, it appears that, in fact, time spent online actually increases depression and a sense of social isolation.[49]

Mood Dysregulation

Emotional (or mood) dysregulation is one of the end products of all these disturbed pathways and mechanisms, and it is nearly always present when a child is chronically hyperaroused. It occurs as the fight-or-flight response causes shifts in mechanical, chemical, and electrical systems (such as blood flow, brain chemistry and hormones, and overstimulated networks) and is compounded by poor sleep. Mood dysregulation is characterized by poor frustration tolerance, tearfulness, irritability, mood swings, and meltdowns or aggression. Aiden becomes extremely emotionally volatile immediately following video game play, and then he continues to feel irritable and anxious for days and weeks afterward. If you've ever felt like you "have to walk on eggshells" around your child, then it is likely you are all-too familiar with this phenomenon.

For a summary that pulls all the pathways, mechanisms, and potential consequences together, see the table in appendix A, "Table of Physiological Mechanisms and Effects of Interactive Screen-Time." In fact, bookmark this page to remind yourself why your child's brain needs a reset!

Chapter 2 Take-Home Points

- The brain does not discern between real or perceived threats, and artificially intense stimulation from electronic screen media produces a psychological and physiological fight-or-flight reaction, regardless of content.
- These reactions have both immediate and cumulative effects, which eventually cause damage.
- Screen devices interface with your child via the eyes, brain, and body, triggering changes in blood flow, brain chemistry, electrical excitability, and hormones.
- Since the eyes are a direct extension of the central nervous system, they provide a pathway for overstimulation of the sensory system as well as for unnaturally bright light to suppress melatonin (the sleep hormone) and desynchronize the body clock.
- Numerous mechanisms, including disturbed sleep, reward/addiction pathways, brain-blood flow shifts, intense sensory experiences, and engaging content precipitate and perpetuate an ongoing stress response.
- Electronics-related sleep disturbance, in and of itself, creates a vicious cycle of exhaustion, compromised mood and cognition, more stress because of dysfunction, more insomnia, and craving for more stimulation.
- Examining the known effects of chronic stress and hyperarousal can assist in envisioning how screen-time may affect your child's behavior, mood, and social skills.

CHAPTER 3

INSIDIOUS SHAPE-SHIFTER

How ESS Mimics a Wide Variety of Psychiatric, Neurological, and Behavioral Disorders

The system of nature, of which man is a part, tends to be self-balancing, self-adjusting, self-cleansing. Not so with technology.

— E. F. Schumacher, *Small Is Beautiful*[1]

For a list of all the ways technology has failed to improve the quality of life, please press 3.

— Alice Kahn

Historically, certain infectious "agents" have become infamous for their capacity to randomly invade a victim's nervous system, lending them an uncanny ability to mimic various neurologic and psychiatric disorders. In fact, both syphilis and Lyme disease have been nicknamed "the Great Imitator."[2] Not surprisingly, both illnesses are also considered to be sources of misdiagnosis as well as misguided treatment.

Other classes of mental health offenders demonstrate a similar nature. Food intolerances, such as gluten or dairy sensitivity, are capable of inflaming the brain and body and causing symptoms ranging from irritability and hyperactivity to fatigue and brain fog. Abuse of street drugs, like cocaine and methamphetamine, can cause wildly variant presentations; symptoms range from mild anxiety or depression to personality changes and overt psychosis. All of the above offenders — infections, certain food proteins, and illicit drugs — are known to cause widespread dysfunction and wide-ranging symptoms in some, and more "classic" symptoms in others, creating challenges for diagnosis and appropriate treatment.

It is, therefore, not such a stretch to imagine that if screen-time is capable of irritating the nervous system in general, that its corresponding syndrome would be capable of imitating or secretly amplifying more specific conditions. ESS "shape-shifts," such that clinicians and parents may think they are seeing one thing when in fact ESS is the real villain. To make matters even more confusing, the way ESS presents itself depends not only on a child's underlying constitution but also on his or her current environment and stage of development, and thus it sometimes morphs into different entities even within the same child. In other words, regardless of the nature of your child's issues, it pays to be on the lookout for ESS.

The Shape-Shifting Nature of Electronic Screen Syndrome

This chapter categorizes and describes the ways in which ESS can either exacerbate or imitate various mental and neurological health problems. This covers a lot of ground, and you may want to turn first to the sections covering the types of dysfunction that you know apply to your child, and then read the chapter more thoroughly later. I have based these findings on my own and others' clinical experience with patients, on what we already know about the brain and body, and on relevant, emerging research about electronic media and these conditions. In other words, this chapter presents the sum of what we see, what we know, and what we're finding out about screen-time's effects. Note that for some conditions, such as tics or psychosis, there remains a paucity of formal research, but the findings described here are nevertheless supported by peripheral research (for example, by screen-time's impact on dopamine), published case reports, surveys, therapeutic effects from the fast, and anecdotal reports from patients and parents. No doubt we will improve our understandings in time.

Although pediatric mental health disorders are notorious for symptom overlap across differing diagnoses, for organizational purposes I have grouped symptoms and conditions into six categories: moods, cognitive concerns, disruptive behaviors and social issues, addiction, anxiety, and neurological dysfunction (including tics and autism). Some children exhibit numerous symptoms from different categories, and some only a specific one or two. Some symptoms may be directly related to interacting with electronic screen devices, while others may be indirect as a result of poor sleep or stress reactions. For some symptoms or disorders, ESS may only exacerbate but not mimic; for instance, autistic symptoms would (theoretically) not be mimicked in a typically developing child. But for most disorders, ESS can either mimic *or* exacerbate them. For example, ESS might mimic the symptoms of ADHD in a child without ADHD, or ESS might exacerbate symptoms in a child who does indeed have ADHD. In spite of these variations, a common ESS combination of symptoms is irritability (mood), attention issues (cognition), and immature or defiant behavior (behavior/social). Hopefully this chapter provides both a "big picture" sense of ESS as well as ways to specifically identify how it may be presenting in *your* child. Think in themes rather than absolutes, and remember most psychiatric symptoms and diagnoses occur on a spectrum.

Luckily, despite its shape-shifting nature, ESS is relatively simple to diagnose. Like food intolerances, the gold standard is simply to remove the potential offender — in this case, screen devices — and observe the child for symptom and function improvement. While this chapter describes most of the ways screen-time might impact a child, the swiftest and most accurate way to figure out if or how ESS is affecting yours is to follow the Reset Program and observe what happens.

Moods and Meltdowns

Mood symptoms are nearly always present in ESS. They can take the form of irritability, depression, mood swings, an inability to calm down, tantrums, or even outright aggression. These mood changes are likely produced by screen-time's impact on dopamine and other brain chemicals, sleep, the sensory system, and the stress response. Interestingly, I've noticed that some children and even teens with screen-related mood symptoms will destroy a screen device by smashing, throwing, or "drowning" it, as if they know on some level it is hurting them. (Remember Ryan, the eight-year-old son of my work colleague, whom I mentioned in the Introduction? Ryan smashed one device and later drowned another in the tank of a toilet during his spiral into screen-related depression.) As I advise all parents, if a device gets destroyed in the throes of frustration, do not replace it! Your child's behavior is telling you something.

Figure 4 below depicts how altered physiology from screen interaction can translate into mood symptoms and difficulty functioning, setting the stage for an apparent mood "disorder."

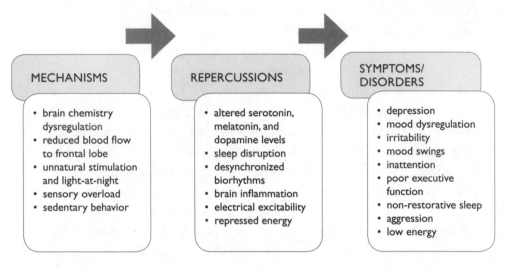

Figure 4. How screen-time effects translate to mood symptoms

Irritability

Irritable moods — along with attention difficulties — are among the most universal symptoms of ESS. In a younger child, irritability often results in frequent meltdowns or even rages over seemingly minor frustrations. These meltdowns, as we saw with Aiden in chapter 2, can be severe enough to disrupt an activity, an entire day, or even the functioning of an entire family. Severe tantrums or meltdowns are frequently the catalyst that brings a parent to my door, but they can also be what motivates a family to make a drastic lifestyle change.

In teens and young adults, ESS-related irritability can present as mood swings or meltdowns, or it may take the form of defiant behavior, withdrawal from the family, or extreme disrespectfulness. Not surprisingly, determining whether irritability is a problem in a teen can present a dilemma for parents: we expect teens to be moody, withdrawn, and even rude to a certain extent, so how do you know if something's really wrong? Trust your gut and ask yourself if your teen's irritability seems out of the norm, chronic, is associated with destructive impulses, or is severe enough to affect daily functioning and quality of life.

Regardless of age, irritable mood is no doubt related to all the factors outlined in figure 4, and most parents can readily appreciate how poor sleep can result in an irritable child. Less obvious, however, is the dopamine connection. When a child is irritable immediately after, for example, video game play, it's likely due — at least in part — to the rapid rise (during play) and fall (upon stopping play) of dopamine. This is not the natural rise and fall you'd see associated with a healthy stimulating activity, like playing a competitive sport. Rather, it's similar to the pattern that occurs with older dopamine-releasing medications (short-acting stimulants) that work quickly but wear off in a few hours. When dopamine rises and falls suddenly — whether from game play or short-acting stimulants — the child can become weepy, impulsive, or angry.* It's as though the sudden fall in dopamine causes the brain to short circuit; every little demand on the child becomes stressful. Since dopamine is needed to execute tasks, when it's suddenly low, every task becomes overwhelming, setting the stage for a meltdown. No wonder the child fights getting off the device — it's uncomfortable!

Aside from this "relative withdrawal" of dopamine levels following screen activity, irritability may also be related to dopamine depletion and desensitization of dopamine receptors that studies show develop over time with excessive screen-time.[3] Unfortunately, it is literally impossible to "taper" going from screen to no screen, from virtual world to real world, so the transition cannot be gradual and smooth. The rapid and extreme drop in stimulation levels is one reason that even *occasional* bouts of video game play are capable of causing dysregulation in some children and why moderation doesn't always work. Our systems simply aren't meant to handle such extremes.

One teen admitted to me, "You know, I do notice I'm always yelling at my parents when they say *anything* to me when I'm on the computer. It makes me snappy." A friend and father of three boys quipped: "We call it 'game-head' when the boys are playing video games and then one of them loses it and smacks the other upside the head." And a grandmother with custody of her two grandchildren related, "When the kids get mouthy, we know it's the electronics. It's like it jumbles up their brains, so we remove them when the kids get out of line." Many parents report crying, emotional sensitivity, and

---

* This is one reason why long-acting stimulants are now prescribed almost exclusively in preference to short-acting ones, to imitate the natural rise and fall of dopamine more closely.

irritability or anger surrounding their child's or teen's game play or computer usage, especially when use is prolonged.

Closely related to irritability is difficulty *regulating* arousal levels. As mentioned in chapter 1, this symptom is one of the hallmarks of ESS. A chronically hyperaroused child may have trouble *recovering* from being angry or sad, as we saw with Aiden. Instead of experiencing an outburst and then calming down, the child continues to be in a state of distress for a prolonged period. In general, the greater the stimulation — in the form of changing scenes, vivid colors, rapid or sudden movements, multitasking, or multimodal sensory input — and the more often that stimulation occurs, the harder it is to regulate arousal, and the more irritable the child becomes.

Depression

The evidence linking overall electronics use and depression is substantial,[4] and virtually all types of interactive screen-time have been implicated: Internet usage is directly correlated with depressed mood, withdrawal or isolation, loneliness, and less parent-child interaction, and the highest users show the most severe symptoms.[5] Use of social media such as Facebook is a risk factor for depression and dissatisfaction with one's life.[6] "Light-at-night" studies demonstrate an association between electronics use at or near bedtime and increased depressive symptoms, suicidal tendencies, self-injurious behavior, and physical complaints like headache and leg pain.[7] Multitasking and smartphone use have been linked to adolescent depression.[8] And excessive gaming is associated with depression, anxiety, and hostility.[9] Tellingly, in a large study that followed more than three thousand children over a two-year period, researchers found that youths who became pathological gamers tended to become more depressed and anxious, while those who stopped gaming in a pathological manner became less depressed and more socially competent.[10]

Note that generally speaking, in children and adolescents depression can present as irritability with or without a depressed mood. In a younger child with screen-related depression, the child may cry a lot, lose interest in activities, become chronically irritable, and withdraw. The child's parent often says things like, "My son seems to have lost his spark," or "She's lost her natural curiosity about life." In teens and young adults, screen-related depression can become quite serious, as it did for Dan, whose case is described below. Regardless of age, frequently the child will have some underlying social difficulties — due to shyness, odd mannerisms, or a difficult temperament — leading the parents to become overly permissive with screen privileges, which sets the stage for a vicious cycle. Psychologically, the child becomes more and more dependent on screen-time for stimulation or a feeling of connection, or to escape from what is an otherwise boring, unfulfilling, or perhaps even painful life. Eventually, even the *thought* of living without screen devices may cause the child to feel highly anxious — as though in an existential crisis. Meanwhile, the child's identity can become so fused with his or her virtual cyber life that normal development is stunted or interrupted; teens who are heavy screen users often make statements such as, "My phone is like my brain. I can't live without it." Or, "Being on the computer is the *only* thing that makes me happy... it's my *life*." In older children and teens, role-playing games may serve as an escape and a place they can control their image and actions, but this can be true for children of any age, who can become obsessed with certain video games or cartoon characters as a substitute for real relationships. As social support erodes, the depression worsens. Studies suggest that children or teens with shyness or social anxiety are at higher risk for screen-related depression.[11]

Alongside these psychological changes are physiological ones, including dysregulation of dopamine and other neurotransmitters (brain chemicals), compounding depression and a sense of isolation. While dopamine is the "feel good" chemical linked to positive moods, another relevant brain chemical is serotonin. Serotonin is important for socialization, stable mood, a sense of well-being, and coping with stress, and it is low in depression, anxiety, and aggression. Serotonin levels are highest in the mornings, and its production is thought to be boosted by bright morning sunlight and physical activity. Lack of morning light and sedentary daytime behavior may therefore blunt serotonin, contributing to depression, anxiety, aggression, and even suicidality.[12] Light-at-night may further depress mood, both because serotonin is made from melatonin (which is suppressed by light), and because sleep disturbance itself is linked to mood issues. As dopamine and serotonin become more and more dysregulated, the child starts to seek out screen stimulation to temporarily boost mood, and screen-time literally becomes a form of self-medication.

Dan: A Curious Case of Depression

Dan was a twenty-year-old young man with mild social anxiety and ADD who — despite a genius-level IQ — was failing out of college. His social life had gone from being fairly active to nonexistent, his sleep-wake pattern was almost completely reversed, and he rarely left his room. Although not actively suicidal, Dan reported he often felt he'd be "better off dead" and didn't "see much point to life." What was happening?

Upon graduating from high school, Dan had continued living at home. But without the eight-hour school days and no job to go to, he suddenly found himself with a lot of extra time on his hands. His electronics' use skyrocketed. Even when his college classes began that fall, Dan continued to spend anywhere from six to twelve hours a day on the computer, playing games, chatting, or reading articles. Dan barely scraped by the first two semesters. By the end of his third, Dan had dropped one class and was getting Fs in the other two. Despite his high IQ, he was struggling to keep up.

He'd also lost a lot of weight, even though he was thin to begin with. Dan's mother reported that he'd stopped going to the kitchen to get food or water, and he was dependent on her to nag him into eating and drinking. By the time Dan came to me, he was gaunt and pale, and his muscles had literally atrophied from sitting and lying down so much.

To see this in a young male was shocking. Dan complained of fatigue, joint pain, back pain, shortness of breath, depressed mood, trouble sleeping, and feeling "flat." His mother had made the rounds to numerous medical specialists and therapists — for both physical and psychiatric complaints — but to no avail. By the time I consulted with him, Dan was taking three psychotropic medications plus a pain medication, and he had been tried on numerous other "psych meds" but found them all ineffective. Not one person ever suggested he remove the computer and other devices from his bedroom, despite this being a standard-of-care intervention for sleep disturbance.

Naturally, when I suggested an electronic fast, Dan resisted. As is often the case with youths over eighteen, his treatment providers and his parents had been reluctant to force *any* screen-time rules upon him, which only escalated the problem. I, however, viewed his situation as an emergency; his behavior was showing us he wasn't able to care for himself. Fortunately, his mother — who had been suspecting that the computer was part of the problem — readily agreed that imposing the fast was warranted, and she removed all the electronics in the home that same day.

Initially, Dan became even more isolated. Most days, he stayed in bed and didn't speak much at all. Because he was so depressed, we decided to extend the fast for at least six weeks, and this proved to be prudent. Right around the six-week mark, Dan started coming alive again. He got out of bed each day, made spontaneous conversation with his mom, and began going to class. His interest in physics and history revived, and he joined some academic clubs. Initially, we maintained the fast except for school-related work, but as time went on, his mother and I established strict rules for personal use and continued to actively moderate his usage, in part by requiring his schedule be structured. Dan got a part-time job, made friends, and started getting As and Bs in school. Slowly, Dan put on some weight and started walking and stretching regularly with a family friend. As he regained his strength and energy, it became clear that all Dan's physical ailments stemmed from deconditioning (being out of shape), depression, and stagnant blood flow — not some mysterious medical disease.

Dan's case underscores the seriousness of electronics' role in mood disorders, highlights the risk that social anxiety can bring, and demonstrates some of the physical effects that can occur with electronics overuse. Other individuals at high risk for screen-related depression are those with autism spectrum disorders, particularly after graduating from high school (for more on autism and ESS, see page 99). Suffice it to say, it is not enough to address depression in young people solely with conventional psychotherapy and perhaps an antidepressant. Even if screen-time is not the primary cause, it is virtually always a contributing factor.

Bipolar Disorder

Bipolar illness is a mood disorder characterized by severe high and low mood states. While "low" refers to a depressed mood, "high" can refer to a state of either euphoria *or* irritability. In adults these swings tend to be relatively discrete episodes, but in children, bipolar episodes are less distinct, and both the "highs" and "lows" can be associated with irritability — making the disease mimic a lot of other mental disorders. Thus, the diagnosis can be missed in those who truly have it, but it also tends to be overdiagnosed in children with other difficulties.

When I first began my "Mental Wealth" blog for *Psychology Today* a few years ago, I wrote a post entitled "Misdiagnosed? Bipolar Disorder Is All the Rage!" in which I proposed that the large increase in pediatric bipolar disorder diagnosis was due (in part) to children who were overstimulated from video games and other screen-time who raged, and thus "looked" bipolar.[13] I received emails from mothers all over the world — including the United States, Europe, Canada, South America, and the Middle East — telling me their child had been diagnosed as "bipolar" because he or she was exhibiting rages. Typically, the email would reveal that the mother had long suspected video games were the real culprit, but that the notion had always been shot down by whoever was evaluating the child. When these mothers read my article, however, the sense of validation they felt prompted them to follow their instincts — and out went the electronics. Story after story poured in about how a child's rages had resolved or at least become manageable when they followed this simple intervention. Although I'd seen this in my practice hundreds of times, it was validating for me to hear that mothers around the world were using the intervention effectively.

However, behind the satisfaction loomed something more ominous. How many children were receiving psychotropic medication unnecessarily? How many were labeled as "bipolar" when they were simply overstimulated and unable to regulate themselves? As I mention in the introduction, the diagnosis of childhood bipolar disorder has increased dramatically in recent decades, and a new diagnosis was created in 2013 — Disruptive Mood Dysregulation Disorder — precisely out of concern that children are being inappropriately diagnosed with bipolar disorder and receiving unnecessary medication. In my experience, disruptive children are sometimes given a "bipolar" diagnosis by a pediatrician during a routine ten- to fifteen-minute visit, while in other cases a teacher or therapist suggests to parents that their child "might be bipolar" and "might need medication," or worse, "can't come back until he's medicated." Often, a child need only exhibit aggression or explosive rage to get this label slapped on by a well-meaning but misinformed clinician. In some instances, a mother will read a description of pediatric bipolar disorder, feel her child fits the description, and then convince herself and others that bipolar disorder is the correct diagnosis. Of course, childhood bipolar disorder can and does exist (with or without ESS), and it's not a diagnosis you want to miss — early treatment improves prognosis. But it is relatively rare, especially if there is no family history of the disease (or no genetic predisposition).

So, what is it about ESS symptoms that prompt this mistake and create what seems to be a bipolar "picture"? In addition to rages and mood swings, ESS symptoms can include severe insomnia, impulsivity, distractibility, and, in certain vulnerable individuals, hallucinations or vague paranoia. Especially together, these symptoms can take on a very convincing bipolar persona. The misdiagnosis of bipolar disorder is even more common in children for whom ESS amplifies other difficulties, such as existing learning disorders, intellectual delays, ADHD, attachment disorder, sensory integration issues, and autism spectrum disorders. These children's nervous systems are already more vulnerable to environmental assaults of all kinds, and they are more likely to become impulsive or aggressive under stress. For instance, say an eight-year-old boy has learning difficulties and ADHD. Both of these disorders will affect functioning of the brain's frontal lobe, which governs planning, judgment, prioritizing, and emotional regulation. Now, if this boy is repeatedly overstimulated from electronics, this will further reduce frontal lobe activity, disrupt sleep, shorten attention span, and worsen mood. Now the boy will have even *more* trouble processing his environment, and very minor frustrations will be experienced as uncomfortable. You can see how a child like this might become explosive and have mood swings, or how he could be calm and loving after getting a good night's sleep but be a wreck again the following day. His hyperarousal and poor processing might also mean he barely remembers his outbursts, and so he acts as though they never happened. These are all patterns that can occur when ESS compounds or mimics other disorders, and they are the same patterns that contribute to misdiagnosis.

Finally, of course, ESS can and does occur alongside true childhood bipolar disorder. ESS can easily make things worse for such a child, since bipolar illness is exquisitely sensitive to lack of sleep: staying up all night can induce mania, while inducing sleep is an important part of managing acute mania. If a child truly does have a serious mental illness like bipolar disorder, an electronic fast can help clarify the diagnosis, and it may help manage symptoms, both directly (by helping to regulate mood) and indirectly (by improving sleep). Either way, it may help reduce the need for medication.

For parents witnessing serious mood disturbances and dysregulation that appear to take on a life of their own, it may be hard to appreciate the link with electronics, and at first they often dismiss screen-time as a serious or central issue. But a child's diminished ability to self-soothe or regulate mood due to of ESS will prolong and worsen the episode, all while creating a hair-trigger response to stress. Then, when the usual treatments don't improve symptoms, parents become even more exhausted — and almost invariably children are allowed even *more* screen-time. This creates a vicious cycle of stress and dysfunction that can further overshadow the role of electronics. The bottom line is that ESS needs to be both ruled out and addressed before tackling whatever lies underneath.

Lily: When a Smartphone Isn't Smart

A bright young girl, Lily was sixteen when I met her. By then, Lily had already been kicked out of school because of her rages and emotional instability, and she was being homeschooled. She had also been diagnosed with bipolar disorder, and because of the prescribed medications she was taking, she'd gained nearly thirty pounds. Her mother initially brought her to me for a second opinion on her medication regimen. Instead, as I discovered the amount of computer time Lily devoted to gaming and chatting on anime sites, I suggest that they do the Reset Program.

After much convincing, Lily's mother agreed, but Lily was furious. During the first few days of the fast, Lily screamed and cried, pleaded, slammed doors, threw things, and generally gave her mother hell. "It was like taking someone off heroin," her mother told me. "She swore up and down and cursed you and me both." I told her mother that this behavior was expected, and I encouraged her to hang tight and continue the fast. When Lily and her mother returned to my office several weeks later, Lily was smiling and admitted her mood was better since the fast, even though she was initially "mad as hell" at me. Her mom described Lily as "more even-keeled" and noticed she was sleeping a lot better. Eventually Lily returned to school, and we were able to greatly reduce her medication doses — which in turn helped her lose weight. Because Lily was a lot more pleasant to be around, she began making friends.

Lily continued to improve over the next several months, and we were able to wean her off all her medications with the exception of a mild mood stabilizer that didn't cause weight gain. During this time, she and her mother decided Lily would try attending a very strict and structured boarding school, which emphasized fitness and developmentally based learning. The school did not allow any electronic screen devices — no cell phones, no television, no computers — and it had a psychiatrist on site who would monitor Lily closely. For the next year and a half, Lily did wonderfully: not only did she lose the thirty pounds she'd gained, but she lost ten more; her mood was relaxed and happy; and her self-esteem and social skills greatly improved.

In April of her second year at school, however, I received a frantic call from her mother stating that Lily's mood swings had suddenly returned and that she was suicidal and had to be brought home. When Lily came in, I tried to find out what stressors may have triggered a mood episode, but could find none. Lily claimed she hadn't used any computers, even when she had been home over that recent spring break. On the surface, it looked like Lily was "cycling," or experiencing a bipolar episode, perhaps because of her reduced medication regimen. But I kept digging — and eventually I uncovered that when Lily had turned eighteen in March, she'd been allowed phone privileges, and her parents had given her a new smartphone.

Lily admitted to texting incessantly, playing electronic games, and accessing the Internet on her phone throughout the day. She also admitted to using her phone at night, texting while in bed, and sleeping with the phone under her pillow. Thus, despite the fact that she was still restricted from television and computer use at school, she had ramped up her interactive screen-time over a very short time period and was exposing herself to light-at-night, which, as mentioned earlier, has been linked to depression and suicidal thinking. Lily's sleep was disturbed, her mood had become dysregulated, and her grades had fallen.

To me, this was a no-brainer: the culprit was the phone. Although neither she nor her mother agreed that the phone could possibly be the trigger, they agreed to a fresh electronic fast — which included handing over the phone — since they were both reluctant to increase or add medication. Lily quickly stabilized.

As with Dan, Lily was now a legal adult, and some might argue that she had the "right" to own a phone. This may be true, but if excessive smartphone use could put her in the hospital, did we really want her have one? Did she really need it? In the end, her mother bought Lily a simple flip phone with no texting, games, or Internet capabilities, and Lily was able to return to school successfully. My opinion is that Lily was indeed somewhere on the bipolar spectrum, but screen-time clearly dysregulated her already vulnerable brain and made it nearly impossible for her to succeed in life.

Cognitive Concerns

As opposed to mood or behavior, *cognition* relates to thoughts and thinking. Cognitive problems associated with ESS run the gamut, from trouble concentrating and diminished creativity all the way to paranoia and even hearing voices. The influence of interactive screen-time on cognition is thought to be due to dopamine imbalance, blood flow shifting from higher to lower centers of the brain, mood disturbance, and stress chemicals and hormones associated with hyperarousal (see figure 5). Furthermore, cognitive effects are compounded by screen-time's effects on sleep. Light-at-night studies confirm that children suffer immediate and lasting impairment of cognition and sleep quality from *any* amount of interactive screen-time after bedtime.[14]

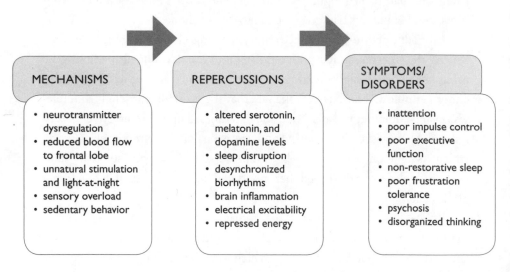

Figure 5. How screen-time effects translate to cognitive symptoms

Attention, Executive Functioning, and Learning

Children with *attention* problems generally have difficulty sustaining and shifting attention, and they have trouble initiating and completing goal-oriented activities — particularly if the activity is experienced as difficult or tedious. Inseparable from the ability to pay attention are two other abilities: *executive function* — that is, the ability to "get things done," which includes planning, prioritizing, organizing, revising, strategizing, attending to details, and managing time and space — and *working memory,* that is, "seeing in the mind's eye," or the ability to hold and manipulate incoming information in the mind. Difficulties with attention and executive functioning, which are largely governed by the brain's frontal lobe, have a profound impact on quality of life — affecting everything from academic and career achievement to the success of relationships.

Attention and executive functioning are largely dependent on dopamine and another brain chemical (or *neurotransmitter*), norepinephrine. These two neurotransmitters are the same chemicals that attention-deficit drugs seek to increase. Our brains need not just an adequate supply of these chemicals, but they also require them to 1) be active in the appropriate areas, 2) bind to adequately sensitive receptors, and 3) strike a balance with other brain chemicals, such as serotonin. These functions are sensitive to stress of any kind and can also be impacted by lack of proper sleep.

Whether related to ESS or not, what do attention difficulties look like? The child or teen with poor executive functioning...

- has difficulty with multistep directions and executing tasks that require planning and prioritizing, like school projects or applying for college or a job.
- loses homework even when completed or forgets to turn it in.
- has trouble keeping track of things, including time and personal belongings.
- is easily overwhelmed and becomes frustrated by small demands.
- exhibits paralyzing procrastination and avoidance of chores, and will have a "hard time getting started" on homework (especially "busy work") and paperwork in general.
- has trouble staying on task, perhaps even with tasks or routines he or she is familiar with, like getting ready for school or bed.
- displays a lack of attention to detail, such as completing chores or homework in a sloppy or haphazard manner, keeping his or her

room "like a disaster zone," or shoving everything into a backpack and never cleaning it out.

- appears "lazy" or "unmotivated" and can't tolerate delayed gratification.
- tends to be impulsive, acts before thinking things through, and disregards consequences of actions.
- often will not perform up to his or her academic potential, particularly in later school years.

It's critical to understand that anything that impacts attention also impacts executive functioning. Attention difficulties are, of course, the hallmark of attention deficit disorder (ADD) and attention deficit hyperactivity disorder (ADHD*). Because screen-time affects dopamine regulation, frontal lobe activity, sleep, and stress levels, ESS can look *exactly* like ADD — and will almost certainly worsen ADD if it preexists. Furthermore, children with attention symptoms are drawn to electronics precisely because they are stimulating; I've yet to meet a child with attention problems who doesn't love screen devices. The two tend to go hand in hand.

Here is a very typical example: Suzanne, a friend from high school, once contacted me about her son, Justin. Justin had become moody, was struggling academically, and was disruptive and defiant in the classroom. Suzanne reported that Justin didn't seem to enjoy playing anything but video games anymore; he had lost his natural "sense of curiosity" and "thirst for knowledge." Justin's teacher and his dad both felt Justin had ADHD and wanted him to see a psychiatrist. Suzanne, however, wanted to first get rid of the video games and other electronics before even considering medication, and she convinced his dad to wait while she tried the electronic fast.

Sure enough, within the first week of the fast, Suzanne noticed that Justin's mood improved. By the end of the month, her son had turned things around at school and was playing healthy activities again, and all discussions about Jason having ADHD were dropped. Eventually, Suzanne let Justin play video games again on a very limited basis, but she learned to immediately pull them back if she noticed mood or attention changes.

---

* Individuals can have attention deficit disorder ("ADD") with or without the hyperactivity component ("ADHD").

Video Games and Learning: The Attention Paradox

Parents often wonder, "Why is it that my child can pay attention to a video game — but to nothing else?!" Likewise, when I tell parents that gaming worsens focus, they often respond, "But I thought video games *improved* his attention." Why the confusion?

Attention is interest-based and driven by stimulation. Children with attention issues are drawn to video games and screens precisely because they can focus on them; the games provide sufficient stimulation for a dopamine surge, and thus gaming may be considered "self-medicating."[15] In fact, studies have shown that ADD medications actually curb cravings for and amount of video game play,[16] presumably because these medications raise dopamine levels.

But what about using the attention-grabbing stimulation of video games and other screen-based methods to *enhance* learning in the classroom? The excitement about using electronic media to engage students has led to a rush to implement electronic learning tools, despite their poor track record in studies. Essentially, what teachers are finding is that they work — until they don't. Soon enough, the novelty wears off, and more and more stimulation is required for focus. Meanwhile, the added stimulation contributes to dysregulation and a worsening of attention in general. When a child reports finding non-screen activities "boring," this should be a red flag to parents and educators — it means the child's brain has become used to an unnaturally high level of stimulation.

Further confusing the issue of attention, learning, and gaming is the highly touted finding that gaming can modify *visual attention*.[17] This is different than the executive attention issues we've been discussing related to "getting things done." An example of visual attention would be scanning an environment and visually picking out a target. Both the scientific and lay media have speculated that playing video games could "improve surgical skills," and that better visual attention skills could perhaps boost the potential to "become a pilot," "be a sharpshooter," or "improve driving skills."

But I would argue that it doesn't matter if gaming improves visual attention if it also worsens executive attention, impulse control, and frustration tolerance. Overgeneralizing and overemphasizing the visual attention effect is dangerous and misleading. The idea that gaming might improve the driving skills in teenage boys is laughable — not to mention inconsistent with research, which finds that gamers tend to be more reckless drivers.[18] And someone who can shoot well but has poor impulse control is not welcome in the military, for obvious reasons. Finally, aside from the fact that pilots and surgeons are a fraction of a percent of the population, you can bet that to persevere in career paths with such long and intense training, pilots and surgeons virtually always have highly superior executive functioning.

There now exists a large body of research implicating screen-time in the development of attention problems, and the earlier the exposure, the stronger the effect.[19] Although many of the studies have focused on television, more recently video games and Internet use have been implicated as well.[20] As I've said, interactive screen-time seems to have a much more potent detrimental effect on attention and executive functioning than passive screen-time, perhaps because the interactivity promotes higher levels of arousal, and because the proximity of the screen causes more severe melatonin suppression and circadian disruption. (EMFs may also be a factor; see the appendix.) Several studies support this distinction. A 2007 study conducted in Germany that allowed children an evening of either excessive television or computer game use found that the gaming group suffered significantly altered sleep patterns and impaired cognition when measured the following day, while the television group showed some sleep inefficiency but no change in cognitive performance.[21] Similarly, a large study published in 2010 that followed children over a two-year period found that total screen-time predicted attention problems, but that video game playing was more predictive than television viewing when the factors were looked at separately.[22]

It is also becoming increasingly clear that the relationship between screen-time and attention problems is one of *causation* — not mere *association* or "self-selection." In a landmark study, researchers followed more than three thousand Singapore children and adolescents over a three-year period and found there was actually a *bidirectional* relationship between gaming and poor attention.[23] In other words, it appears that gaming causes attention problems, and that children who are inattentive are more likely to game. This finding held true even when the researchers controlled for earlier attention problems, suggesting that screen-time as an environmental factor worsened attention whether or not the child had previous genetic-related attention problems. The authors also found that while violent gaming added slightly to the risk, the "dose" or total time spent was more important. Another study found that the association between screen-time and attention issues persists into adulthood.[24]

Research suggests that screen-time causes *immediate* effects on attention as well. As mentioned earlier, a 2011 study found that viewing a fast-paced cartoon — in this case *SpongeBob SquarePants*, a not particularly violent cartoon — for just nine minutes produced deficits in executive function in four-year-old children.[25] Another study tested children's attention before and after playing a video game and found that those with higher levels of daily computer use performed more poorly compared to those with more minimal use.[26] In other words, higher levels of overall screen-time appears to potentiate short-term attention effects.

Aside from attention, other aspects of cognition seem to be negatively affected as well. Consistent with "poor time management" complaints heard from parents, a 2006 study demonstrated that players experience time distortion when gaming, whether they're novices or experts.[27] (And who hasn't lost track of time while on the computer?) Other research suggests decision making is impacted. In 2009, researchers concluded from a series of studies that players exhibited increased risk taking after playing an auto racing game — the so-called Racing-Game Effect.[28] This finding lends credence to the concern that gaming can precipitate reckless behavior by glorifying and rewarding risk taking.

As I've mentioned, a growing body of research implicates the use of screen devices at night as a negative influence on daytime functioning, cognitive ability, and memory performance.[29] Studies also show that light-at-night causes higher nighttime core temperature and heart rate and lower melatonin levels,[30] markers associated with poor sleep and high stress. Lastly, numerous studies on multitasking — think Skyping and texting while doing homework — show it reduces efficiency and worsens performance.[31] One 2013 study found that students who checked Facebook just once while studying tended to have lower GPAs.[32]

One of the most compelling studies to date has come out of Denison University, where researchers demonstrated that video game ownership can interfere with reading and writing skills in boys.[33] Here, in a move that effectively eliminated any self-selection bias, researchers randomly split sixty-four boys ages six to nine who had never owned a video game into two groups. The children and families in the study were told only that they were receiving a reward for their participation — a video game console. One group received the console at the beginning of the four-month trial, while the control group received it at completion. The two groups were then compared in terms of academic achievement and behavior. The results showed that the boys receiving the console at the beginning of the study tested lower in reading and writing assessments, had more teacher-reported learning problems, and spent less time doing homework. Similarly, a 2010 study examined data collected on 150,000 middle school students in North Carolina and found that introducing a home computer had a negative and persistent impact on reading and math scores.[34] The same conclusion was found by another 2010 study on low-income Romanian students, which compared the grades of those who had acquired a new home computer via a government-sponsored voucher program and those who had not.[35]

Likewise, various experts have made disturbing observations regarding technology's effect on reading and learning. Dr. Leonard Sax, author of *Boys Adrift,* notes that in comparison to girls, boys are "falling off the curve" in terms of academic achievement and that the "gap" between boys' and girls' reading ability is growing; he cites video games as the second of five major contributors.[36] Nicholas Carr, author of the critically acclaimed *The Shallows,* contends that the Internet is changing the *depth* of our reading and thinking. Carr writes, "The kind of deep reading that a sequence of printed pages promotes is valuable not just for the knowledge we acquire from the author's words but for the intellectual vibrations those words set off in our own minds. In the quiet spaces opened up by the sustained, undistracted reading of a book...we foster our own ideas."[37] How can one reflect on or make new associations from written material at the same time one is skimming large amounts of information from the Internet — or having to process excess stimulation, for that matter?

In short, it is not an exaggeration to say that technology is "dumbing us down." Screen-time makes us less attentive and less able to learn, remember, and think for ourselves.

Cole: Making the Grade

Cole, a young adult patient of mine with learning disabilities and ADHD, provides a dramatic example of screen-time's effect on attention and learning. When he first came to see me, Cole declared that he wished to work on his reading skills and had recently taken placement tests at a local college. Academically, Cole had tested at a fifth-grade level in both reading and math. Fifth grade, interestingly enough, was the same year his teachers had introduced him to a computerized reading program. "They were all excited about it," he said, "but then they gave up on me when it didn't work." In light of these goals, and because his mood and sleep patterns were dysregulated, I asked Cole if he was willing to give up a handheld video game of his that had practically become a new appendage. After a forty-minute discussion, Cole decided to leave the game in my office. A few days later, Cole's brother left a voicemail stating that Cole's mood had evened out almost immediately. Shortly after this (and much to my delight), Cole's game console at home broke — he was now video game–free. A couple of months later, he was retested at the college for placement.

The results were nothing less than shocking: in math, which he'd always claimed he was good at, Cole now tested at a high school level, and his reading score had climbed four grade levels. I wouldn't have believed him if he hadn't shown me the actual testing results. Clearly, screen devices had been hindering this young man for many years, and his brain was now functioning at a level much more representative of his true capacity — making his literacy goals much more achievable. Indeed, as I'll cover in chapter 11, research shows that screen-time use in general makes literacy achievement more difficult and that reading from a screen hinders reading comprehension.

Green-Time and Attention Restoration: A Cure for Aggression?

Appreciating the link between attention fatigue and tantrums, meltdowns, and more serious aggression is key to putting a stop to this type of unwanted behavior. Children with attention difficulties are at much higher risk for aggressive acts[38] — not surprising considering inattention is associated with low frustration tolerance and an inability to check impulses. Meanwhile, restoring a child's mental capacity for focus reduces risk. *Attention restoration theory* posits that while stress depletes attention, sensory input or stimulation that lowers the stress response ("easy attention") restores the ability to focus.[39] Studies show green environments reduce aggressive acts and improve attention, impulse control, and academic performance.[40] Greenery draws the eye but lowers heart rate and blood pressure, thereby restoring focus and our ability to tolerate stress. Even pictures of greenery and viewing nature out of a window help, but time spent outdoors in nature is most powerful. Thus, in addition to the numerous ways screen-time contributes to aggression via hyperarousal, the fact that time spent indoors reduces exposure to the restorative effects of "green-time" is equally important!

Psychosis

Perhaps the most frightening repercussion of electronic devices is the emergence of psychosis, in which there are abnormal thoughts or thought processes. This can take the form of hallucinations (hearing voices or seeing things that aren't there), delusions, paranoia, or confused thinking. In the cases I've witnessed, psychosis triggered by screen-time has occurred in individuals with underlying vulnerabilities, such as intellectual delays, a mood disorder, autism, or a history of neglect or severe abuse, especially sexual abuse. The vast majority of the time, the psychosis resolves or dramatically diminishes with the electronic fast. Often, in contrast to an individual with an "organic" psychosis, the person often knows what he or she is experiencing is imagined: the voices are heard but don't feel "real," the sense that others are talking about them doesn't jive with reality, the nagging fear that someone is outside the window watching them at night seems silly during the day. Treating these cases can be very rewarding, because in addition to relieving symptoms, antipsychotic medicines can often be avoided, or if they've already been started, they can be reduced or even discontinued. This can lead to other pleasant by-products like weight loss and other health improvements.* Additionally, when a person's psychosis resolves, he or she may suddenly become capable of attending school, holding down a job, or engaging in a romantic relationship.

On the other hand, if an individual is genetically predisposed to psychotic illness, such as schizophrenia or severe bipolar disorder, screen-time may represent the proverbial straw that breaks the camel's back. It can trigger a "first break" — the initial episode in which an individual experiences a break from reality. In one sad case, a thirteen-year-old boy was allowed a substantial increase in his video game play during the aftermath of Hurricane Sandy. After several weeks of playing up to ten hours a day, the child started acting out scenes from his favorite game, and at times he seemed to believe he was actually in the game. Eventually he began acting out scenes in his sleep — a visible sign his brain was completely imprisoned, not to mention that sleep was not offering any relief. While searching for answers, his mother came across an article I'd written about screen-time and psychosis and promptly removed all video games as well as his computer. When she contacted me for a consultation a couple of months later, the worst of his symptoms had resolved, but the boy was continuing to hear voices, and he wound up requiring antipsychotic medication. In the months that followed, it became clear that the boy had a budding mental illness, likely schizophrenia. There was no family history of the disorder, but the child did have some vulnerabilities — learning disabilities and social problems — that, when combined with excessive gaming, was enough to create a tipping point.

When I first wrote about screen-time-related psychosis in *Psychology Today* in 2012,[41] I received a backlash of criticism and skepticism from several neuroscientists. But the first case report was published in 1993 (involving a Nintendo game), and multiple cases involving computer games and Internet-related psychosis have been reported since.[42] More recently, researchers have become interested in *how* excessive technology use might trigger psychotic symptoms. In 2013, an extensive report was published on so-called Game

---

* Antipsychotic medication used to treat psychosis often causes weight gain, and it can raise cholesterol and blood sugar.

Transfer Phenomenon, a process in which gamers experience game-related visual hallucinations during real-life situations.[43] It may be that these visual hallucinations — thought to be a sensory imprint of sorts — are more "benign" than other forms of psychosis I mention here. They are certainly more common and, for the most part, don't cause distress. (When the article came out, I was shocked at how many of my male friends admitted to having experienced them after long bouts of gaming.) Nevertheless, gamers and parents should interpret the presence of *any* psychotic phenomenon as a cautionary red flag.

How might screen-related psychosis occur? One factor likely at play here is dopamine regulation. Drugs and medications that increase dopamine (stimulants) are capable of producing psychosis, and many medications used to treat psychosis block dopamine. As you now know, gaming releases dopamine. Other factors may be sensory overload and the brain's inability to discern a virtual environment from the real one — especially as gaming environments become increasingly vivid and lifelike. This last factor may particularly be true for a child's brain and psyche, which are not yet solidly formed. Unfortunately, we are seeing an increased incidence of violent crimes in which young people act out particular video game scenes or role play a video game character. The perpetrator is often in a semi-dissociative state, which has been initiated and perpetuated by repeated exposure to virtual environments for years. Many of these cases don't "make the news" because the incidents involve minors, but they're occurring much more often than the general public realizes.

Because the consequences of psychosis can be so dire, parents should take extra screen-time precautions in a child with the vulnerabilities mentioned above, particularly if the child has trouble separating fantasy from reality, has a history of violent behavior, or has a family history of serious mental illness such as schizophrenia. Most physicians and mental health clinicians will not suspect video games or computer use when a patient reports psychotic symptoms, so it's likely that this screen-related phenomenon is largely underreported — which is a horrible shame, considering that it's treatable with strict screen elimination.

Disruptive and Defensive: Behavior and Social Issues

Behavior is essentially the outward manifestation of all the other issues we've been talking about. Typically, it's a child's *behaviors* that drive parents and teachers to the edge of the proverbial cliff — leading a parent to seek treatment. Socially, a multitude of important issues exist in relation to electronic media usage, such as identity development, sexting, and cyberbullying, to name a few. Here we'll look primarily at the impact of electronic media on behavior and social skills in the context of ESS — in other words, at how the physiological effects of screen-time translate to social problems in your child. With its core components of hyperarousal and mood dysregulation, ESS can affect relationships with peers and family, stunt social development, and diminish capacity for empathy and intimacy. Figure 6 below shows how this might occur.

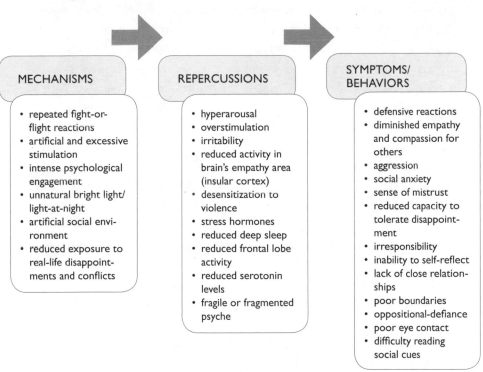

MECHANISMS

- repeated fight-or-flight reactions
- artificial and excessive stimulation
- intense psychological engagement
- unnatural bright light/light-at-night
- artificial social environment
- reduced exposure to real-life disappointments and conflicts

REPERCUSSIONS

- hyperarousal
- overstimulation
- irritability
- reduced activity in brain's empathy area (insular cortex)
- desensitization to violence
- stress hormones
- reduced deep sleep
- reduced frontal lobe activity
- reduced serotonin levels
- fragile or fragmented psyche

SYMPTOMS/ BEHAVIORS

- defensive reactions
- diminished empathy and compassion for others
- aggression
- social anxiety
- sense of mistrust
- reduced capacity to tolerate disappointment
- irresponsibility
- inability to self-reflect
- lack of close relationships
- poor boundaries
- oppositional-defiance
- poor eye contact
- difficulty reading social cues

Figure 6. How screen-time effects translate to social dysfunction

Oppositional-Defiant, Argumentative, and Impulsive Behaviors

"I say black and he says white."

"I could say, 'The sky is blue,' and she will start arguing with me."

"When we ask him to do something, his whining and arguing is so annoying that we just wind up doing it for him."

"When we enforce a consequence, she becomes so enraged that she wears us down and we give in."

"He doesn't listen and just does what he wants."

These are comments frequently expressed by parents in my office, and research suggests that there's a link between amount of media consumption and such disruptive behaviors.[44] Although "oppositional-defiant disorder" is an actual diagnosis listed in the DSM, in practice these symptoms are virtually always related to something more specific, such as ADHD or trauma.

Opposition and *defiance* are strategies children will use to exert some control over their environment when they feel stressed or inept in some way — it's a sign of a disorganized state of mind. These behaviors are often secondary to attentional or learning issues, hyperarousal, overstimulation, or poor sleep. Saying "no!" harks back developmentally to age two, when a child realizes that saying no gives him or her power over caregivers. Even as adults, when we feel overwhelmed, we might interrupt someone with a knee-jerk "no" before the person can even finish the question. *Arguing* is another common behavior indicative of poor attention or irritable mood* that's made worse by interactive screen-time;[45] arguing is a major source of parental frustration and exhaustion. Arguing may actually be a way for an unfocused child to raise arousal or dopamine and norepinephrine** levels, plus it serves to engage the parent — which can help a disorganized child feel more anchored. When a parent complains that a child is oppositional, argumentative, and irritable, especially if these symptoms seem to be worsening over time, my "index of suspicion" for ESS is very high.

In a classic example, a mother was telling me how her six-year-old twin boys weren't watching cartoons in the morning anymore; she and her husband had decided to get rid of cable TV to save money, and she knew that cartoon watching could affect attention. But their hectic morning routine had become a daily nightmare when it came to getting the boys ready for school. They'd argue and stall, refusing to dress themselves, put on shoes, or brush their teeth, crying, "I *can't!*" — all while refusing any offer of help. Inadvertently, the mother mentioned that because they weren't getting up to turn the

---

* Argumentativeness is also common in autism spectrum disorders.

** Recall that norepinephrine and dopamine are the two main brain chemicals (neurotransmitters) involved in attention and executive functioning.

television on anymore, she and her husband were able to sleep in a little longer in the mornings, despite the fact that the kids continued to get up earlier than they did. "So what do the kids do instead of watch cartoons?" I asked. "We let them play on our phones," she replied. Mystery solved! The boys' daily fifteen or twenty minutes of phone play was enough to disorganize their nervous systems and set the tone for the day. She and her husband began taking turns getting up early, stopped the phone play, and smoother mornings soon followed.

Another ESS behavioral symptom we've already touched on is *poor impulse control*. Impulsiveness refers to the tendency to act without thinking, such as hitting a sibling without regard for consequences, running into the street without looking for cars, continually interrupting others, and so on. Children with attention problems and hyperactivity are typically impulsive as well, and thus they tend to engage in more risk taking, resulting in more frequent accidents. Consistently, impulsivity has been found to be a risk factor for problematic gaming and Internet use,[46] and it seems to be a product of them as well. That is, just as there is a *bidirectional* relationship between gaming and poor attention, impulsivity and video games have been found to be mutually reinforcing. Violent games may pose an additional risk for poor impulse control.[47]

Violence and Delinquency

Violent aggression and delinquency are serious behavioral issues that are linked to excessive electronic media, particularly with violent content,[48] but also with screen-time in general[49] and with disturbed sleep.[50] I have already discussed this connection in several places, and how the mood dysregulation, hyperarousal, and attentional fatigue that occur with gaming can lead to meltdowns and aggression. In general, aggression and delinquency are associated with poor frontal lobe functioning, which is a clear consequence of excessive screen-time.

These links have been demonstrated no matter what content is viewed. Importantly, research suggests that total time spent gaming is a stronger predictor of aggression than the level of violence in the games played.[51] As with ESS in general, "It's the medium, not the message." That said, violent games pose a unique risk, and studies suggest that both violent and competitive games increase the risk of aggression compared to prosocial games.[52] This risk is especially strong in violent games where players team up to face a common enemy.[53] There's something about the social nature of these games that makes them risky for both aggression and addiction.

While content is not the most important factor in the development of ESS, because of their highly stimulating nature, violent games are likely to cause more severe ESS symptoms. I used to believe that parents already realized that violent games were harmful, and therefore I didn't spend much time driving this point home. What I didn't realize was that many — if not most — video games (including those made for younger children) *are* violent. More than 90 percent of games rated as appropriate for children ten and older are violent, and the majority of boys play mature, or M-rated, games.[54] Parents may be in the dark about how violent games really are, and ratings for video games are unreliable. Furthermore, many video games don't display any sex or violence on the cover or in their advertisements, masking their true nature. Violent games also often portray female characters in a degrading manner and can contain sexual violence (including rape) and racist content. Thus, it's advisable that parents watch or even play a game in order to screen it.

At this point, six decades of research have solidified the connection between acts of violence and aggression and exposure to media violence in television and movies,[55] while the past decade has seen an explosion of research on violent gaming in particular.[56] Do not be fooled by studies claiming there is no connection or that it's inconclusive; an overwhelming majority of evidence tells otherwise, and there is a strong consensus not only within the medical community but among researchers whose work is unbiased and non-industry-affiliated. Violent video game playing is associated with poor school performance; increased aggressive thoughts, feelings, and behavior; increased physiological arousal; and decreased empathy and prosocial behavior.[57] One reason for this is *desensitization* — that is, a blunting of our mental and physiological aversion to violence, whether real or virtual. Studies of violent video games have documented desensitization by measuring brain, cardiovascular, skin, and empathy responses.[58] Disturbingly, one study showed the desensitization response occurred after just twenty minutes of play.[59] As one young man explained to me, "I don't know if I'm addicted, but I tell you one thing, it's true what they say about violent video games and desensitization.... I don't feel any reaction *at all* to seeing violence.... I mean *nothing*. [Laughs] I could see someone get torn apart by a machete and it's the same to me as looking at someone walking down the street."

Children with mental health issues — especially boys — who play violent games and those who have addictive tendencies are at high risk for aggression, as are children who have a poor sense of reality or who have a tendency to attribute hostile intentions to others.[60] Newer, more technologically advanced games are more strongly linked to aggressiveness than older games, a trend researchers attribute to more realistic and vivid graphics and heightened "feelings of presence" (the sense that you are actually there).[61] Indeed, each generation of games creates higher levels of risk for both aggression and addiction than the one before: lifelike realism creates higher levels of arousal, hyperarousal is linked to both addiction and aggression, and addicted players are more likely to be aggressive.

In regard to other delinquent behavior, studies suggest that excessive screen-time (including smartphone use) in teens and preteens is associated with risky behaviors such as school truancy, experimenting with drugs and alcohol, and having unprotected sex — behaviors consistent with poor impulse control.[62] Interestingly, one study found that higher amounts of computer use was a stronger risk factor for delinquent behaviors than high television or video game use.[63] Lastly, research shows that poor sleep — which goes hand and hand with technology use — is in itself a risk factor for high-risk behaviors.[64]

Aside from the obvious safety issues surrounding aggressive acts, aggression is a leading reason why children are placed on psychotropic medication, misdiagnosed as having bipolar disorder, suspended or expelled from school, and charged with criminal activity. Needless to say, it's important to create environments that reduce this behavior, especially in high-risk populations.

Arrested Social Development

Children who experience *social anxiety* — feeling discomfort or distress in social situations — or who are socially incompetent are particularly at risk for developing dependence on electronic media. This is true whether the preferred agent be the Internet, video games, or a smartphone.[65] The more a child hides behind a screen, the more socially awkward he or she becomes, creating a self-perpetuating cycle. In contrast, a shy child who continually works at overcoming social anxiety is likely to overcome it. In the past, the strong desire to belong to a social group during adolescence helped override resistance to social interaction, which would lessen over time simply due to practice. Nowadays, socially anxious or awkward children and teens aren't forced to practice face-to-face and eye-to-eye interaction because some of their social needs are met online. Thus, in socially anxious children, the ability to tolerate the physical presence of others never builds, and "walls" are erected instead to keep the child feeling safe. An adolescent with somewhat poor social skills in high school can easily become reclusive as a young adult, spending more and more hours online and less and less time interacting in real life. This pattern makes it increasingly harder to make and keep friends. Relationship problems show up at home, too; research indicates that the more time a child spends using the Internet, the less healthy the parent-child relationship becomes.[66] Thus, social incompetence and screen-time represent another bidirectional relationship.

Interacting with young people with screen-related social anxiety can be awkward or even irritating: they tend to make poor eye contact, seem distracted or "not present," or squirm with discomfort. Often, they seem apathetic and demonstrate passive body language, like a weak handshake. They can take long pauses before answering questions and may be unable to engage in meaningful, reciprocal conversation. When they do open up, they may not be able to follow longer or more nuanced questions because of a shortened attention span, they may not give others the sense of being "heard," and they often can't seem to "resonate with" or "mirror" the other person's emotions.

A few years ago, I had a very enlightening conversation with my then sixteen-year-old nephew about this very issue. We were sitting together at his sister's high school graduation. The previous time I'd seen him, just six months earlier, he'd been his usual self — friendly, talkative, and high energy, but not able to pay attention to anything for more than a few seconds. If your question was too long, you lost him. Forget about sharing something with him — he wasn't listening. As we sat there, I was struck by a change in him. We were having a great conversation: he was listening to me, making eye contact, and responding without going off topic. At first I just thought, *Wow, he's really matured.* However, as we talked about football, which he'd played that year for the first time, my nephew shared that his coach had instructed the team members to stop playing video games because he felt it affected their ability to focus during games and could negatively impact grades — and therefore their eligibility to play sports. My nephew said at first he only cut back. Then, after realizing the difference it made, he quit completely. He said one of the first things he noticed was that he was suddenly able to talk to adults more easily, and he was speaking up more in class. He said that although he'd felt shy around his peers before, he'd found himself speaking up more in groups. Needless to say I was excited: here was a teen without a psychiatric disorder who'd quit playing video games on his own and was able to verbalize the changes in himself. His capacity for meaningful interaction had expanded dramatically.

Interestingly, my nephew then told me about one of his friends who was diabetic and sometimes faked being sick in order to miss school, either so he could play video games all day or because he'd been up late the previous night playing. (My nephew could "see" online when his friend was logged in to the game.) After quitting himself, my nephew became appalled by his friend's behavior, especially when he realized that during those long gaming sessions his friend's blood sugar would go way up. As he finished telling me this story, my nephew said, "His handshake is really weak. It's like a dead fish." After imitating it, he said, "I mean, come on, who'd hire a guy like that?"

He'd hit the nail right on the head. Impressions are made in the blink of an eye, and young people with poor social skills will have trouble getting ahead in life. Conversely, as my nephew's social skills improved, so did his awareness of their impact. This ability to self-reflect is part of what helps children not just survive but thrive.

In school-age children, social impairment related to ESS can manifest as poor sportsmanship when playing games, acting bossy or controlling, or being super competitive. (It doesn't help that many video games reward competitiveness.) Kids with ESS often have a low frustration tolerance that results in meltdowns and a tendency to blame everyone but themselves. They may also hold grudges or attribute hostile motives to others where there are none, such as assuming a peer purposely bumped into them. All of these behaviors drive other children away.

Because social skills and mood regulation are dependent on good frontal lobe function, children with ESS often act much younger than their years, and they may be teased, bullied, or ostracized because of outbursts. This occurred to Billy, a ten-year-old boy I worked with whose story I tell in chapter 4 (see page 117). In part, this dynamic occurs because screen-time creates a false experience of ease and success: electronic media offers immediate gratification, endless (and effortless) stimulation and entertainment, the ability to control one's environment or one's image, and the opportunity to be a hero — features that don't reflect how things work in the real world. Real life is much more difficult. Screen-time makes children less able to tolerate disappointment and boredom, more entitled, and less willing to work — whether it be for school, at a job, or to improve a relationship.

Disconnected: Empathy and Intimacy Issues

As I've already described, both violent gaming and excessive Internet use have been linked to a diminished capacity for empathy. Indeed, brain imaging studies of adolescents with Internet gaming addiction show damage to the *insula*, an area involved in empathy that helps integrate bodily sensations with emotion.[67] Empathy is different from sympathy; empathy is the ability to resonate with another's state of mind and actually feel what the other is feeling. It helps us bond because the other person "feels felt," and it fuels compassion and social responsibility by allowing us to feel others' pain. These characteristics make empathy fundamental to enjoying a fulfilling emotional and social life. But violent gamers and Internet-addicted individuals aside, what about today's children in general? Does time spent behind a screen impact one's ability to relate face to face?

Mounting evidence suggests that it does. A study examining empathy score trends of college students from 1979 to 2009 found scores to be falling, with a particularly sharp drop after the year 2000[68] — right in line with the first generation of children who were born into the age of video games and computers. Much of social competence is learning how to read subtle cues in body language and facial expressions, and studies show face-to-face contact is highly correlated with social well-being, while media use and media multitasking correlate with the opposite.[69] I've seen this firsthand: children who complete the Reset Program invariably display improved social skills, and their emotional competency grows quickly in the absence of screens. A 2014 study came to the same conclusion: preteens who spent five days at a wilderness camp in which screen media was completely restricted showed an enhanced ability to accurately interpret others' facial expressions.[70] Interestingly, one way we develop empathy is by unconsciously imitating the physical actions of others, so the freedom to move one's body while viewing others' bodies — something that being screen-free affords — appears to be important as well.

Eye contact is another element important in determining the quality of our social relationships. Eye contact is an essential part of the bonding process from birth onward. It reflects our capacity for intimacy, and an inability to tolerate sustained eye contact often translates to shallow relationships. Capacity for eye contact is likely related to the amount of an individual's current screen-time habits, the total years of screen-time, the age at which screen devices were introduced, and the quantity and quality of past and present face-to-face time — which is, of course, related to parental screen-time, too. Note that when a child operates with a defensive nervous system (from frequent fight-or-flight and less face-to-face interaction) on a regular basis, he or she will be less able to tolerate eye contact without unconsciously interpreting it as a threat — much like wild animals do — and will thus avoid it until the absence of screens forces the child to build tolerance.

Nowhere is the capacity for eye contact more critical than in romantic relationships. Although as a parent you may or may not be concerned about your child's romantic relationship potential at the moment, it'll be important at some point, usually starting in adolescence. A child's ability to form close friendships, to be honest and open about feelings, to empathize by putting themselves in another's shoes, and to communicate during conflict without becoming defensive will dictate the quality of his or her relationships, starting with friends and family and later with romantic interests as well. I see a number of young adult males with screen-time issues in my practice, and many of them want a girlfriend but have no clue about "live" interaction. Others begin relationships only to see them end quickly when their partner senses intimacy limitations and moves on. It takes a lot of hard work and resources to work on these issues as an adult — it's much easier to prevent them from developing in the first place.

In short, the same stress or fight-or-flight reactions that affect mood and cognitive symptoms also impact social relationships. Extreme shyness, poor sportsmanship, limited empathy skills, and reduced tolerance for intimacy are all made worse when face-to-screen replaces face-to-face. A defensive nervous system in survival mode cannot trust and therefore cannot form close relationships, and a poorly functioning frontal lobe cannot delay gratification, tolerate disappointment, or self-reflect. Aside from predicting relationship quality, these are essential ingredients for becoming a responsible adult with a strong moral compass.

Hijacked: Addiction and Reward Pathways

Addictions occur on a spectrum, and screen addiction is no different. However, when I work with patients, I don't like to focus on screen or tech addiction per se because it undermines the fact that ESS can be triggered by even "regular" use. Although severely screen-addicted individuals will virtually always have ESS, individuals with ESS aren't always or even usually addicted to screen-time. Furthermore, teens and young adults often find the term *addiction* off-putting, which can create roadblocks in treatment. Thus, I feel the most accurate and helpful term is "problematic," since it includes the child who experiences screen-related symptoms but whose screen habits are not necessarily excessive or addictive in nature. Nevertheless, the terms "pathological," "excessive," "overuse," and "addiction" are all used in the scientific literature, so for purposes of discussion here, they may be used interchangeably.

In reality, if the average school-age child is consuming four to six hours and the average teen is consuming seven-plus hours daily,[71] then the majority of children have screen habits that should be considered "excessive" — especially considering that we don't yet know what the long-term effects will be. Terminology notwithstanding, the findings in screen addiction research dovetail nicely with those observed in ESS, including biological, psychological, and behavioral aspects. If ESS and screen addiction are part of the same spectrum, then addiction research highlights the need for aggressive screen management — to "head it off at the pass."

Screen addiction or dependence can be psychological (causing anxiety or distress with lack of screen access), physical (causing brain changes and a true "withdrawal syndrome" similar to drug withdrawal), or both. In developed countries worldwide, an estimated 5 to 15 percent of people have screen-time addictions, making it an epidemic.[72] The silver lining behind the enormity of the problem is that because the problem is more widely recognized, a robust body of literature now exists that didn't a decade ago.

As I've said, electronics overuse bears a striking resemblance to stimulant abuse and addiction. Like amphetamine abuse, focus and mood may seem — and indeed may be — enhanced by the stimulation of screen-time. However, over time and as usage increases or accumulates, the "user" will begin to experience mood changes, sleep disturbances, shortened attention span, irritability, depression, defensiveness, an inability to tolerate stress, and a general worsening of functioning. Other similarities between screen addiction and stimulant addiction include decreased interest in other activities and feeling anxious if forced to be "without." Also, as with drug abuse, electronics use or abuse "just on the weekends" can still produce significant issues.

As with drugs, people are drawn to interactive electronic media for its ability to provide immediate gratification and intense stimulation. Marketers exploit these tendencies and thus "up the ante" with every new game, gadget, or application. Each new version becomes more stimulating, titillating, or rewarding — and thus more addicting — and the hijacking begins. Both physiological arousal and "feelings of presence" are factors known to promote and maintain engagement in video game play, and these factors are enhanced with newer games.[73]

Although there has been considerable media hype about the ways in which technology may be rewiring our brains, the bigger concern is that excessive video game and Internet use is causing actual brain *damage*. Numerous brain imaging studies have shown abnormalities in both brain structure and function similar to damage caused by drugs, such as in heroin, cocaine, and alcohol addiction. As discussed in chapter 2, research has demonstrated brain shrinkage in processing areas (gray matter), including the frontal lobe; loss of integrity in connection pathways (white matter); reduced cortical thickness (higher brain areas); and more impulsive but less accurate cognitive processing. When video game addicts are shown cues that induce "craving," their brains light up in the same areas that drug-addicted brains do. Finally, dopamine receptors may become desensitized, effectively requiring larger amounts of dopamine to do the same job.[74]

Interestingly, one group of researchers summarized the literature on pathological Internet use in a way that described the mood, attention, and behavior traits seen with ESS: "Taken together, these findings indicate that internet addiction disorder is associated with structural and functional changes in brain regions involving emotional processing, executive attention, decision making and cognitive control."[75]

Other research has looked at risk factors and outcomes. A study that followed more than three thousand children over a two-year period found that pathological gamers were at higher risk for subsequent depression, anxiety, social difficulties, and lower grades, while risk factors for becoming addicted were more time spent gaming, poor social skills, and impulsivity.[76] Not surprisingly, having ADHD poses a risk for both video game and Internet addiction.[77] As with other addictions, boys are more likely to be addicted to gaming and Internet use than girls — but the ratio is much more even when it comes to pathological smartphone use. Indeed, the explosion of smartphone and tablet ownership has pushed screen addiction to a new level. Though the screen may be smaller, the ease of accessibility, the shorter distance from the screen to the eyes and body, and the fact that devices are often snuck into bed and used after "lights out" makes them very risky.[78] Numerous studies have shown that smartphone addiction is similar to other tech addictions in terms of the associated psychopathology — depression, anxiety, physical complaints, social withdrawal, attention issues, and aggression have all been linked.[79] Again, these symptoms echo the range of ESS presentations.

Because screen addiction is so difficult to treat once it takes hold, you want to nip this in the bud — the sooner the better. It's *much* easier to prevent than treat. In fact, in terms of the Reset Program, whether your child is truly addicted or not is almost a moot point; by doing an electronic fast and restricting usage afterward in ways your child can best tolerate, you will begin to address potential addiction issues that may exist. That said, there are certain red flags that can indicate whether screen usage is possibly becoming addictive. Review the list below; you may notice some overlap from the ESS quiz presented at the start of chapter 1 because they share some of the same behaviors surrounding screen-time, and because some ESS symptoms are due to addiction or reward pathways being activated in the brain.

RED FLAGS FOR SCREEN ADDICTION

- Lying about device use or length of time used, or sneaking to use devices (such as in bed after lights out or while on screen restriction)
- Preferring to use electronics over every other activity, losing interest in other activities, or losing one's natural sense of curiosity about the world

- Becoming increasingly socially isolated, and/or using screen activity to escape from stress or avoid others
- In older teens and young adults, an inability to voluntarily cut back on amount or frequency of use (children and most teens shouldn't be expected to cut back on their own)
- Continued use despite adverse consequences (whether social, academic, or health), or escalating use
- Excessive negotiating when play is restricted, or becoming inappropriately angry or devastated when screen limits are imposed or even merely discussed (such as threatening suicide or becoming assaultive)
- Lack of improvement in ESS symptoms after three weeks of being screen-free, or immediate and severe relapse of ESS with very small amounts of use following the electronic fast
- Signs of physical deconditioning, such as shortness of breath, muscle weakness or wasting, weight gain, or fatigue
- Poor reality testing (such as trouble discerning game from reality), or dissociative tendencies (feeling unreal or that surroundings aren't real)
- Excessive or escalating use of multimember online role-playing games (MMORPGs) or using them as primary source of social interaction

Antonio: When Play Becomes Addiction

Antonio was a troubled older teen who was referred to me by a colleague who was seeing Antonio's family for therapy. Antonio's gaming began around age five when his mother and stepfather gave birth to a little boy. Along with the demands of a new baby, Antonio's mother experienced postpartum depression, so Antonio was often under the watch of his stepfather, whom he felt "didn't like me and never played with me." In fact, Antonio couldn't recall playing with much else besides video games as a child. In grade school, Antonio was reportedly "hyper" and somewhat disruptive, but he typically got As and Bs. In the mornings, he'd watch cartoons before school, and in the afternoons he'd begin playing video games as soon as he got home.

Around age thirteen, Antonio began playing World of Warcraft (WoW), an online role-playing game. Friends at school also played the game, and

Antonio felt himself drawn more and more to WoW. His grades began slipping, and he became more defiant at school as well as at home, particularly with his stepdad. When Antonio was ready for high school, his parents tried transferring him to a strict military school, but he was soon ordered to leave for not following rules.

So Antonio returned to his old school and old friends, and he began dating a girl who also played WoW. Antonio felt happy in the relationship, but eventually the girl complained about how much time and energy Antonio spent on the game, and she suggested they both quit. Antonio told her he'd feel guilty if he quit and let his "guild," or team, down, and so he refused, prompting a breakup. Antonio was devastated and began smoking pot; he admitted he would "smoke and play games, pretty much every day." Throughout the next several years, according to his mother, Antonio would stay up all night gaming, rarely went outside, and would "hide" when other family members visited the home. Antonio's mother said she herself continued to struggle with depression during this period, and that her husband distanced himself from parenting completely. She felt helpless to control Antonio, while Antonio felt no one noticed or cared what he did.

By junior year of high school, Antonio's truancy became such an issue that he decided he'd rather work. He got a job at a grocery store and seemed to thrive for a while, but eventually he was fired for not showing up. Now, without any school or work obligations, Antonio would hole up in his room, blinds drawn, and play WoW all day and night. As his friends graduated high school and went off to college, Antonio became increasingly socially isolated and began to experience dissociative feelings. He noted, "Sometimes I'd feel like, 'Is this real? Am I real?'" When he wasn't gaming, he'd fantasize about violence, like eviscerating or slicing up zombies, and he was continually trying to incorporate aspects of the game into his real life. Finally, after a particularly bad row occurred with the stepfather, the whole family was referred for treatment by social services, and Antonio admitted to both feeling depressed and being afraid he'd seriously hurt someone.

Unfortunately, Antonio refused to believe the gaming played any part in the way he felt or how his life was going, and with his parents either unable or unwilling to take action, it was never addressed. Antonio continued treatment with his therapist for a couple of years and was even able to quit smoking pot, but he continued to game and remained unemployed. Eventually, and unfortunately, I learned he was facing serious criminal charges.

This is a sad case, but it shows how disabling gaming addiction can be. The longer it goes on, the more entrenched it becomes in the individual's brain and mind. This story also illustrates some common dynamics associated with tech addiction: a lonely child using gaming for stimulation, social interaction, and as a means to escape; a lack of solid early relationships setting the stage for inadequate coping skills; and the association of screen addiction with delinquency and other addictions.

Which brings us to an important point: addictive behavior during adolescence sets up the brain for addiction later in life.[80] During this period, the frontal lobe is very sensitive to environmental input, and its development can be compromised or permanently damaged, which can lead to self-medicating, poor choices, and poor impulse control. If addiction pathways in the brain are hijacked by electronics, this may set the stage for other types of addiction; preliminary data on video game dependence and other addictions support that they may be mutually reinforcing.[81]

Anxiety and Apprehension

Anxiety, like ESS itself, comes in a variety of shapes and sizes: Panic attacks can cause dizziness, shortness of breath, or a racing heartbeat. Trauma-related anxiety can be experienced as nightmares, emotional numbness, or in children, as hyperactivity. Obsessive-compulsive symptoms take on the form of intrusive thoughts combined with compulsive acts to keep the thoughts at bay. Generalized anxiety manifests as excessive worry about everything. And anxiety seen in autism can present as rigid or inflexible thinking or as an increase in self-stimulatory behaviors. Like ESS, anxiety symptoms are born from an overly aroused nervous system.

Obsessive-Compulsive Disorder (OCD)

Of all the entities mimicked or triggered by ESS, I've received the most emails about screen-related OCD, perhaps because it can emerge so dramatically and seemingly out of nowhere. Since OCD is intimately related to dopamine regulation, its development may be particularly sensitive to screen exposure. In OCD, there is too much dopamine in brain areas involved with movement. Interestingly, I know of a number of cases that have been triggered by the Wii, an exercise video game ("exergame") in which players wave a wand and otherwise move to control play. Since dopamine levels rise during exercise, and exercise obviously involves movement, the link between exergames and OCD is not surprising. Many parents believe exergames to be healthier, so this connection is important to appreciate.

What happened to Jack, my colleague Mary's son, provides us with an example. Several years ago, Mary reported to me that six-year-old Jack had suddenly developed what she thought were tics: repetitive movements in his hands and arms that seemed to have no purpose. When questioned about it, however, Jack told his mother that he "couldn't stop touching things" and that it bothered him all day long. Mary had never let her children play a lot of video games, but when the family received a Wii gaming system as a gift, Jack started playing every day, eventually to the exclusion of other activities. Mary suspected the Wii was the source of his symptoms and asked me if I thought this was possible — *Of course!* I replied. Mary took it away, and Jack's symptoms resolved within a couple of weeks. One month later, Mary reintroduced the Wii, but the symptoms reappeared immediately. She then gave Jack a much longer break — about four months. Eventually, she figured out that he could tolerate play about once a month for thirty minutes — and that was it. Interestingly, Jack himself was so disturbed by his symptoms that he didn't mind his games being taken away and in fact avoided video games when they were around.

In 2012, I told Jack's story in a blog post,[82] prompting a mother to email me about her three-year-old son, Emory, who developed similar symptoms after playing games on the iPad. The mother related that initially she'd allowed her son to play educational games only, but that she'd eventually permitted an action game his older brother had been playing. Soon after, Emory began touching things compulsively. One night, Emory's mother asked him why he kept touching and rubbing his arms all over his headboard before lying down to sleep. He replied, "I don't *want* to. I just can't stop!" His mother stopped the action games immediately, but she felt conflicted about stopping the educational games. She told me Emory's symptoms hadn't gone away, and that she wasn't sure what she should do. I assured her that there is no proof that educational apps or games give children an "edge," but that there is lots of proof otherwise — especially in the very young — and that she could stop those games too with a clear conscience. She agreed to stop the iPad use altogether, and Emory's compulsions resolved shortly thereafter. (Note that while it was the action games that immediately preceded the compulsive behavior, it wasn't enough to restrict the action games. All iPad use had to stop to reset this child's brain.)

These might seem like unusual cases, but they provide vivid examples of how ESS takes the brain hostage and presents as the spitting image of a specific mental disorder. In other OCD cases, the child or teen already has the disorder, but the symptoms worsen or become immune to treatment when electronics are added to the mix. In these instances, restricting electronics may not be the *only* treatment, but they are a *necessary* part of treatment. I've seen cases where traditional OCD therapy has been applied unsuccessfully for years, but then it moves forward once screens are out of the way.

Rarely, gaming may trigger the onset of OCD that is not easily reversed. In one case I consulted on, a nine-year-old boy developed severe, disabling OCD following a period in which he'd been playing video games up to twelve hours a day. The family had moved to rural North Carolina in July, leaving the boy with lots of unstructured time and no one to hang out with. His parents, who were fairly strict about screen-time, felt guilty about transplanting their son during a time of year when it would be difficult to make new friends, and they uncharacteristically allowed unrestricted access.

By the time they called me, his mother had already stopped all video games for a month, but the OCD seemed to have taken on a life of its own. The boy was so afraid of touching something dirty that he'd literally become immobilized and cry that he couldn't make a move. This child required medication, intense therapy, and no electronics for many months before his symptoms were under control. Thus, electronics can create, exacerbate, or perhaps even "flip a switch" to trigger OCD that may or may not become chronic.

Obsessive Thoughts and Rumination

Obsessive or ruminative thinking can occur in children and teens with anxiety, depression, or autistic spectrum disorders. Youths with these tendencies may experience an increase in obsessive thinking when exposed to even moderate amounts of screen-time. In some cases, very little screen-time is needed to trigger an increase in obsessiveness. Typical manifestations of this in teens or young adults include a worsening fixation on a romantic interest, obsessing about a real or perceived rejection by someone they admire, or becoming preoccupied with past relationships. In depressed patients, screen-time can worsen rumination regarding past failures, regrets, and painful shame or guilt. Children on the autism spectrum (including Asperger's) — who by nature have limited interests — may become more obsessive regarding certain movies, songs, or cartoons. In high-functioning autistic teens or young adults, romantic obsession can become quite serious or even delusional when combined with excessive screen-time.

Because dopamine can reinforce obsessive "loops," electronics worsen these symptoms. Further, preclusion from real-world interactions worsens internal preoccupation. Teens or young adults often describe this state as "I can't get out of my head." Regardless of the child's primary diagnosis, when electronics are removed, many parents report a decrease in the level of their child's obsessiveness.

Fight, Flight — or Freeze?!: Other Anxiety Symptoms and Syndromes

Aside from fight-or-flight, the third choice for an individual in survival mode is "freeze" — like when an animal plays dead. In humans, the freeze state can be experienced as "paralyzing anxiety," feeling helpless, or being "afraid to make a move." In ESS, this kind of immobilizing anxiety occurs more often in children with a history of trauma, attachment issues, intellectual disabilities, and autism, though it can happen in children without such histories, too. Particularly in girls, ESS may present as anxiety (stress directed inward) as opposed to meltdowns (stress directed outward), and it may arise from seemingly innocuous screen activities. Let's look at a few examples.

SEPARATION ANXIETY AND FEARFULNESS

A six-year-old girl developed sudden, severe separation anxiety whenever her mother dropped her off at school. A behavioral intervention did not help, and there were no other identified stressors or problems at school. Careful history revealed that for several months the child had been playing some educational games on a Leapster every day for about thirty minutes at a time. Removal of the Leapster device allowed the behavioral intervention to succeed. In another case, a fellow physician approached me about his five-year-old son's escalating fear of the dark, which had begun affecting other activities besides bedtime, like going into movie theaters. The family had bought an iPad eight months before. Despite the fact that they'd set usage limits of thirty minutes or less per day, the iPad proved to be the culprit.

Panic Attacks

An adolescent girl with sensory sensitivities began having sudden episodes of extreme anxiety and a fear of strangers. In the past, the child had been unable to tolerate medication or even herbal remedies, and she had been unwilling to participate in therapy. We were at a loss about what to do, until we discovered that she'd been drawing on an iPad every day for several months. This was enough to put her more vulnerable brain in a state of fight-or-flight — or in this case, "freeze." After removal of the iPad, she still had some anxiety, but the disabling panic attacks resolved.

Trauma and Attachment Disorder

An adopted seven-year-old boy with a history of abuse and neglect complained of nightmares and of seeing and hearing monsters. His parents reported he'd "go into a trance" when watching cartoons or playing video games, and he tended to act out scenes from these rather than engaging in imaginative play. Eager to promote healthy bonding with their adopted child, his parents readily removed all video games, which are often used as an escape in children with attachment issues.* Because of trauma, this boy's baseline state was fight-or-flight, and even thirty minutes of video game play on the weekends caused setbacks. We had to be extra careful about eliminating stimulating screen sources — including cartoons — but eventually this strict screen management allowed the family's attachment work to move forward and the boy's creative play to emerge.

In another case, an eighteen-year-old young woman with a history of sexual assault was referred to me for repeated aggressive acts toward her male peers at a special-ed school-work program they all attended. She'd already been prescribed five medications, three of them antipsychotics, in an

---

* Children with attachment issues are at very high risk for screen addiction and are "primed" for arousal dysregulation, so extra diligence should be given to this population.

effort to control the aggression, and she had been in therapy for years. As it turned out, the staff at her program were rewarding her with computer time, which amounted to two to three hours of screen exposure every day. Once we stopped this practice, her aggression ceased, and she eventually became gainfully employed. An added bonus was that living in a more relaxed state allowed her to work through her past trauma more effectively in therapy.

In other cases, gaming creates a picture that looks similar to post-traumatic stress disorder (PTSD) in someone with no trauma history in real life. Recently, I consulted on a case in which an eighteen-year-old boy had attacked a friend while in a dissociative state. As I reviewed his psychiatric records, I was struck by impressions that the boy had suffered trauma and severe neglect in early childhood; the symptoms and themes were similar to the ones I saw in children I'd worked with who'd been living in foster care. When I interviewed him, however, he reminded me instead of the veterans I'd once treated during my residency days. He literally seemed like someone who had gone off to war, someone haunted by violence of epic proportions. Yet I couldn't find any history of substantial trauma. His family was stressed, but loving and kind, and there was no abuse history. I knew from his records that he was an avid gamer, but it wasn't until he began talking about the game Warhammer that I suddenly realized that his likeness to a war veteran was because he'd been immersing himself in that world for years. Warhammer is a strategic role-playing war game, and he'd been playing for hours on end daily since age twelve. Not only had his nervous system been affected, but his *psyche* had been damaged: he was convinced that some of the characters in the game had invaded him — and in many ways, he was right.

NIGHT TERRORS AND NIGHTMARES

A bright nine-year-old boy with a long history of night terrors had been free of them for about eight months after completing the Reset and then continuing to be game-free. On Christmas Day, his mother let him play a video game for several hours while she cooked and entertained guests. That night and the next, he experienced severe night terrors that kept her and the boy's father awake most of the night. Over the next year, it became clear that even occasional play could cause the night terrors to return.

Night terrors are due to a large, sudden surge of fight-or-flight chemicals released during deep sleep, so it makes sense that they can occur with ESS. A child experiencing a night terror will often sit up in bed and appear terrified, screaming, crying, or thrashing around, but typically he or she won't remember the episode in the morning. Night terrors tend to occur more often when a child is stressed. Not surprisingly, they're extremely disturbing to parents, and living with a child who has them can be exhausting.

Nightmares, on the other hand, occur while in the dreaming stages of sleep. Like night terrors, nightmares are related to stress, but they are much more common. Indeed, they are a normal part of life. However, if a child complains about nightmares on a regular basis and has developed other anxiety symptoms, such as headaches or stomachaches, it's certainly worth trying the Reset Program to see if the symptoms improve. Research suggests that TV shows, movies, and games with scary content can cause bad dreams even if viewed during the daytime, and both TV and gaming close to bedtime are associated with nightmares even when the content is nonviolent.[83]

Tics, Quirks, and Jerks: Neurological Dysfunction

One very tangible way that we know screen-time irritates the nervous system is because it can provoke neurological phenomena, such as tics, seizures, and migraines. Other neurological "side effects" of electronics are precipitation or worsening of sensory integration issues and autistic symptoms.

Tics, Tourette Syndrome, and Stuttering

Tics and Tourette syndrome (which is a combination of motor and vocal tics) are becoming increasingly common.[84] I first learned about some of screen-time's effects by treating these disorders, and these cases remain some of the most rewarding to work with, since prescribing the Reset can be highly effective. As with OCD, it's easy to see when tics get better or worse.

Recently, a study organized by the Association for Comprehensive Neurotherapy surveyed parents of children with Tourette syndrome about which environmental factors were felt to trigger their child's tics. Over two thousand families participated, and the answers were tallied in order of frequency. Out of all the environmental riggers mentioned, video games were ranked sixth and flashing lights tenth.[85]

Like obsessive-compulsive symptoms, tics are thought to be produced by abnormal firing in motor areas of the brain from an overabundance of dopamine. Stimulants and other ADHD medications that increase dopamine tend to make tics worse (and can bring them out in a child who's never had them), while dopamine blocking agents (as in certain antipsychotic medications) are the most effective at reducing them. Thus, it's easy to see why screen interaction can make tics worse. Interestingly, some parents report a quieting of tics when the child watches television but an exacerbation with other screen activities, giving credence to the idea that screen *interactivity* causes dysregulation in and of itself. On the other hand, the same movie watched quietly at home might produce tics if seen in a theater, due to the intensity of sensory and psychological stimulation. Other factors that make tics worse are poor sleep and stress, both of which are worsened by electronics.

In some children, it's very obvious that gaming or Internet use makes their tics worse because they'll experience a large outpouring of tics during or immediately after electronics use. Parents sometimes bring in video of their child ticcing away while gaming or doing homework on the computer. In other children, electronics may cause an increase in overall frequency or intensity, making the screen-time connection less obvious. Regardless of pattern, it is virtually always helpful to aggressively manage interactive screen-time in children with tics.

In one case of Tourette syndrome, the child's family had made some rather drastic environmental adjustments, including replacing their carpeting and eliminating wheat, dairy, food dyes, and preservatives from their child's diet — but they couldn't bring themselves to lose the video games. After an iPad acquisition preceded a bad exacerbation, the parents were finally convinced to do the Reset Program. The tics quieted, but the child's mother wasn't really convinced that the intervention had made a difference until a couple of months later. She let the boy play video games for several hours at a friend's birthday party, and severe tics followed for several days in a row. "He was a *wreck*," she told me.

In another case, the three-year-old daughter of a neighbor of mine developed an eye-blinking tic. Her mother shared with me that throat clearing (a vocal tic) had also developed, but only when the girl watched fast-paced cartoons or other highly stimulating children's shows. A stay-at-home mom with a small baby, this mother wasn't ready to give up the cartoons, as I suggested she try. One morning while in my front yard I saw the little girl and her dad climb into their minivan. I waved to them as they buckled up, then noticed the father give his daughter his smartphone to play with. *Aha!* I was convinced that the phone gaming was probably a bigger culprit than even the cartoons, so risking their annoyance, I brought the subject up again the next time I saw the parents. They agreed to eliminate this habit, and the tics resolved in a matter of weeks. Subsequently, the girl was able to watch cartoons (in moderation) without the tics recurring.

Stuttering has some similarities to tics, in that they both involve motor areas of the brain, both can be triggered by stress or excitement, and both respond to dopamine blocking agents. I've seen a few teen boys whose stuttering completely resolved after giving up video games, although it may be more realistic to expect improvement but not necessarily cessation.

Autism Spectrum Disorders (ASD)

Children with autism and Asperger's are uniquely vulnerable to ESS for several reasons: 1) children with autism spectrum disorders (ASD) tend to have sleep and sensory issues to begin with; 2) electronic media interaction tends to facilitate compartmentalization and inhibit integration of brain areas, a pattern that already exists in autistic individuals;[86] 3) individuals with ASD are not only more drawn to screen devices than other children, they are more likely to become addicted and to exhibit symptoms from relatively small amounts of exposure;[87] and 4) the pathological processes involved in autism development mirror many of the pathological effects found in EMF research.[88] For these reasons, ESS in autistic spectrum children can be particularly severe. In my experience, screen-time can precipitate regression (loss of language or of social or adaptive living skills), exacerbate repetitive or obsessive behaviors, further restrict interests, and trigger aggressive and self-injurious behaviors. Needless to say, screen-time often becomes a source of added stress for parents who are already dealing with challenging behaviors. In fact, since the advent of the iPad, I find myself saying to parents of autistic children: "For your child, the iPad is the devil."

Children "on the spectrum" typically show intense interest in electronic screen devices, be they video games, computers, televisions, handheld devices, and so on, and parents of autistic children tend to use screen-time both to purposely manage behaviors and out of sheer exhaustion.[89] One study found that ASD children spent significantly more time with screen activities than all other non-screen activities combined, that they used them considerably more than their siblings did, and that they displayed more symptoms related to problematic use.[90] Another study looking at ASD boys found they were more likely to have video game access in their bedrooms compared to typically developing siblings, and that attention symptoms and a preference for role-playing games were predictive of problematic use.[91]

Earlier, I described how obsessive behavior can be made worse by interactive screen-time because of dopamine dysregulation. In autistic children this trait often preexists, and it can manifest as repeatedly viewing, verbally repeating, or acting out certain scenes from preferred movies, games, or cartoons. When ESS compounds this trait, the child will have increased difficulty disengaging from a screen activity, often culminating in a meltdown. Many autistic children have aggressive or self-injurious behaviors to begin with, and these tendencies are made worse by the hyperarousal, overstimulation, frustration, poor impulse control, reduced movement, sleep disruption, and attention difficulties that come hand-in-hand with screen-time. Autistic children also typically have abnormal sleep patterns, low melatonin levels,[92] and sensory integration difficulties[93] as part of their disorder, and these too are made worse. Regarding melatonin, one mechanism thought to be a contributor to the development of autism is that there is excess oxidative stress or inflammation in the brain. If melatonin, a potent antioxidant and sleep regulator, is lowered further by electronics, unchecked inflammation could rapidly ensue — both from not having the antioxidant protection and because poor sleep itself causes inflammation.

Regarding social deficits, screen-time exacerbates some of the same dysfunctional behaviors we see in typically developing children: poor eye contact, limited empathy, and emotional outbursts. For autistic children, immersion in screens heightens internal preoccupation and lack of interest in the outside world, including in other people. In short, these kids' brains are ripe for screen hijacking. Ironically, the industry has attempted to exploit this attraction to screens by marketing video games and tech-based therapy "tools" designed to teach autistic children how to read emotion. The fact that these games have no merit apparently doesn't matter because parents and clinicians are desperate.

Autistic regression is a phenomenon that is often seen during the initial onset of autism, and it is sometimes seen again at other times during the autistic person's life. It's unclear exactly why this happens, but experts think there may be a tipping point or perfect storm of environmental and genetic factors (called "insults"). These factors perturb cellular processes and brain pathways and eventually overwhelm repair mechanisms, creating a downward spiral. There is some evidence that screen-time exposure in the first three years of life is one of those factors.[94]

Another screen-related factor that may be contributing to this tipping point is radiation from electromagnetic fields (EMFs). Dr. Martha Herbert, a pediatric neurologist and autism expert at Harvard Medical School and Boston's Massachusetts General Hospital, published an extensive report in 2012 arguing that because pathological processes in autism and EMF damage from wireless communications observed in laboratory research are similar, it is likely that EMFs from electronic devices compound autistic illness.[95] Dr. Herbert feels these effects should be considered a public health threat, not only because of the recent dramatic rise in autism and other mental disorders, but because WiFi is increasingly incorporated into our schools at levels many times stronger than what is in the average home. In the EMF appendix, a special autism section outlines all the different mechanisms that may be involved, which is of extra importance for parents of autistic children to read.

Today, there is considerable pressure on parents of special-needs children to embrace new technologies, both as motivational and as educational tools. While communication devices can certainly be helpful at times, I've also noticed a consistent pattern with autistic children after an electronic device, such as an iPad, is introduced. Often, mothers will report academic gains initially, only to see the child lose those gains and regress even further within a year. At a recent lecture I gave about strategies to minimize psychotropic medications — which naturally included restricting electronics — several therapists who were also mothers of autistic children described regressive behaviors appearing several months after the child started using an electronic communication device. One mother said that her son used the device initially, then regressed and stopped communicating altogether. Others described rages or a loss of language or eye contact. Unfortunately, many therapists trained in applied behavioral analysis (or ABA, an in-home therapy used to improve autistic behaviors) now use video game play as a reinforcer. "They're the only thing that motivates this child!" they'll say triumphantly, often without even attempting to try other reinforcers. All too often the next thing I hear is that the mother has "fired" the agency, finding the therapy or the staff to be ineffective, or even being bothered by male staff spending inordinate amounts of time gaming with the child.

In stark contrast, autistic children who do the Reset Program often show significant symptom reduction fairly quickly, and the changes are maintained when screens are strictly managed. One of the first things to improve in ASD from the Reset is sleep — an element critical to healing. Deep rest supports detoxification processes, which serve to improve mood, anxiety, and attention — a *virtuous* cycle. Another dysfunctional behavior that often improves rapidly is aggression. One ten-year-old patient of mine went from having full-blown rages (including one in which he destroyed an entire classroom, overturning and smashing desks, chairs, and tables) to complete resolution of aggression once video games were removed. Two years later, his behavior reports showed *zero* aggressive incidents. Several mothers I work with have reported noticing an increase in language and creativity and even improvement of empathy and development of abstract thought. Needless to say, witnessing these kinds of improvements in autistic children is extremely rewarding.

With autism, the "dose" of screen-time that can bring on ESS is quite low, especially in boys. If you do decide to use an electronic communication device, use one that is "bare bones," with no games and more natural sensory stimulation (for example, real buttons are better than a lit touchscreen). Watch closely for signs of classic ESS, such as hyperarousal and dysregulated mood, and stop use immediately if you suspect regression. Regarding leisurely electronic device use, finding replacement activities may feel particularly challenging for these children, but it is certainly possible and well worth the effort.

Disordered Development: Sensory, Movement, and Balance

These days, an alarming number of children are having trouble with printing, reading, and mood regulation because of inattention, poor fine and gross motor skills, weak core muscles, and imbalanced sensory systems. In other words, they are displaying problems with sensory integration, which is how the brain makes sense of signals from bodily sensations and the external environment, using the five senses plus the vestibular* system.

What do children require to develop optimally? Kids need several hours of unstructured physical play daily to adequately stimulate and integrate sensory pathways; they need secure attachment (bonding) to caregivers, plenty of touch, and varying levels of environmental stimulation that support calm alertness during the day and restful sleep at night. They also need conversation with adults, contact with nature, and creative outlets, such as music, art, or dance. Screen-time reduces time spent experiencing all of these things, plus it overstimulates the visual and auditory systems, making it difficult to filter relevant from non-relevant stimuli. Vestibular stimulation during screen activities is low, which over time results in a weak core and delayed visual-motor skills needed for printing, reading, and regulating arousal.[96] Children using screen devices are also held less and touched less, and they receive less eye contact from the mother (who may be using a screen device herself). Since long-term brain development is impacted by neglect more than any other factor,[97] any reduction in bonding time is cause for concern. Interestingly, the reward pathways that addictive drugs and activities hijack are the same ones meant to facilitate bonding. Thus, bonding may serve as a buffer, preventing the need to self-medicate with chemicals or stimulating screen-time.[98] Reduced deep touch (such as from being held or hugged or from roughhousing) leads children to be restless and to seek out deep sensory input, which can take the form of hitting, squeezing, or pushing others. Finally, repeatedly viewing a 2D screen does not provide the eye muscles and vestibular system the 3D input they need to develop properly.[99]

Thus, screen-time activity can produce or worsen visual-motor, sensory, and vestibular deficits, creating problems with printing, reading, focus, memory, and difficulty regulating mood and arousal levels. If a child is constantly feeling uncomfortable in his or her environment, the child will act out in order

---

* The vestibular system determines balance, posture, and sense of body position in relation to the environment. It affects muscle tone, particularly core strength, and coordinates with the visual system as well. Its development is highly dependent on movement typically acquired through unstructured play, such as jumping, swinging, bike riding, and playing on the monkey bars.

to get those needs met and won't be able to learn. If screen-time is producing these deficits by affecting how the nervous system develops, then it may be that some of the children requiring specialized services — such as occupational therapy, sensory integration, and vision therapy — wouldn't need these services if screen devices were simply eliminated and the level of active physical play rose by default.

On the other hand, sensory integration work can be quite powerful; it sometimes resolves serious emotional regulation problems when other treatments don't work. I have witnessed children climb several grade levels in a few months' time once sensory issues were addressed — but sensory integration won't work well if the child is still using electronics. ESS is very stubborn in this regard.

Seizures and Headaches

As I mentioned earlier, one of the most dramatic accounts of visually provoked seizures occurred in 1997 in Japan, when several hundred children experienced seizures and vomiting after watching a particular scene in a Pokémon episode with rapidly flashing blue and red colors.[100] Admittedly, this was an unusual event, but the point is that visual phenomenon can trigger enough electrical excitability to cause a neurological event, even in people with no seizure history.

Video-game-induced seizures have been reported since the eighties, but they are considered to be relatively rare. In my practice, I've only seen a handful of *confirmed* cases over the past decade or so. But while the Pokémon episode mentioned above was banned, the type of visual stimulation it contained has only intensified over the years in the effort to make cartoons and games more stimulating — rapid pacing, flashing and abnormally vibrant colors, an overly bright screen, fast zooms, abrupt movements, and changing patterns. This kind of stimulation can quickly overload the visual system, especially an immature one.[101] Furthermore, poor sleep — part and parcel of electronics use — raises seizure risk in general. Does that mean we can expect to see more seizures as time goes on? I expect so.

The problem is, while a generalized "grand mal" seizure is very obvious, other more subtle types of seizures — such as partial complex and absence ("petit mal") seizures — may also occur during screen activities but are harder to detect. These seizures are not as obvious to the observer, and they may or may not show up on an EEG (a test looking at brainwaves for seizure activity). Risk factors for visually induced seizures include a history of autism, ADHD, a previous seizure, and developmental delays. Clinically, these types of seizures are often misdiagnosed because they can manifest as extreme "spaciness," memory problems, depression, rages, fatigue, or losing touch with reality (for example, having conversations with characters on a TV program) — symptoms that mimic psychiatric diagnoses.[102] In some video game seizure cases, the parent will notice the child's pupils are not just dilated but "huge" after gaming, indicating an outpouring of metabolic reactions. Academically, the child with seizures may seem "stuck" at a certain grade level because daily seizures don't allow the brain to process information normally, much less continue maturing.

These symptoms are hard to distinguish from other issues, and there's no easy way to ascertain if seizures are a part of your child's picture. (The most accurate way is probably to have an EEG performed while the child is gaming, but accomplishing this is easier said than done.) Video game seizures are probably not as "rare" as the gaming industry would like us to believe, but they're not as common as some of the other shape-shifting scenarios presented in this chapter, either. Regardless, the electronic fast may provide some helpful information and perhaps some relief if they are occurring. Removing screens (especially video games and computers) may be enough to resolve these types of seizures, but sometimes seizure medications (many of which are mood stabilizers) can provide additional improvements. Occasionally, there will be a large "jump" in intellectual capacity following screen removal plus seizure medication treatment, which suggests that seizures may indeed have been present.

As far as headaches, both migraine and tension headaches can occur as a result of screen activity. Sometimes parents will make the association that a child's headaches began after the arrival of a jumbo-sized TV screen in the living room (since screen size affects arousal levels). Migraines may be precipitated as a result of irritating visual input and electrical excitability, while tension headaches may be from a combination of visual stimulation and muscle tension. Both types of headaches are made worse by hyperarousal, poor sleep, and other stress reactions.

Physical Ailments

Many screen-related physical ailments are the really the indirect consequence of all the mental health issues related to ESS, particularly the stress response and poor sleep. Others are due to low physical activity level, poor blood flow, repetitive movements, or prolonged postures.

When blood flow stagnates from being sedentary, nutrition and oxygen delivery slow, and waste products build. Eventually, this process leads to inflammation, which affects us all the way from the cellular level to the whole-body level. Tissue damage examples include things like neck or back pain, repetitive stress injuries, eye damage, and blood clots. All-over muscle tension is common with screen-time, and it can lead to muscle adhesions, which restrict blood flow even further. Muscle weakness and even atrophy (wasting) can occur as well, from lack of use. Examples of whole-body dysfunction include fatigue, poor posture, weight gain, hormone dysfunction, high blood pressure, and deconditioning. To add insult to injury, the combination of fight-or-flight plus low activity compounds all these issues plus it increases the risk for heart disease and diabetes.

Similarly, the brain too suffers from deconditioning, inflammation, mental fatigue, and tissue atrophy from screen-time. Physical health reflects mental health, and vice versa. Truly, screen-time affects us from head to toe, inside and out.

Chapter 3 Take-Home Points

- ESS can create symptoms and dysfunction that mimic or exacerbate various psychiatric, neurological, and behavior disorders. Effects from screen-time are cumulative, leading to increased risk of ESS over time.

- Mood symptoms are common with ESS and include irritability, depression, mood swings, and mood dysregulation. When ESS produces mood symptoms plus aggression, it is often misdiagnosed as bipolar disorder.

- Cognitive symptoms are also common, including trouble with attention, impulse control, and organization. These symptoms can impact grades, creativity, and curiosity.

- Behavior issues include oppositional-defiance, meltdowns, and poor impulse control. Social dysfunction can look like poor sportsmanship, difficulty making or keeping friends, and intimacy issues.

- The association between screen-time and some types of dysfunction is "bidirectional," or mutually reinforcing. That is, children with certain issues are attracted to screen-time, and those same issues are made worse with screen-time. Examples include inattention, poor social skills, depression, delinquency, and autism.

- There is ample evidence that Internet, video game, and smartphone addiction is both disabling and damaging; screen activities can "hijack" the brain in the same ways as drugs and alcohol.

- Children with attention issues and/or social incompetence are at higher risk for developing tech addiction, as are children with autism.

- Anxiety symptoms are a common manifestation of ESS, such as obsessive-compulsive behavior, nightmares, panic attacks, and excessive worrying.

- Neurological phenomena — tics, seizures, stuttering, headaches, sensory dysfunction — can be triggered by screen-time.

- For all of these issues, the electronic fast can help clarify diagnosis and reduce symptoms, whether underlying disorders exist or not.

CHAPTER 4

THE BRAIN LIBERATED

How Freedom from Electronic Screens Can Change the Brain in Days, Weeks, and Months — and for Years to Come

An 11-year-old today is performing at the level
an 8- or 9-year-old was performing at 30 years ago.

— Professor Michael Shayer, King's College, University of London[1]

When you are facing a dilemma, all it takes to begin
is to ask yourself three questions: What are the consequences of
my decision in 10 minutes? 10 months? And in 10 years?

— Suzy Welch, author of *10-10-10*[2]

In the 1980s, intelligence researcher James Flynn wrote about a curious phenomenon: over the previous century, IQ scores had risen about three points per decade, which had prompted researchers to renormalize the curve every fifteen years or so — the so-called Flynn effect.[3] Since the effect was seen globally in developed nations, experts speculated that the effect was due to socio-environmental factors, such as improved nutrition, more stimulating environments, and educational advances, particularly in special education. During the 1980s and 1990s, though, IQ scores appeared to slow and then plateau in first-world countries, while they continued to rise in developing countries, suggesting that IQs could reach an effective "ceiling" once environmental benefit was maximized.

Then researchers began noticing something equally curious. In 2007, Michael Shayer of King's College at the University of London and two colleagues published some startling research suggesting the trend had actually reversed: a well-tested measure of math and science intelligence had declined considerably from 1975 to 2000, despite peaking in the mid-nineties, and it had continued to decline from 2000 to 2003 in seventh-grade students.[4] The study produced three other interesting findings: 1) that the math-science score gap between boys and girls had disappeared; 2) that although both boys' and girls' scores had declined, the boys' scores had dropped more severely — about double the rate of girls; and 3) that the declines were uniform across both the high and low scorers. In fact, none of the children in the top 10 percent in 2003 scored as high as the children in that same tier back in the 1970s. On average, children were *three years* behind their 1970's counterparts, which prompted Shayer to write the quote that opens this chapter. Since then, other research has suggested similar declines in other IQ measures.[5]

What caused such a trend reversal, and why have scores continued to fall? Why are boys being more affected than girls? No one can say for sure, but various experts have speculated that the growth of television viewing spurred the initial decline and that growth of video games and computer use has perpetuated it. Experts have also speculated that lower activity levels, less time spent reading, and less imaginary play may also account for the difference. That is, either directly or indirectly, much of the decline may be attributed to screen-time and everything that comes with it.

IQ doesn't measure brain health per se, but it can act as a sort of yardstick for developmental maturity. As we've seen in the last couple of chapters, in the short term screen media imprisons your child's brain and impacts functioning in all areas of life. In the long term, observation and research suggests that screen media creates *drag* on development itself, causing stunted growth, plateaus, or even regression. Conversely, removing screens is like reinvesting the dividends in a good stock: the gains compound over time, so much so that a child who grows up with little to no interactive screen-time may eventually surpass a brighter child with "typical" screen exposure in terms of emotional-cognitive development and level of functioning.

This is the flip side to chapter 3: liberation from screens seems to provide not only a myriad of mental health benefits but also developmental benefits that are realized over time. When screen-time is removed, brain chemistry re-balances and circadian rhythms resynchronize. Overstimulated networks are quieted, stress hormones ebb, and blood flow is redirected back to the frontal lobe. These changes begin with the removal of dysregulating influences, and they are reinforced by better sleep. At the same time, in a beautiful synergy, these effects are multiplied by what takes place instead. When screen-time is eliminated, it most often gets replaced with the very activities and inter-actions children need for healthy development: families bond, and children engage and play in the natural world around them.

Indeed, the mission of the Reset Program itself and of mindful screen management thereafter is to optimize your child's mental health now as well as his or her development down the road. While the steps to accomplish this are discussed throughout the rest of this book, in this chapter, I want to show you what screen liberation looks like, so you have a picture in your head, and so you'll realize and appreciate why the Reset gives you so much bang for your buck. First, I'll explain how mental health is defined in terms of features — which happen to be the same features that optimize development — and I'll describe generally what the brain requires to behave in such a fashion. Then, I'll describe the benefits themselves, both as a result of the Reset and over the months and years that follow when screen-time is strictly limited.

Toward Integration: Mental Health Defined

When it comes to mental health, we tend to seek symptom relief without defining what we want to move *toward*. We know a lot about what can go wrong in the brain, as well as how mental disorders manifest in symptoms and dysfunction. Indeed, in the last two chapters I've broken down what can go wrong into bits and pieces, so you can appreciate how screen-time affects us adversely by a variety of mechanisms and at a variety of levels. But while illness is about how things break down — both in function and in description — health is about integration. No matter what the condition, the goal is to move toward making the brain more *whole*. We want it to function as more than the sum of its parts — whatever those parts may be. The more inte-grated the brain is, the more resilient and capable it becomes.

Child psychiatrist Dr. Dan Siegel, a pioneer in the study of the neurobi-ology of mindfulness and healthy attachment, uses the analogy that mental health can be thought of as a flowing river, with one bank representing chaos and the other bank representing rigidity. The goal is to avoid either extreme and to flow nicely down the river, exerting more control when needed and letting go when stuck. Individuals who navigate the river well tend to have a more integrated brain, reflected by certain features, for which Dr. Siegel offers the acronym FACES —*flexible, adaptive, curious, energetic,* and *stable.*[6] Thus, we want children to be flexible, not rigid; adaptive when encountering stress, change, or challenges; curious about the world around them and about themselves and others; energetic, not depleted; and stable or self-regulated, not dysregulated.

So what are the conditions that support optimal integration? First, the brain cannot become healthy if it is under constant stress. While we encounter stress every day, and small amounts can be tolerated and even helpful, chronic stress is detrimental, as I've shown. Second, the brain requires adequate downtime, or rest, to recuperate from daily stress and to process information and emotions. Third, the brain requires nurturing, in the form of parent-child interactions, which include eye contact, talking and sharing of feelings, touch, being held or hugged, having basic needs met, and being understood. Fourth, the brain needs a variety of stimulation but in appropriate amounts at appropriate times; this is most easily achieved by the child interacting with and learning from the natural environment, along with periods of low stimulation. Lastly, the brain needs the body to move and feel, to obtain both gentle and rigorous exercise, to move in rhythmic ways and in different directions, and to experience a variety of sensory experiences, including deep pressure, in order to integrate the entire nervous system.

Many of the above factors are related to *right-brain functions.* Fittingly, the right brain is the more holistic side of the brain, and right-brain stimulation heals us both psychologically and biologically. Bonding, movement, creativity, emotion, and abstract thought all stimulate the right brain, and they also help integrate the entire brain, including the frontal lobe, as well as help connect the brain to the body. The left brain, on the other hand, is much more literal. It likes information. When you read a story in this book, your right brain takes it all in and makes sense of it; when you read about dopamine or melatonin, your left brain remembers the details. In general, because screen-time is information packed, it tends to overstimulate the left brain and understimulate the right, which makes the entire system more fragmented and less connected.[7] Thus, when the nervous system begins to dysregulate, we need to emphasize right-brain activity to get back on track.

We all have an intuitive "knowing" of what it means to be whole. Our language reflects this: When we speak of someone's ego or psyche being *integrated*, we might describe him or her as "so together," "resilient," or "with it." But if an individual's ego is easily fragmented, we might say, "She falls apart so easily," or "He can't handle any stress. He just comes apart at the seams." When a child's mind is *organized*, it's easier for that child to complete routines, like getting ready for school. We might refer to that child as "being on top of things," while a disorganized child "can't get themselves together."

Clinically, we know wholeness, too: When an individual's psyche or ego is strong but flexible, we know it can withstand stress, while a weak one "fragments." When the brain's hemispheres and the body's sensory-motor system are well-integrated, the child will learn easily, thrive in new and stimulating environments, and demonstrate synchronized motor movements. The child with sensory integration dysfunction, on the other hand, easily becomes overstimulated and disorganized and will demonstrate inefficient movements and a dysregulated mood. In fact, our bodies also have an intuitive knowing, as integration and synchronization can occur at every level, from the cell to the nervous system to the psyche. At the cellular level, when circadian or body clock cells are in sync with nature, *all* cells throughout the organism are more synchronized, and hormones and organ functions follow suit. Similarly, when stress hormones are low, the heart produces coherent electrical rhythms, and the brain's rhythms become coherent as well.

Nature abhors a vacuum. Holistically, there is nothing that occurs in isolation, and *integration at any level helps create virtuous rather than vicious cycles*. Thus, once the brain is liberated from the stress of screen-time, once it's had a chance to rest, rejuvenate, and reset, then the entire system becomes more organized, integrated, and whole. So long as adequate screen limits continue, our systems tend to keep going in that same direction, finding the middle of the river more often.

The Screen-Liberated Brain

Let's look more specifically at the health trajectory that freedom from screens provides to a child's brain in days, weeks, months, and years. These are changes based on what I've observed with patients and others I've worked with, what the research shows, and what we know about how the brain works and responds to environmental cues, reductions in stimulation and stress, deeper sleep, and so on. These lists are meant to capture *typical* gains, but of course there is variation, and of course life can throw us curveballs along the way. Every child and every circumstance is different: some children respond faster than others, some children are dealing with more stress outside of screen-time than others, and some families have to contend with more screen-time outside of the home — such as at school — than others. At the same time, more severe symptoms or dysfunction may take longer to reverse, and older teens and young adults may require longer stretches of time to see the same benefits as younger children, particularly if they've been logging in many screen-time hours for years. Nevertheless, these are changes that tend to occur in children more often than not, roughly in the time periods outlined below:

WITHIN DAYS

- The child's initial negative reaction to the plan — tearfulness, anger, arguing, and so on — subsides.
- The child's mood, attitude, and compliance begin to improve.
- The child begins to sleep better, and may go to bed earlier.
- Play begins to become more creative and more physical.
- The child's initial preoccupation with restoring screen-time diminishes (especially with younger children), though negotiations over this may linger.

WITHIN WEEKS

- Meltdowns become less frequent or less severe, or both.
- The child's mood becomes brighter and more stable.
- The child's attention improves, sometimes dramatically, and the child stays on task more easily.
- Grades noticeably improve.
- Sleep deepens and becomes more restorative, promoting the healing process and allowing the brain to reset biochemically.
- The child's body clock (or circadian rhythm) resynchronizes to daylight hours, which helps normalize the sleep-wake cycle, stress hormones, the immune system, and serotonin levels.

- The brain reclaims lost cellular energy due to decreased inflammation.
- The blood flow in the brain shifts from primitive/survival areas to higher learning centers, including the frontal lobe.
- Increasingly, more homework is completed, and in less time, and doing homework becomes less "torturous" for both parent and child.
- In interactions, the child's eye contact improves, conversations are longer, and the child "listens better."
- The child exhibits better sportsmanship and better manners in general.
- Sensory processing often improves, such that the child becomes less sensitive to environmental stimuli and is less likely to become over-stimulated.

WITHIN MONTHS

- Meltdowns diminish further and may resolve completely, and mood stabilizes further.
- Grades may markedly improve.
- The child progresses more quickly when learning attention-sensitive subjects, such as math and reading.
- Learning new information solidifies or "sticks" better.
- Signs of social improvements become more apparent, such as enhanced empathy, increased tolerance for sustained eye contact, and a stronger social network.
- Self-reflection improves, particularly in teens and young adults.
- The child's ability to accurately read others' emotions and actions improves, and the child is less likely to inappropriately attribute hostile motives to others.
- The child becomes more self-aware; some (but not all) will attribute feeling or functioning better to being screen-free, or will realize gaming makes them "feel bad."
- The child may prompt friends to engage in screen-free activities or may prefer friends who rarely use screens.
- Coordination may improve as motor-sensory-vestibular systems integrate.

Long-Term Benefits

Before I list the benefits that can occur over years as the child develops, it bears mentioning that it inherently becomes more difficult to tell what changes are due to screen liberation and what are due to maturation from simply aging. Over long stretches of time, some benefits will be easier to discern by comparing the child to his or her peers, since the reality is that most children are screen-bound. For example, in years past, your child may have been relatively emotionally immature compared to peers, but over time your child may catch up to or even surpass peers in this realm. Or your child may have struggled with reading comprehension in earlier years, but in later years your child may like to read books and talk about them much more than his or her friends do. Not that development is a competition; in fact, competing is part of what's creating the overuse of technology in the first place. Nor do we want to rush development, for every child is different. Rather, over the course of years, comparing the development of your child with other, similar-age children can make the appearance of certain attributes and traits more obvious. You may realize your child is becoming more mature in certain areas or ways in which others might be stunted. Similarly, it may dawn on you that your child is closer to where you or *your* peers were when you were that age, and others, including teachers and grandparents, may make remarks about your child being particularly mature, responsible, or caring.

OVER YEARS

- The child's self-direction increases; that is, he or she thinks of the future, makes plans, and acts accordingly.
- Empathy and compassion are noticeably enhanced; that is, he or she shows more concern and consideration for others' welfare and can imagine how others feel.
- The child's sense of self becomes more rounded, and the child demonstrates a rich variety of interests and activities.
- The child is more likely to seek out mentorship or ask others for help and guidance.
- The child's ability to process negative events and emotions, like loss, grief, and disappointment, is more developed, and negative emotions are less likely to cause setbacks.

- The child is better able to learn from mistakes and is less likely to blame others.
- The child prefers and chooses healthier peer groups, with similar attributes and interests, and may "drop" friends who are excessive screen users.
- The child may recognize screen-related dysfunction in those who are heavy screen users.
- The child completes household chores with less resistance and with better attention to detail.
- The child has a stronger sense of responsibility and more respect for authority figures.
- The child continues to develop self-awareness, including strengths, weaknesses, hopes, fears, and areas for improvement.
- When interacting socially, the child becomes increasingly capable of having extended conversations and making sustained eye contact, and demonstrates an ability to reflect on what's been said.
- The child reads more and processes material more readily and deeply.
- The child often becomes more health conscious and self-disciplined, and he or she may be more likely to follow through on efforts to eat right or exercise more often.

Billy: Breaking New Ground

Let's turn to Billy, a boy I mentioned in chapter 3. This was a case I consulted on when I first began writing this book, and his story nicely demonstrates the powerful changes in maturity and development that are possible in a matter of months.

When I first met Billy, he was ten years old and getting straight As in school. The son of two Ivy-League-educated engineers, Billy was quite bright, but his parents were concerned because he seemed socially immature. He was a poor sport, and he frequently lied and cheated when playing board games, playground activities, and team sports. If he lost at anything, he'd have a major meltdown and blame everyone but himself. He hung out with a circle of friends he'd known since kindergarten, but as the children had grown older, their patience with Billy had worn thin. Billy essentially had to "rotate" whom he spent time with, and his parents were worried that if this continued, he'd eventually be ostracized. Billy had no insight into his behavior, and he couldn't see how his actions might be off-putting to others.

On the surface, Billy didn't appear to be suffering from concentration problems, since he was a straight-A student. He also had no mental health history, and nothing concerning enough to warrant any other kind of professional evaluation in the past. When his parents told me what they'd been observing, I naturally asked about video game play. I've found that with particularly bright children, they can develop ESS and still maintain their grades.

Billy's parents said he played a handheld Nintendo DS every day on the school bus, and after school he often played computer games as well — including MMORPGs, or multimember online role-playing games, which are known to be particularly addictive. In addition, Billy's parents reported they'd caught him "sneaking" play during restricted times. To Billy's parents, none of these screen-time behaviors seemed unusual or out of the ordinary compared to his peers, but to me, Billy's reactive mood swings told me his nervous system was overstimulated and hyperaroused, and the "sneaking" suggested that cravings and dopamine dysregulation were at work. I also wondered if Billy's immaturity was because his frontal lobe development was being suppressed. After discussing these concerns, Billy's parents agreed to try the Reset Program.

When informed of the plan, Billy apparently cried, but his mother reported that he also appeared relieved. I spoke to his parents again approximately one month later.

"We were shocked," his mother told me. "His mood seemed better almost immediately, within a few days it seemed. He just seems happier overall. He still is having trouble losing at games on the playground, but in general he's not having complete meltdowns over minor things like he was doing before."

After continuing the program for the next couple of months, Billy's parents decided to let Billy play a computer game for thirty minutes on the weekends. Immediately after his first time playing, Billy picked a fight with his mother out of nowhere and sobbed uncontrollably, yelling at her that he hated her. Two days later, Billy seemed to have re-regulated and his mood stabilized. He didn't play computer games again for another month, when again his parents allowed him thirty minutes. This time, not only did he pick a fight with his mother, but he lashed out at his father. Billy then ran down the street over to a friend's house and got into a physical altercation — totally new territory for him.

Because of these two incidents, Billy's parents decided to maintain their strict no-gaming policy for a while, since he seemed so sensitive to the electronic screen trigger.

Six months later, they reported that Billy had decided to run for class president, for which he had to give a speech — something that previously would have terrified him. Billy had never shown leadership skills before; this was an unexpected development. Additionally, he spontaneously and successfully organized an elaborate neighborhood game of hide-and-seek. His friends were no longer avoiding him, and his sportsmanship had improved markedly. Billy's parents reported feeling "blown away" by the changes in Billy. "He's matured in leaps and bounds," his mother told me.

Billy's new behaviors — leadership, organization, planning, communication, and initiative — are all aspects of healthy frontal lobe development, an area Billy had clearly shown a lag in before. Were these changes mainly due to the electronic fast? We can't say for sure, but the sequence of events makes it look that way. It is certainly not unusual for parents to notice "spurts" in maturity, but Billy went from being socially and emotionally immature to doing things that are mature for any child his age. This was more like a quantum leap — and certainly a larger than expected jump for normal development. It was as though his frontal lobe went from being suppressed to being nourished. Billy's natural intelligence and formerly suppressed strengths and leadership skills had been liberated.

Sometimes parents will ask me: "If my son games a lot, but is getting straight As, is it really a problem?" Good question. Is it? Is it a problem if a child is fairly successful in multiple realms of function — but is perhaps not meeting his or her potential? This is the concern that Michael Shayer and the IQ studies raise, which is that for some reason children today are not developing the same way that they used to. In the larger picture, don't we want *all* children to maximize their potential, whether they have psychological or developmental issues or not? Indeed, it's not just the children exhibiting major dysfunction who will benefit from screen liberation; in terms of optimal development, *all* children will benefit from removing screen-time's drag on development. Often, though, the reason parents ask those questions is because they're wondering if their child is suffering in some other area, such as friendships. For better or worse, it's the parents of children who are struggling in one way or another who will be the most motivated to make lasting change.

The Screen-Liberated Family

When a child struggles, it negatively impacts everyone in the family, and when a child flourishes, the entire family becomes less stressed. Naturally, the positive effect on how a family interacts is even more pronounced when parents become more mindful of their own screen-time. I see marked changes in family dynamics when families follow the Reset Program and remain committed to very limited screen-time, and I observe similar traits in families who are conservative with screen-time to begin with. The following list describes traits or dynamics in these families:

- The parents are (or become) less worried about the child's future, and they have more trust that the child will achieve milestones like going to college, getting a job, and living independently.
- The family members spend more quality time together, both one-on-one and as a unit, and tend to talk more.
- The children are less likely to complain that parents don't spend time with them, or that a parent is "on the computer all the time" or "always on the phone."
- The parents are less stressed and are less likely to "avoid" family time through overwork or other activities.
- The parents are less likely to undermine each other's authority, and they are better at communicating with each other when parenting styles differ.
- Family members are less likely to mock one another or put one another down.
- The children are more likely to tell their parents if they're worried about something or if something bad happened (and less likely to broadcast problems on social media).
- The children are less likely to report feeling as though the parents have "no idea what I do" or "no control over me."
- The parents don't "walk on eggshells" around their children, they aren't afraid to discipline, and they aren't afraid to say no.

- The parents are (or become) unconcerned with "keeping up with the Jones's" regarding technology.
- The children expect to earn privileges rather than feel entitled to them.
- The children have a better sense of how money works, and the parents are more likely to implement "earning" money or allowances rather than just giving it regardless of behavior or giving it "when they need it."
- The siblings are more likely to look out for one another's well-being and are more aware of and in tune with their siblings' inner emotional lives.

Though it may seem a stretch to attribute all the positive family dynumics listed above simply to good screen habits, research supports these observations. Studies regarding television and Internet use show that higher levels of screen-time have a negative effect on parent-child interaction,[8] and that video games that emphasize role-playing can contribute to children developing pathological attachment styles, including dissociative tendencies that create emotional barriers.[9] Other research has shown that families talk more when they don't watch television during dinner, and that children in families who eat dinner together without screens on a regular basis have better grades, higher self-esteem, and a lower likelihood of getting into trouble.[10] If we combine these findings with what I've already shared about how screen-time impacts emotional regulation, empathy, and impulse control, it's not hard to see how a screen-liberated family will function in a much healthier manner.

Boys to Men: Two Long-Term Case Studies

The question of what benefits we can attribute to limiting screen-time is an important and difficult one. It's much easier to quantify and confirm the negative effects of too much screen-time than the positive effects of very little screen-time. To help illustrate the difference, here are two long-term cases involving boys I treated from the age of nine or so into adulthood. Though both have psychiatric disorders, one of them initially had more severe psychiatric problems and a relatively lower IQ, but he wound up with superior organizational, emotional, and relational skills.

James: Failure to Launch

I began seeing James when he was nine. He was an extremely bright, attractive child who had ADHD mixed with some anxiety and depression. Extremely shy, James felt anxious in social situations and was drawn to the computer, where he felt proficient and in control. In elementary school, he was described by his teachers as "an angel," and he was frequently rewarded for good behavior with computer time. Throughout his school years, James was continually praised by teachers, therapists, and other adults for his excellent computer skills, though he showed other academic aptitudes as well. At the age of thirteen, James got his first cell phone. Although he continued to struggle making male friends, his good looks attracted girls, and he began having "texting relationships" with several of them. Nearly every night, James stayed awake texting girls until the wee hours of the morning. He'd wake up exhausted each day and complain he couldn't sleep.

During middle and high school, James was relatively more social compared to his younger years, but he also spent more and more time at home on the computer, playing video games, surfing the Internet, and barely interacting at all with his family. His depression, which had been fairly mild before, became dark and stormy, and James eventually was diagnosed as having mild bipolar illness. However, getting him and his family to comply with medication was difficult, and my attempts to establish a regular sleep-wake routine, which is an essential aspect of treatment for bipolar disorder, proved to be futile.

My efforts to remove video games and limit computer use were thwarted by both his parents and his teachers, who felt his computer use represented a strength for him and that video games were an "outlet." When James began to have romantic relationships, his girlfriends would complain about him "not talking" during face-to-face interactions, and eventually they would break up with him. James was devastated by these breakups; he clearly craved emotional closeness. During high school, he obtained various part-time jobs, and his bosses typically reported he was a good worker. However, despite these good reports, James got fired from multiple jobs for either showing up late or missing work altogether because of getting the schedule mixed up.

After graduating from an alternative high school with fairly decent grades, James repeatedly missed deadlines to apply for community college.

By the age of nineteen, he could build a website — but he couldn't hold down a job, keep a girlfriend, register for school, or develop meaningful friendships with same-sex peers. He became increasingly depressed and suffered from low self-esteem. At home, his relationship with his parents went from bad to worse. In particular, tension with his mother reached a boiling point: he regarded her prompts to "get his act together" as nagging criticism, while she perceived his angry responses as displaying utter contempt — a dynamic that resulted in ugly screaming matches.

James's mother also complained that James never helped around the house, and when he did, his work was "really sloppy." James's mother became increasingly resistant to taking away privileges like phone or computer use because she was afraid he'd "hate me even more" and because "he's an adult now." She felt helpless and wished he would "just learn to listen" and "make good choices." By this point, James's father had pretty much checked out and avoided getting involved.

James, meanwhile, only increased his computer usage and continued to become more isolated. His bitterness toward his mother grew, and James blamed her for his lack of success, while his relationship with his father was nonexistent. When I last contacted James, he was twenty-three and living in the basement of his parents' house, ostensibly looking for work, but he didn't have his driver's license and rarely left the house. He and his mother were barely speaking to each other.

James is generally liked, and he is often described as having a "sweet spirit." His IQ tests in the ninety-fifth percentile. He doesn't drink, smoke, do drugs, or commit crimes. But clearly, he's stuck, and his emotional and cognitive potential are tragically stunted. Is this due entirely to screen-time and gaming? Perhaps not, but clearly it's contributed, both directly and indirectly. Unfortunately, we can only guess how much better his life might be without it.

Liam: Nurture Over Nature

Like James, Liam was nine years old and had ADHD when I first evaluated him. But Liam also suffered from learning disabilities, bipolar disorder, and obsessive-compulsive disorder. Furthermore, he'd been exposed to methamphetamine in utero, making his brain particularly sensitive to environmental stimuli. His parents had adopted Liam when he was two, and when they came to me, they were at their wits' end. His explosive behaviors and compulsions took up hours of each day. They were so stressed they were ready to place him in residential treatment to get some relief. Liam's parents reported he was "climbing the walls — literally!"

Clearly, Liam was overstimulated and unable to regulate his moods. Initially, we focused on getting his parents more support so they could better manage the stress. Liam's mother was a teacher, and she used to tell me she could pick out the kids in her class who were gamers, so she was readily on board with my suggestion of no screen-time. In fact, over the years, Liam's mother never allowed him to get a cell phone or Facebook account, nor did she allow a TV or laptop in his room: "He's got too many problems already without adding those into the mix," she'd say.

When I started working with him, Liam was virtually friendless because of his extreme hyperactivity, but over the years Liam calmed considerably and developed a core group of friends. Liam and his mother were religious about keeping a regular sleep-wake schedule, even on the weekends. During adolescence, Liam experienced a couple of manic episodes for which he was hospitalized, but over time he became more adept at regulating his mood and anxiety. Previously crippling compulsions to repeat tasks over and over again faded as he was able to implement coping skills learned in therapy.

Despite needing special education, Liam graduated from high school with all As and Bs. He enjoyed many friends of both sexes with whom he'd go to the beach, out to lunch, and to amusement parks. He was likeable, respectful, charming, and could converse with adults while maintaining good eye contact.

I recall a moment early on in his treatment when his mother broke down in tears, afraid that Liam would never be able to leave home and live on his own. But by age twenty, Liam was attending junior college, balancing his own time, and taking steps to learn good money management. By twenty-two, he'd moved out of his parents' house, and his volunteer position at a pet shelter had turned into a paid job with benefits. Today, he leads a full, active, independent life. He goes on road trips, hikes and camps with his friends, is successful at work, and is pursuing school part-time. In fact, he recently turned down an offer for a managerial position in order to continue his education. He does a minor amount of texting, doesn't email much, finds Facebook "a waste of time," and plays zero video games.

THE BRAIN LIBERATED | 125

Can we *know* that it was screen liberation that allowed Liam to overcome his developmental and psychological challenges and succeed in his life? Without question, Liam benefited from other factors: his loving and supportive parents, his therapy, his teachers, and so on. What of his improvement, then, can we attribute to his lack of screen-time? How do we *know* that, in the absence of screens, Liam slept better over the years than he would have otherwise, that his dopamine was better regulated, that his frontal lobe developed more optimally because it wasn't overstimulated? How do you *prove* that? Perhaps screen-time simply displaces healthier activities, and therefore it's more a matter of increasing healthier activities than it is reducing screen-time. Perhaps this trajectory happened because Liam simply exercised more or had healthier parents. Perhaps all the benefits were indirect.

Perhaps, perhaps not. I'd bet my bottom dollar that they're not all indirect. For Liam and for all children, *all* the changes — direct physiological ones and indirect ones — combine to manifest the wide-ranging benefits we see with screen liberation. As I mentioned earlier, these changes become synergistic: the frontal lobe gets freed up, and it then tends to choose right-brain activities, which integrates the entire brain, and so on. But the truth is, if an intervention helps a child, does it really matter why it works? A 2014 obesity-prevention study showed that when parents monitored media and reduced total screen-time that kids got more sleep, performed better in school, were more socially cooperative, and less aggressive.[11] Let the researchers tease out how much influence can be attributed to direct versus indirect mechanisms. But for clinicians, educators, and parents, it doesn't matter much. Both direct and indirect effects result in improved frontal lobe function, which in turn improves functioning in all realms of life. Better is better, and worse is worse.

Dr. Siegel's work on attachment shows that an integrated brain with good frontal lobe functioning means not just better mood regulation and executive functioning but enhanced empathy, compassion, and capacity for love.[12] Despite James being blessed with keen intelligence, good looks, a sweet personality, and a wish for closeness, the suppression of his frontal lobe development has left him handicapped. And despite Liam being dealt a rough hand in life, his brain and frontal lobe have developed optimally, providing him with emotional maturity and pushing his functional capacity far past our expectations.

The power of screen liberation should not be underestimated.

Chapter 4 Take-Home Points

- Going screen-free produces benefits almost immediately, and long-term changes are profound in terms of social, emotional, and cognitive development.
- Virtually all positive changes are attributed to improved integration of the brain in general and the frontal lobe in particular, which governs executive functioning and emotional regulation.
- The goal of screen limits is not merely to get rid of bothersome symptoms but to optimize a child's development over time. All children benefit from screen limits, which have a compounded effect on functioning later in life.
- In a matter of days of being screen-free, the child will typically exhibit improved mood and attitude and start to sleep better.
- In a matter of weeks, the brain starts to function better cognitively and is rejuvenated because of restored energy. The child is better able to regulate mood and tolerate stress.
- In a matter of months, outward signs like improved grades and relational skills become more apparent, and "leaps" in maturity can be observed.
- Over years, screen liberation significantly improves the maturity level of a child or young adult, so they exhibit more responsible, thoughtful, and empathic behavior.

PART TWO

THE RESET SOLUTION

A Four-Week Plan
to Reset Your Child's Brain

CHAPTER 5

WEEK 1: GETTING READY

Set Your Child Up to Succeed

*Let our advance worrying
become advance thinking and planning.*

— Winston Churchill

Part 2 describes the four-week Reset Program, which typically consists of one week of planning and three weeks of an electronic fast. While I've seen parents plunge right into the electronic fast without planning and still succeed, most families benefit greatly from planning in terms of ease and compliance. Even a poor plan is better than no plan, as the saying goes, and parents who don't anticipate and prepare often wind up missing something crucial that undermines success, like forgetting about a device the child rarely uses, failing to provide adequate replacement activities, or not making sure other caregivers, like the babysitter, know the rules.

This chapter guides you in the planning process, which can take shorter or longer than a week depending on your motivation and situation. I find that when parents are ready for change, they often manage to arrange things quite quickly — in a few days — while others might take longer (though sometimes this is more due to stalling than active planning). Plan to spend at least a weekend and up to one week preparing for the three-week electronic fast.

Preparation for the fast consists of defining problem areas and setting goals, forming a strong support team, deciding how you will replace screen devices and activities, structuring the three-week schedule, and informing your child of the plan. Each step is important, and actively strategizing now will help strengthen your commitment and lessen stress later. Ultimately, a successful Reset largely depends on how strict you are with the fast. If you do the Reset half-heartedly, it won't be effective, and you may be robbing your child of an opportunity to heal and grow. I've broken down Reset preparation into ten steps, which are followed by two other considerations: television and school. The only supplies you need are a notebook and a monthly calendar you can post on the wall.

Ten Steps to Prepare for a Fast

1. Define problem areas and target goals
2. Get your spouse and other caregivers on board
3. Set a date and create a schedule
4. Inform relevant adults in your child's life
5. Obtain toys, games, and activities to replace screen-time
6. Schedule breaks or treats for yourself
7. If possible, enlist a playmate's parents to join you
8. Inform your child and involve the entire family
9. Perform a thorough "screen sweep"
10. Set your intention

Step 1: Define Problem Areas and Target Goals

It's important to define the problems that you hope to solve with a Reset. How do these issues manifest in your child's life, and what would you like to see instead? Articulating clear goals helps keep everyone focused on what's most important — healthy functioning. Additionally, fleshing out specific problems and goals will make the Reset feel more tailored or relevant to your child's particular needs. Studies show that, in general, goal-setting helps people stick to programs and realize the gains they hope to see.

EXERCISE *List and Prioritize Problem Areas*

First, brainstorm all the areas that are causing dysfunction or distress in your child's life. Consider also what your spouse, your child, and your child's teacher would consider to be problematic: Is your child disruptive in class? Defiant? Alienating friends? Your list should answer the question: "Why am I doing the Reset in the first place?"

To help you define your child's areas of difficulty, I've created a table with five categories: emotional, behavioral, school-related, social, and physical. Circle whichever items in table 1 seem most relevant to your child. The table lists common examples, but feel free to rephrase these to fit your child's specific issues and also add any issues in the appropriate category. If there are no problems in a given category, leave it blank. Also, for now, if a problem is relatively minor or seems appropriate given your child's age, don't list it. (If you're not sure if a problem or symptom is "normal" or age appropriate, and it's causing you or your child significant distress, go ahead and list it.) Focus on the major issues that are causing the most stress. After the fast, when the more pressing problems have hopefully been resolved or at least lessened in intensity, it may be helpful to return to this table and the list you made before the Reset to see what progress has been made and what work remains.

Now, once you've made your list, *prioritize* these issues. Most parents name a number of problems, but you can't fix everything at once (nor do you need to), and it's impossible to track everything. So pick the *top three problems* to target, and choose the issues that bother you most or cause the most dysfunction. Don't pick three from each category, but the top three overall. Ask yourself which of these problems would bring the most peace if they were resolved. Why only three? Because more severe problems are easier to track, and because their reduction will bring more relief. Furthermore, when the "worst of the worst" gets dealt with, other problems have a funny way of disappearing, too — or at least becoming much more manageable.

EMOTIONAL	BEHAVIORAL	SCHOOL-RELATED	SOCIAL	PHYSICAL
Meltdowns	Oppositional	Forgets homework	Poor sportsman-ship	Headaches
Irritable mood	Defiance	Easily distracted	Blames others	Stomachaches
Depressed mood	Argues a lot	Disruptive in class	Annoys peers	Migraines
Fearfulness	Yells/screams	Trouble learning	Lacks empathy	Body aches
Nightmares	Aggression	Poor concentration	Can't read others	Back/neck pain
Separation anxiety	Defensiveness	Fights reading	Inconsiderateness	Low energy
Isolative, withdrawn	Hyperactivity	Struggles in math	Poor eye contact	Out of shape
Doesn't enjoy activities	Can't stay on task	Procrastination	Avoids face-to-face	Overweight
Easily frustrated	Messy room	Under-achievement	No/few friends	Craves sweets
Compulsiveness	Refuses chores		Immaturity	Tics/stuttering
Obsessiveness	Impulsiveness			Trouble sleeping
	Can't "get ready"			Oversleeping

Table 1. Examples of problem areas

EXERCISE *Set Your Goals*

Once you've chosen three (or even two) problematic areas to focus on, assign related goals for each. For example, if the three biggest problems are *meltdowns*, *forgets to turn in homework*, and *trouble falling asleep*, your goals might be *fewer meltdowns*, *turns homework in more often*, and *falls asleep earlier*. If possible, quantify the problem and make the goal to reduce the intensity or frequency. Completely eliminating the problem is usually unrealistic in the short-term, and it can be self-defeating to target specific reduction amounts if the chosen amount or level is not met. (Rest assured, however, I wouldn't be writing this book if the Reset didn't produce improvements that are significant, if not dramatic.) So, while you might be counting and measuring to determine if there's been some improvement, the actual goal should be just a reduction of some kind. Table 2 below provides an example of what problem-related goals might look like; as you can see, some goals lend themselves to being measured in a quantitative way, while others will need to be measured in an impressionistic or subjective way.

TOP THREE PROBLEM AREAS AND CURRENT SEVERITY	RELATED GOALS

1. Meltdowns
   Frequency: 1–2/day
   Typical length: 30 minutes
   Typical intensity: rated 8/10
	Less frequent (less than daily)
	Shorter length (less than 30 minutes)
	Less intense (rated less than 8/10)

2. Homework
   Forgets to turn in about 50 percent of
     completed work
	Turns in more than half of work
	Homework score improves

3. Trouble sleeping
   Complains of tiredness in morning
   Fights going to bed
   Has dark circles under eyes
	Answers "yes" to "Did you sleep okay?"
	Goes to bed earlier or more readily
	Looks rested, has more energy

Table 2. Examples of targeted problem areas and goals

Some people find goal-setting confusing, overwhelming, or annoying. Keep it simple. In fact, tracking only one or two areas works just fine. If the mere thought of writing down all these issues and then picking three overwhelms you, or if you and your spouse start arguing about what's more important, just pick one problem area you can agree on and go from there. Once you've identified what you will track, start measuring, counting, or rating the problems the week before the fast begins, in order to create a baseline for evaluating gains. During the fast you'll collect data, and you'll reassess the problem areas again upon completing the fast. If you need help, you can find it in chapter 7, which covers tracking in more detail, but the important thing is to track *something* to help you remember why you're doing the Reset in the first place. Goals help keep your eyes on the prize, so to speak.

Step 2: Get Your Spouse and Other Caregivers on Board

As with any parenting issue, it's important to approach the Reset — and screen management in general — as a "united front." If your child senses that the adults in charge have differing views, or that one parent is clueless about what the restrictions are or will "give in," you can be sure that he or she will take advantage of this — that's one of the things children do best! Even worse, this dynamic can cause parents to fight, which makes it that much harder to keep the Reset on track.

If you live in a two-parent household, your spouse can help brainstorm and plan activities, and he or she can provide emotional support and accountability throughout the program. Some parents choose to enlist other friends or family members to fulfill different aspects of planning, support, or implementation. For example, in one family I worked with, the dad helped police the new rules, while a grandmother — who happened to be a former teacher — brainstormed activities with the mom and helped her stay accountable with daily phone calls. Despite the division of labor, the family members were aware of each person's role, and they were thus able to back one another up. Whatever you do, make sure everyone is communicating with one another.

In order for the Reset to go as smoothly as possible, both parents should be able to appreciate *how* interactive screen-time contributes to mental health issues, and should understand not just what the fast entails but the rationale behind it. Have your spouse read this book or visit the website (www.Reset YourChildsBrain.com) to understand the basics. Parents who are more involved in the education and planning stages are more likely to stay involved throughout the Reset and beyond.

The Unique Impact of Dads

Generally speaking, when it comes to parenting, dads sometimes report that they feel left out or that their opinion doesn't count. Yet research shows that when dads do get involved, children do better in school, they form more trusting relationships, and they enjoy better physical and mental health.[1]

In fact, involved fathers impart unique contributions to development. For example, research suggests that while moms are somewhat more likely to set boundaries, dads are more likely to *enforce* boundaries and consequences and to not feel guilty for doing so. Additionally, the amount of time a father spends with his child directly correlates with the child's capacity for empathy as an adult,[2] and these two findings may be linked. As gender studies expert Dr. Warren Farrell explains, "Teaching the child to treat boundaries seriously teaches the child to respect the rights and needs of others. Thinking of another's needs creates empathy." Moreover, the type of roughhousing and physical play that dads tend to engage in teaches children social and cognitive skills. Farrell writes, "[Dad] uses a different style of play — one that encourages risk taking and competition, pushing the child's boundaries of physical and mental skills, leading the child to win more and lose more (and, therefore, laugh and cry more); and, through the play, he is teaching the child to improve her or his skills and focus, and to deal with losing without cheating or becoming vindictive or violent."[3] These attributes — empathy, frustration tolerance, focus, and respect for boundaries — represent some of the skills dysregulated children need most, and they are the same ones that have become harder to build in today's immediate-gratification world.

Thus, a father's involvement in the Reset, in screen management in general, and in play and in bonding provides benefits that go way beyond just having another warm body around to do work. We all would do well to be more aware of dads' worth.

If Your Spouse Resists

Not uncommonly, one parent will be ready to do the Reset, but the other resists. Often, it's the mother who's ready and the father who's reluctant, though of course it happens the other way around, too. This may be simply because statistically the mother is more likely to be the parent managing health and school issues, so she's the one motivated to find an answer and take action. Often, however, I find that moms presume it's a foregone conclusion that the child's father will refuse to go along with the fast or will refuse to read anything, so she won't make much of an effort to talk to him about it — which becomes a self-fulfilling prophecy. As I say, a father's involvement is uniquely important. Further, research shows that with humans and with mammals in general, fathers step up their role in child rearing when they know they're needed, and they become less involved in that role — or they disengage completely — when they feel unneeded.[4] Thus, dads need to feel valued, and they need to know specifically how they can help.

These issues aside, when dads resist hearing about or participating in the Reset, it is often due to a reason that can be resolved. Why might Dad resist? A common reason is that he enjoys gaming himself, and he particularly enjoys playing video games with his kids. Further, if there are boys in the family, Dad may consider gaming to be a "male bonding" activity, which only adds to the feeling that the request to give it up feels unfair or unjust. If this is the case, when discussing the fast, acknowledge that you (the mom) realize that Dad enjoys the activity and that the program requires a bit of a sacrifice, but that shared gaming can simply be replaced with other activities. Have suggestions ready, like playing a board game or cards, building something together, or simply throwing the ball around outside. Another source of resistance is that Dad may interpret Mom's request to do the electronic fast as a criticism of his own screen-time behavior, whether that be gaming, computer use, or vegging in front of the TV. To buffer against this reaction, it's important to emphasize that the request is not a critique or complaint, but a call to action that will hopefully solve problematic behavior in your child and improve quality of life for the entire family.

What if Mom is the one holding back? A common reason Mom might resist while Dad is ready is out of fear the program will create more work for her. This can be solved by giving moms prescribed breaks (as discussed in Step 6) and by divvying up child-care responsibilities. Moms often need to hear specifically how and when Dad will help, which is another reason to have both parents actively involved in the planning stage. Writing down who will do what and holding each other accountable helps both parents feel commitments will be taken seriously; accountability strategies are discussed below.

Another reason a spouse might resist (which happens with both moms and dads) is if the prospect of removing extraneous devices produces some unease or anxiety. Obviously, this is more likely to occur with parents who engage in screen-time or rely on devices throughout much of the day and evening for work, leisure, or both. Parents who use computers all day at work often have numerous laptops or tablets lying around, and they may feel inconvenienced or even regard the suggestion that laptops be removed as a personal affront: "Well, *I'm* in front of the computer all day, and I'm fine." Alternately, a spouse might protest and say he or she needs certain devices available at all times for work purposes. Parents who are heavy social media users may resist the fast as well; a typical scenario is a mom who has a hard time not checking Facebook repeatedly in the evenings or on weekends. Taken together, these issues affect many if not most families, but they can be worked around. The rest of the steps will help you address and manage them, particularly the section "Parental Screen-Time and Accountability," page 147.

Not uncommonly, considering and discussing screen-time effects and the fast raises buried issues and emotions. Suggesting that a fast is necessary may produce anxiety or deep-seated guilt about past or ongoing screen-time allowances, so a parent may minimize, rationalize, or deny the problem rather than face these uncomfortable feelings. Parents may also silently recognize that their own computer or social media use isn't healthy and feel anxiety about having to pare down usage. Intimacy issues or conflicts that have been avoided may also come to the surface, so family members may resist because they realize they won't be able to hide behind screens anymore and will be forced to spend more time interacting with one another. Whatever the case, if your spouse or anyone in the family is resistant, attempt to uncover the reason why, validate the feelings behind it (which is different than validating the reason itself), and educate him or her with this book's material as much as possible. It can also be helpful for parents to sit down and do a cost-benefit exercise together, which I discuss more fully in chapter 8, but the exercise will be much more meaningful if the education piece is already in place.

If your spouse refuses to listen or read any of the material, try phrasing the proposal for the electronic fast like this: "I know you don't believe that electronics are part of what's going on with our child, but I was wondering if you'd be willing to just humor me and go along with the plan for three weeks. I'll set it up and show it to you, and I'd appreciate your help orchestrating it. You don't have to agree with it; you just need to go along with it for a few weeks to see what happens — it's an experiment."

In my experience, even parents who are steadfast non-believers will say yes to this. Framing the request as a favor and as an experiment effectively side-steps any arguments about whether the premise behind ESS and the Reset are true, and it takes the focus off of trying to predict whether the new rules will be in place "forever." Of course, with a resistant spouse, it's extra important to spell out all the rules for the fast (per this chapter and chapter 6), to avoid any arguments or excuses later, like, "Oh, I thought we were stopping only *gaming*, not using the iPad during car rides...." Also, if your spouse agrees to try the fast but hasn't read the book, he or she will surely ask, "What happens after the fast?" Simply explain that it will depend on what kind of effect the fast has. Once the fast is over, together you can decide the best way to handle screen-time in the future. Post-Reset considerations are the subject of chapter 9.

And finally, don't give up on trying to educate your spouse throughout the process; getting him or her to read something during or even after the fast is still helpful. Men in particular often want to see "hard science"; if they resist reading the book, it may be helpful to print out a few research papers or articles to persuade them. Some good choices are Dr. Aric Sigman's 2012 presentation on screen-time to the European Union, "The Impact of Screen Media on Children"; Dr. Douglas Gentile's 2012 research paper "Video Game Playing, Attention Problems, and Impulsiveness"; and my article summarizing brain-scan research in excessive video game and Internet use, "Gray Matters: Too Much Screen-Time Damages the Brain," which includes full references. You can find links to these articles in the book's endnotes.[5]

Coordinating Other Major Caregivers

Of course, for an electronic fast to be "clean" and most effective, you'll need the cooperation of all of your child's caregivers: relatives, neighbors, babysitters, staff at after-school programs, and so on. Enlisting support is discussed in detail in chapter 8, but in brief, I suggest that you approach everyone you know your child will spend time with or be supervised by in a typical (or the coming) month. Start by simply telling them you're trying out a new program based on evidence that interactive screen-time can exacerbate behavioral or emotional issues because it's overstimulating, and ask if they're willing to cooperate with the rules. As with a reluctant spouse, you don't need others to accept that ESS is valid; they just need to agree to do what you ask and go along with the program.

If you don't trust that a particular caregiver will respect the fast's restrictions, see if you can just "rotate them out" for the three weeks of the fast. The last thing you want is to put in all the effort to follow strict guidelines at home, only to have the Reset sabotaged because a relative or neighborhood friend allows your child to play video games at their house.

If You're a Single Parent

Doing the Reset as a single parent is a mixed bag. On the one hand the entire burden of orchestrating and enforcing the electronic fast falls on you, but on the other hand you won't be undermined in your own home by a parent who doesn't take the program seriously. However, try to enlist another primary caregiver, close friend, or relative to help you, even if it's someone, such as a grandparent, who only phones to check in every other day to provide emotional support and keep you on track. Having someone else be aware of what you're doing makes it more likely you'll stick to the program.

If you're divorced and your child splits time between you and the other parent, try to get your ex-spouse to work with you as much as possible. I get a lot of emails about this issue, and it's not easy. As above, explain what you've learned about ESS and how it may be affecting your child, and share this book with them. If your child is struggling, your ex-spouse may not be as resistant to a fast as you might think. I discuss this issue further in chapter 8, but the take-home point is to not let an ex-spouse's resistance stop you. Do the best you can.

Step 3: Set a Date and Create a Schedule

For the electronic fast, it's very important to plan ahead: pick the soonest start date you can, and then structure your child's time to minimize or eliminate downtime that would typically be filled with screen activities. I suggest getting a monthly wall calendar, writing everything on it, and posting it where everyone can see it, such as on the refrigerator. Any type of monthly calendar will do, but it might be worth buying a magnetized, one-month, dry-erase calendar at an office supply store.

When is the best time to do a fast? In general, you want to "strike while the iron's hot." There will never be a "perfect time," so I recommend starting the Reset as soon as you finish reading parts 1 and 2, when it's all fresh in your mind. Some parents try to avoid doing the program during holiday vacations or summer because there's more unstructured time, but from my perspective, these can be good times, since you don't have to worry about schoolwork contributing to screen-time. That said, if you know of a trip or event coming up that you can't control — such as a vacation with cousins or friends where you know there will be lots of gaming — wait to start the fast until after it's blown over. Then, set a firm start date and start preparing.

Typically, most people find it's easier to start on a Monday. That way, you can get ready and finalize plans the weekend before, and by the time the next weekend arrives, you'll already have five detox days under your belt. Figure 7 below is an example of what a four-week Reset might look like.

Make a special effort to plan activities for days that have a lot of unstructured hours, particularly weekends. You can write down all the activities in any given day — like homework, school sports, church activities, and so on — or leave these out if they're a given and only highlight whatever is special.

MARCH

Sunday	Monday	Tuesday	Wednesday	Thursday	Friday	Saturday
						1
2	3 **Prepare:** tell spouse	4 **Prepare:** tell other caregivers	5 **Prepare:** brainstorm and plan activities	6 **Prepare:** Lego's, board games, books	7 **Prepare:** art supplies, find Reset partner	8 **Prepare:** inform child
9 **Prepare:** screen sweep	10 **FAST**	11 **FOR**	12 **THREE**	13 **WEEKS**	14 → game night	15 → football with Dad
16 → chess with Mom, brownies	17 →	18 →	19 → dinner date with Mom	20 → library trip	21 → spend night with Grandma	22 → dog beach
23 → family hike and picnic	24 →	25 →	26 → ice cream outing with Dad	27 → game night	28 → movie and popcorn night	29 → art and music night
30 → skate park	31					

Figure 7. Four-Week Reset Calendar (example)

You don't need to schedule something for every day, but make sure you have several fun things on the calendar your child will look forward to.

Think of a range of activities or events: physical activities as well as creative activities, family time with everyone and one-on-one time between parent and child. Most of all, by planning fun events and doing things together as a family, you send your child the message that the electronic fast is not meant to punish. The point is to improve everyone's health, in brain, mind, emotions, and body, which means doing less of the things that harm us and more of the things that heal or help us. In addition, putting in the effort to plan interesting activities demonstrates that you're an active partner in the Reset, too, and that you want to spend time with your child. Many children today feel ignored by busy and preoccupied parents and long to spend more time with them. Finally, once you inform your child of the plan, they are likely to feel anxious at the loss of screen stimulation. Having already arranged replacement activities will help ease some of that anxiety, and then you can also invite your child to come up with his or her own ideas.

Of course, as the weeks progress, your schedule may change. As other parents of friends hear about the Reset, they may be happy to jump in and help arrange screen-free get-togethers. On the other hand, once your child's brain is free from overstimulation, he or she will naturally return to more natural, physical, or creative play — even when nothing is "set up" to entertain them. With each new week, you may find you don't have as much planning and orchestrating to do.

Here are some examples of easy-to-do activities to get the brainstorming wheels turning:

Exercise and Community Activities

Go on family bike rides, hikes, or picnics. Play catch, tag, Frisbee, or handball outside. Take your child and a friend or two to the park, to a swimming pool, or to play basketball. After dinner, take a walk together. Try out climbing gyms, explore nearby parks, or have a dance party at home. Check your town's parks-and-recreation department for affordable classes or lessons, like swimming, tennis, racquetball, sewing, cooking, chess clubs, and so on. Investigate retail stores: grocery stores sometimes host cooking classes, Home Depot offers a free parent-child project class once a month, and arts and crafts stores often run classes on a regular basis.

If it's cold out, bundle up your kids and get them outside anyway. Moving around to get the blood flowing is essential to healing, and sunshine replenishes Vitamin D, of which nearly all children are depleted.

Family Time

Each week, plan special family times or outings that involve everyone. An easy one is to make an event of dinner: Cook the meal together and then have a "dress up" dinner. You can have a theme or simply have a candlelight meal. One family I know was forced to do this during a blackout. They ordered takeout, lit candles, and wound up having a fun night playing board games after weeks of stress, tears, and yelling — and afterward made this a weekly ritual. Indeed, family time doesn't need to be any more complicated than having "game night." Other good ideas are doing a home-improvement project together, going fruit picking in season, visiting the zoo, and so on.

One-on-One Time with Each Parent

Aside from family time, schedule some one-on-one time with your child. Kids thrive from having a parent's undivided attention. Bonding helps children feel grounded while calming the nervous system and engaging the right side of the brain, and one-on-one interaction facilitates sustained eye contact and nurturing touch, which is crucial to optimal brain development. One-on-one time doesn't have to always be with a parent, either; have the child spend the night alone with a grandparent or other relative. If visiting relatives is typically done with siblings, this provides the child with a special experience of individual attention (and can be done with the other siblings, too).

Whatever you do, make your child feel special. Make them your focus. Dragging your child along while you grocery shop or run errands doesn't count. A once-a-week parent-child "date night" is a highly effective and underutilized way to achieve focused bonding time, and it lets your child know they're important to you. Also, commit to ignoring or turning off your phone during these times. (Even better, leave it elsewhere so you won't be tempted to sneak a peek.) Doing so strengthens the message you're sending and ensures you're listening. Think of these dates as precious time you'll never get back, ones your child will likely remember into adulthood.

Step 4: Inform Relevant Adults in Your Child's Life

The more people who know about the electronic fast and support you, the more likely the plan will succeed, and the less likely that opportunities to cheat will present themselves. As I discuss in more detail in chapter 8, talk to any relevant adults who interact with your child, such as teachers, coaches, grandparents, and so on. Coaches can be particularly helpful, as most of them *hate* the idea of kids being inside playing video games! Of course, who you tell and when entirely depends on your situation. Some people, like caregivers, you probably want to talk to *before* you tell your child, while others it may be more appropriate to reach out to *after* you've informed your child.

Step 5: Obtain Toys, Games, and Activities to Replace Screen-Time

As I mention in Step 3, you don't need to schedule activities for every waking second of every day. Don't be afraid of unscheduled, unplanned time, but prepare for it by collecting a range of non-screen items your child can play with. Boredom is an essential instigator of natural, creative play. Remember, creative activities, movement, and exercise will stimulate and engage the underused right side of the brain, as well as support whole-brain integration.

So, during the week before the fast, go through your closets, borrow from friends, and buy whatever toys, games, puzzles, drawing pads, magazines, and activities you think your child might find interesting. Gather a variety, find a few surprises, and think "old school" — certain games are classics for a reason. Think about what you did when you were a kid, or what your child *used* to be interested in before screens took over. Your child will become interested in these things again once the electronics are gone. Legos, books, models, jewelry-making, art, comic books, and so on are all helpful to have around.

You may hear your child say, "Board games are boring." But present them with classic strategy games like Battleship, Stratego, and Clue or puzzles like the Rubik's Cube and both boys and girls will be intrigued. One of my teen patients told me she and a group of kids found an old Monopoly game at school and started playing every week. Checkers, chess, backgammon, card games, dominoes, and mancala* remain popular with children and teens. As for toys or activities that kids can play or do on their own, anything they can build or make with their hands is good. I also like anything that provides kinesthetic input, like working with clay, playing marbles, juggling, arranging sand trays, and anything that promotes physical movement, such as a swing or trampoline. Below is a list of good items to have on hand.

IDEAS FOR SCREEN-FREE TOYS AND ACTIVITIES

- Clay or Play-Doh
- Legos
- Magnetic building sets**
- Models
- Jacks
- Marbles
- Art supplies
- Musical instruments
- Train sets or Hot Wheels tracks
- Solitaire card games
- Solitaire peg board games
- Rubik's Cube or Pyramid
- Jigsaw puzzles
- Jewelry-making kits
- Knitting, crochet, or macramé supplies
- Books or comics
- Bikes, skateboards, or skates
- Dolls and action figures
- Jump rope
- Yo-yo

Step 6: Schedule Breaks or Treats for Yourself

One of the reasons — perhaps the biggest reason — parents don't like to give up screens is because they act as an electronic babysitter. I get it: when kids are occupied and quiet (at least while playing), Mom and Dad can get things done and have a little peace. Many parents protest that screen-time is "the only time when *all* the kids are quiet." Thus, removing screens may mean

---

* Mancala is an ancient "count and capture" game, played with a board with shallow "pits" and beads or other objects (such as seeds or beans) that players move. Note: Pretty glass beads or natural objects make pleasing and rhythmic clicking noises that tend to engage children for longer periods than plastic pieces.

** Consisting of magnetic balls and sticks, this is perhaps my favorite toy of all time: it's appealing to all age groups, both genders, and the "connect" aspect is kinesthetically satisfying and psychologically therapeutic.

more work for you, at least initially. So, just like you're replacing your child's video game with healthier games, you need to replace the breaks you've been getting through screen-time with other types of breaks. Self-care is very important and is essential for avoiding burnout. Try to schedule in "me" time at least once a week. Do something that you used to enjoy before the kids came along. Date night with a spouse or an adult evening with friends certainly qualifies, but schedule some "alone time" as well, whether that's attending a yoga class, going to a café and reading a book, or indulging in a scented bath.

Busy moms are notorious for taking care of everyone else's needs first, but this practice can keep a family from moving forward. One exhausted mom avoided doing the Reset for months because she felt she couldn't survive without the breaks she got during her child's screen-time. Her husband was supportive and spent a lot of time with their son, and he even babysat to allow her free evenings, but instead of going out and having fun, she would run errands. One night, though, she decided to invite some girlfriends over to drink wine and play Bunco instead. This glimpse of fun opened a door in her mind and made her realize she felt less stressed — and therefore parented more lovingly — if she had something to look forward to each week. She also started drawing again, something she'd given up years before, and she eventually felt rejuvenated enough to try the Reset with her son. She continued her good self-care habits during and after the fast and was able to manage screen-time much more effectively thereafter.

Step 7: If Possible, Enlist a Playmate's Parent to Join You

Enlisting the parents of one of your child's friends to do the Reset with you can be exceedingly helpful. It's not necessary, and you may not know a family who would make a good partner, but it can be a great strategy when your child has one or two close friends he or she plays with on a regular basis. When families do the Reset together, they can share the burden of scheduling activities and can support one another with self-care. Each family can take turns with activity days — allowing the other to have a break. Organizing screen-free play dates is a win-win for everyone.

If you're unsure who to approach or how to raise the topic, remember that you will need to talk to *all* the parents whose homes your child plays in to make sure they will be willing to follow no-screen rules for your child during the fast. This provides an opportunity to explain what ESS is, the types of issues your child is dealing with, and how you hope a fast will help. If other parents seem open and interested, take that moment to ask if they want to join you in the Reset. Don't rule someone out just because they let their child play video games all day — parents may not be aware of the harmful effects of screen-time, or they may want to cut back but don't know how. On the other hand, if you talk to parents and feel they can't or won't comply, avoid having your child spend time at that friend's home, especially during the fast.

Step 8: Inform Your Child and Involve the Entire Family

Chapter 6 will cover in more detail how to talk to your child when presenting your decision to do the fast. It describes the best ways to explain your decision and the common reactions children have, in regard to hearing about the fast and during the fast itself. Here, we'll stick to more general logistics.

However you present the fast to your child and the rest of the family, you should be crystal clear with all the practical details. Depending on how upset your child is upon hearing the news, you may not want to discuss everything in the first conversation, but eventually your child will want and need to know the exact parameters: Tell your child the start and finish date, tell them exactly which devices they cannot use, and explain whether (and if so, how much) TV or movie time will be allowed (for more on this, see "Television Viewing During the Reset," page 156). Show them the calendar of fun activities you have created and the toys and games you have gathered that will replace screen-time. Let them know who has been told of the electronic fast, including other caregivers, relatives, parents of friends, and so on.

You can give your child the start and end date, but make no firm promises about which, if any, electronics will be returned once the three weeks are over. That isn't a decision you want to make until after you see the effects of the electronic fast. As we've already seen in several case studies, some children can return to a modest amount of screen-time or gaming, and some can't seem to handle any at all. (For more on how to approach electronics after the Reset, see chapter 9.)

Finally, you need to explain the screen-time rules that the rest of the family will follow during the fast. You should also tell your child that you (the parents) will be accountable for holding up your end of the bargain (see "The Accountability Act" below). Letting children know they aren't doing this alone, and giving them some control within the situation, helps "balance the scales" and provides a sense of fairness.

Parental Screen-Time and Accountability

An electronic fast involves everyone who lives in the house. Per the next section, siblings should have the same or very close to the same restrictions (at least at home), and parents should be mindful of their own screen-time, too. To what degree you as a parent want to fast is, obviously, up to you, but there are several important reasons to try to limit screen-time as much as you can: by removing devices and eliminating unnecessary screen-time at home, parents will model good habits, demonstrate respect for the child's needs, and remove temptation. In fact, parents benefit mentally and physically from reduced screen-time in the same way children do (see "Six Reasons to Reduce Your Own Screen-Time During the Reset," page 149).

Although not every rule applies to parents, the "house rules" detailed in chapter 10 are a good guide for curbing parental screen-time. The critical rules are to keep all electronics out of the bedroom and to be screen-free during meals and any family or one-one-one activities. It's helpful — not to mention more efficient — to corral all your computer "errands" like answering emails and paying bills into one or two designated time periods during the day (rather than scattered throughout) and to designate a single place (such as a family workstation or home office) to do them.

I also recommend parents consider giving up social media during a fast, as well as other types of "leisure" interactive screen-time, though in reality it's tough to get parents to agree to this. If you don't want to give up screen-time entirely at home, consider making this a point of negotiation in which children can name some terms: perhaps that parents must match their screen-time with playtime with the kids or with time spent exercising (per the "house rules"), or that Mom and Dad have to be off their devices during certain hours. With fairness and healthy habits in mind, it's helpful to ask your child if he or she feels you spend too much time on your phone, iPad, computer, and so on. How does your screen-time make your child feel? Validate what your child says without justifying or rationalizing your use — including for work reasons. If your child feels ignored, apologize and emphasize the changes *you'll* make during the fast.

This conversation helps shift the Reset from a behavioral issue to a family issue. Also, by joining in the fast as much as is practical, parents show that they are invested in the plan and believe in the benefits of limited screen-time. But another important aspect of this is accountability: *parents need to follow through on the things they promise to do*, especially spending more time as a family and playing one-on-one with a child. Often, when a family is in my office discussing activities, the child will say to the parent, "You say that you'll play with me, but then you never do." That's why I like posting all the planned activities and outings on a calendar — it's a visual, concrete reminder.

THE ACCOUNTABILITY ACT

A highly effective way to make sure parents keep their end of the bargain is to create what I call "The Accountability Act." This is an agreement drafted with the child that specifies that the parents must pay a "tax" when they forget to do something, violate their own screen-time limits, or cancel a planned activity at the last minute. This tax can be almost anything, but in fact, monetary credit is very useful; the tax should be a sum that makes a difference to the child and that "hurts" enough to encourage the parent not to make the same mistake again. For instance, say Mom has agreed to play chess on Sunday at 3 p.m. with her son. However, on Sunday, she forgets about the chess date and spends all afternoon grocery shopping. By the time she gets home, there's only time for dinner, homework, and then bed. Since Mom was the one who "flaked," she owes a tax: a twenty-five-dollar credit for a new Lego set. Why a "credit"? This avoids handing cash to a child and lets the parent control what he or she spends it on.

An alternative is to put the money in a tax jar that goes toward family outings (such as pizza night, baseball tickets, and so on). The tax could also be for bonding activities like a ten-minute back or foot rub, extra stories at bedtime, or sitting together in a rocking chair. Brainstorm with your child about what the consequences for various mistakes and slip-ups should be. Kids like to "make deals," and this practice really does help make everyone accountable. It helps reassure the child that the fast won't be torture and that everyone's involved.

Six Reasons to Reduce Your
Own Screen-Time During the Reset

Being strict about your own screen-time greatly improves the odds that you'll be able to implement your child's Reset successfully, and it will give you a leg up on healthy screen management afterward. Why? Because in addition to setting a good example, *you* will feel better, function better, and sleep better.

Child rearing is harder than ever, and parenting a child who's having serious problems can produce stress that's "off the charts." Ask yourself if you have a tendency to use a mobile device throughout the day or while in bed at night as a means to escape from that stress. The activities may seem innocent enough, like reading on a Kindle, sharing funny family pictures on Facebook, or reading blog posts about parenting. But screen-time affects an adult's frontal lobe, too, so it can cause a parent to become disorganized, exhibit poor impulse control, lack self-discipline, and have trouble following through on goals, including establishing healthy screen management. Screen-time also affects an adult's body clock, melatonin levels, and physical health. Just as with children, these effects are more likely to occur if a parent is stressed, not sleeping well, or has difficulty in those areas to begin with. Thus, there are numerous reasons to cut back. In fact, doing the electronic fast *with* your child can be a powerful healing experience for everyone.

In short, here are six reasons why it's worthwhile for parents themselves to put down those devices:

1. *You'll model good screen habits.* Parents' own screen habits closely correlate to their children's, and joining a fast with your child helps build mutual respect.
2. *You'll be more aware.* Screen-time is distracting, and it diminishes how in touch we are with our environment. You'll be more aware of how your children are doing during the fast and more vigilant about any attempts to skirt the ban.
3. *Your executive functioning will be enhanced.* Everyone's frontal lobe functions better with less screen-time, so planning and

problem-solving will come more easily. You'll also be more creative, which makes activities more enjoyable — for you and your child.

4. *You'll be much more likely to finish the Reset Program.* Improved frontal lobe function helps us sustain efforts and be self-disciplined.

5. *You'll be more emotionally attuned.* Your in-the-moment awareness and sense of emotional connection will be enhanced — and your child will notice.

6. *You'll be more rested.* Reducing your own levels of hyperarousal will help you sleep more deeply, improve your ability to tolerate frustration, and give you more energy.

Are Siblings on the Plan, Too?

Parents handle this issue differently, but I recommend that what goes for one child goes for all others, particularly if the children are close in age. Explain that the Reset Program is a family plan that *everyone* will be participating in. Some parents choose to have siblings follow the same rules and give up all screens entirely, and some decide that siblings will give up screens at home, but they can be allowed screen-time at school and at friends' houses. If the siblings are older, it may be more appropriate to simply have them follow the house rules in line with what the parents are doing. Consider what seems fair, but also consider how difficult it will be to monitor everyone; the most important objective is to get a handle on the child you're worried about.

In my experience, involving siblings doesn't usually become a major issue. Either siblings are indifferent to giving up screens because they're not as drawn to them, or they become upset, in which case they're probably too attached and could use the break anyway. The child doing the Reset is most often bothered by a sibling who continues to game when he or she is not allowed. Thus, focus your sibling restrictions on that aspect and whatever else makes sense for your situation.

A sibling will sometimes object and ask, "Why do I have to stop playing? I'm not the one causing problems." Acknowledge the sacrifice the fast entails and validate their frustration, but explain that everyone in the family needs to work together to help things run more peacefully for everyone. If the sibling protests that it's not fair, you can point out that what would be *really* unfair is to ask that "your brother give up gaming while you continue to play right in front of him." In fact, this kind of family support is similar to what is recommended when a child with obesity or diabetes needs to be on a special diet — the whole family needs to follow the diet or it won't work.

Step 9: Perform a Thorough "Screen Sweep"

The day before the fast begins, start your screen sweep by removing any and all screen devices. I suggest making another round on the first day of the fast because inevitably you'll find devices you missed. Devices need to *removed* — not just hidden. I recommend taking devices to work and stashing them in a drawer. I can't tell you how many times I've heard stories of kids finding video games that Mom "hid" in a closet, or who reconnected games and computers that the parents swore they'd disabled, or who figured out or got around passwords locking Internet use. If a child wants to play a video game or use the Internet badly enough, he or she will sniff out a device and set it up, I promise you.

From your child's room, remove all electronics, including games, computers (including desktops), mobile phones, e-readers, laptops, tablets, digital cameras, and iPads. Be sure to remove even those e-readers that utilize e-ink, like the Kindle and the Nook. Also remove any television sets and DVD players, since any allowed TV or movie watching shouldn't be done in the bedroom. Check under the bed, in the closets and drawers, behind curtains, and so on. Then inspect every room in the house, top to bottom. Search through piles of "forgotten" toys in a playroom or basement, scour the garage, and remove any gadgets from your cars. In addition, I suggest you disable all social media accounts your child has: Facebook, Instagram, Twitter, and so on. Then, even if a child sneaks a device, these accounts won't be accessible, which lessens the temptation to cheat.

Finally, do not make the mistake of believing that merely telling your child not to use certain devices will be enough to do the trick. Whether because they don't want to go through the hassle of unplugging, disabling, and hiding devices, or because they truly trust their children (or want to), parents sometimes think that simply telling or asking the child not to play on a device will be enough. But remember that a child's frontal lobe is not fully developed, and thus even a trustworthy child who promises not to play anymore (and really, really, *really* means it) can't be expected to check urges or control impulses when temptations arise. Trust me on this one. This mistake is also likely to occur when parents don't take away cell phones during the fast and want to trust that the child won't use them during homework or after lights out, or when they want to allow a child to use a computer in the bedroom for homework. Don't feel guilty that you're not allowing the child a chance to be "responsible." That's putting the cart before the horse.

As discussed below in "Reset Planning and School" (page 158), if your child must use a computer for homework, have your child use a stationary one, preferably a desktop, in a common area where you can see what he or she is doing. Ideally, the whole family will share one computer, which both forces everyone to schedule computer time wisely and reduces the number of computers in the house. If this isn't feasible, reduce the number of computers to the bare minimum, and make them stationary. This may seem hugely inconvenient, but see if you can do it at least for the fast — it'll save you headaches in other ways.

Make sure your screen sweep is thorough:

DEVICES TO REMOVE IN A SCREEN SWEEP

- All handheld electronic devices in the house, including iPads, iPods, iPod Touches, video games, tablets, e-readers (including Kindles), cell phones (including old ones), and smartphones (including old ones)
- All of the above plus any laptops, notebooks, desktop computers, television sets, and DVD players from the child's bedroom
- All laptops in the home
- All handheld games or other devices used in the car
- All video game consoles in the home, including the Wii
- All electronic-screened educational or learning games

Evan: Uncovering Hidden Screens

Evan and his parents first came to see me when Evan was ten years old. He was a highly intelligent boy who suffered from tics, poor focus, and social awkwardness, and his father wondered if Evan had Tourette syndrome. Both he and his wife had observed Evan's tics "going crazy" when Evan sat at the computer playing video games or surfing the Internet, which they allowed him to do often and for long periods, since Evan had trouble making friends. Since screen-time was essentially Evan's only source of entertainment, his parents were initially skeptical when I told them they needed to remove the electronics to get a handle on his tics and attention issues. Because of the sheer amount of time Evan spent on his computer every day, I was 100 percent convinced the parents would see a dramatic improvement if they did a strict electronic fast.

His parents agreed, but two months later, they came back to report that Evan wasn't showing much improvement. They said they'd taken the computer out of his room and that he didn't own any handheld games. Since Evan really didn't have any friends at school, his parents didn't think he was using someone else's games there, either. Believing the fast hadn't worked, the parents decided they wanted to pursue other treatments, and I referred them to an acupuncturist who specialized in treating tics.

I kept thinking about the case, though. Evan had also seemed depressed, and he was clearly isolated, both of which are known to correlate with Internet usage. I felt sure Evan was somehow continuing to use electronics, keeping his symptoms alive and well. On a whim, I decided to call the parents to ask a few more questions and see how he was doing. This time the mother admitted that they'd found an old notebook laptop under the bed in Evan's room and that he'd been using it during the time they'd believed him to be screen-free. She said he'd never really used it before, so she'd forgotten it existed. Then she admitted there was probably a second source: twice a week, Evan's aunt took care of him, and while there, he probably played video games with his cousins. The mother had been reluctant to address this with the aunt, since the aunt was doing them a huge favor by watching Evan.

After finding all this out, I encouraged the parents to give the fast another try. They agreed, and this time they removed the old laptop from Evan's room. They also spoke to the aunt. Since they were hesitant, I suggested that they tell the aunt that Evan's doctor had ordered that he refrain from playing video games because of his tics, so she'd have to completely restrict video games when he was at her house. If that wasn't okay with the aunt, they'd have to find alternative care for a few weeks, but the aunt readily obliged.

With a strict fast in place, Evan's depression lifted considerably and his tics were negligible by the time he visited my office a month later. He was turning in more homework, too. More relaxed and mentally organized, Evan was able to start working on his social skills, including establishing friend-ships. If we hadn't uncovered the hidden screen sources, the family never would have been convinced that screen-time was impacting Evan, and we wouldn't have been able to shift into deeper stages of work — work that was necessary to improve Evan's quality of life.

EXERCISE *Brainstorm Screen-Time Opportunities*

To maintain an effective electronic fast, you need to brainstorm all the ways, places, and times your child might "sneak" screen-time. Imagine every moment of your child's day, write down any and every opportunity you can think of, and then figure out how to eliminate it. Consider *when*: such as in the car (with you or other parents), on the bus, at night in bed, or while a parent is working at home and distracted. Consider *where*: such as at a sitter's house, in school, in an after-school program, or at a friend's or relative's house. Consider *what*: such as video game consoles, handheld games, cell phones, laptops, tablets, iPods, and desktop computers. Consider *how*: such as sneaking off with cousins during holidays or family get-togethers (a very common and easily overlooked source), capitalizing on moments when a parent is or will be preoccupied (such as getting on the computer while a parent is on a conference call), and conspir-ing with friends (such as getting a friend to sneak a video game when adults aren't supervising them).

In essence, assume that any available device will be used if the child can figure out how to get it working and how to get away with it. This is why an electronic fast ideally means no phones (see the box "Hang Up the Phone"), and why a screen sweep means removing all devices from the home. Chil-dren may interpret vague instructions very conveniently: "I thought you just meant I couldn't play my Playstation. How was I supposed to know you meant my friend's DS, too?"

Hang Up the Phone

Until fairly recently, children didn't even have phones, and some-how parents managed to pick them up from school, activities, and the mall. However, expectations are different today, and some parents are reluctant to take away a child's phone during a fast for communication or safety reasons. This is a tricky issue, since for an electronic fast to be successful, even little cracks need to be sealed.

I advise several different strategies, depending on the situation. The simplest solution is to simply survive the next few weeks without your child having a phone. If communication is the main concern, remember that even if your child doesn't have a phone, others around him or her will. If you feel your child must carry a phone, swap out any type of smartphone for a bare-bones flip phone that the child turns in as soon as they walk in the door. No texting is best, limited texting (to you) is next best, and this use still needs to be monitored. I cannot stress enough how risky it is to leave a smartphone in the mix. Even if you delete all preloaded and downloaded games and disable the Internet access, there are often apps and files that are impossible to remove that the child can interact with, and not removing this screen defeats the purpose of the fast. (Really, using a smartphone is the epitome of interactive screen-time.) You don't want to go through all the work of a Reset and have it undone by one device.

Step 10: Set Your Intention

Take five to ten minutes to set a conscious intention to embark on the Reset Program in order to free and heal your child's mind, brain, and body. Review the goals you defined in Step 1 (and perhaps review chapter 4) and meditate on what you want for your child now and in the future. Finally, write down your intention as a mission statement and say it out loud.

An example might be: "My mission is to create a healthy environment for my daughter, such that she feels happy, focused, and loved by friends and family. In the future, I want her to reach her greatest potential in school and work, acquire fulfilling relationships, and develop strong moral character. To this end, I intend to provide a screen-free setting for the next three weeks in order for her brain to rest, heal, and reset, and for me to gain clarity for managing screen-time in the future."

Television Viewing During the Reset

Typically, during an electronic fast, I allow my patients to watch a small amount of television or an occasional movie at home. If you decide to allow this, aim for *five hours or less per week*. See the box "Reset Rules for Television," below, for the complete list of guidelines that should be followed, but the basics boil down to this: no viewing in the bedroom, no viewing on any device other than a reasonable-sized TV set (from across the room), and no cartoons or other content that is violent, fast-paced, or too visually stimulating.

Why is "a little bit" of television okay during the Reset when I otherwise insist on NO video games or other interactive screen-time? Essentially, a modest amount of calm TV viewing doesn't create the same quality or *level* of hyperarousal, agitation, and dysregulation that interactive screen-time does. I describe the specifics for why this is so in chapter 1 (see "Interactive vs. Passive Screen-Time," page 19), but I find that a little TV viewing doesn't undermine the effectiveness of the Reset in the same way that "a little bit" of interactive screen-time can. Additionally, children may whine when limits are set for TV, but they usually accept them — in contrast to the endless rounds of negotiation, anger, and tears that can accompany interactive screen-time restrictions.

Nevertheless, use your child's behavior as your ultimate guide. Plenty of studies have shown that television viewing, especially when begun at a very young age, is associated with subsequent attention problems, depression, obesity issues, and so on. If your child has sleep problems, limit TV to one hour on any given day, and avoid it in the period before bedtime. If sleep problems persist during the Reset, then cut down further, or stop all TV watching entirely. Indeed, if your child seems addicted to television, is struggling with learning how to read, is severely depressed, or gets very little exercise, you may want to consider not allowing television at all.

Reset Rules for Television

Rules for How to Watch

- Aim for five hours or less per week total for TV and movies (and consider weekends only).

- No television in the morning before school or during meal times.
- No television until all homework and chores are done.
- If sleep problems exist, limit to one hour in one sitting, and if sleep problems persist, eliminate TV watching entirely.
- No viewing on a desktop, laptop, iPad, or any other handheld device.
- View the TV from across the room, and aim for a distance of 2.5 to 3.5 times the size of the screen (measured diagonally), or a minimum of eight feet away.
- Use the smallest screen in the house, and if you only have a huge flat-screen TV (that exceeds the viewing-distance dimensions above), consider no TV at all.
- No television watching in the bedroom (and remove TVs from a child's bedroom).
- Don't leave televisions on "in the background."
- Don't flip through channels quickly and mindlessly; don't give your child the remote.
- Consider placing a small lamp or back-lighting behind the television (which helps ease visual stress).
- Lower the "brightness" level of the TV's screen and match the room's brightness level to that of the TV (the more the screen "blends in," the easier it is on the eyes and brain).
- Adjust the TV's color mode to "natural," rather than a super-saturated or extra bright mode.
- Do not stream online content through the TV set via WiFi (which adds unnecessary EMF exposure; see appendix B).

Rules for Content

- No cartoons and no modern animated movies (which are usually too stimulating).
- No violent content.
- Avoid programs that are fast-paced or action-packed.
- Avoid content that is visually stimulating, with frantic editing

and overbright colors (which applies to many live-action children's shows, like *Yo Gabba Gabba!*).

- Focus on nature shows and older live-action movies that are slower paced (such as *The Sound of Music, Benji, Annie, The Black Stallion*, the original *Muppet Movie*, old *Sesame Street* re-runs).

- Older Disney animated movies are fine, since the colors are more muted and the pace slower (such as *Pinocchio, Dumbo*, or *Bambi*).

Reset Planning and School

One of the most common planning questions parents have is whether and how to eliminate computer use that's required for school. In truth, school-related screen-time can sometimes be out of a parent's control, particularly for older children. Thankfully, most of the time, the electronic fast is successful if all interactive screen-time outside of school is eliminated, and two other rules related to homework are followed: 1) schedule computer-related work as early in the afternoon or evening as possible, and 2) require that your child use a stationary computer in a common area where he or she can be seen. However, even if these guidelines are followed, there will be some children for whom the elimination of school screen-time will be necessary for the fast to be effective. In fact, for some children with ESS, school *is* the primary source of screen-time, and thus addressing it becomes necessary.

Today, nearly all kids use computers at school on a regular basis, but the amount varies considerably. How much exposure your child receives is based on grade level, how high-tech the school is or wants to be, whether your child has been assigned to a tech-based pilot program, and the mentality of individual teachers. Indeed, the growing use of technology in education constitutes a host of problems beyond the Reset, which I discuss in chapter 11. But for the Reset itself, whether to eliminate school-related screen-time depends on the following:

- How much interactive screen-time your child receives at school on a daily basis
- How dysregulated your child is, and how sensitive your child is
- How feasible (or how complicated) it is to eliminate it

- How much computer-related homework your child gets, and how much light-at-night the homework adds

For grade-school children, it might be worth observing the classroom to see how much screen-time occurs in a typical day. It's also worth finding out if the teacher ever rewards students with computer time or video games, and if gaming or phone use is allowed at recess or breaks. If any of this is occurring, ask that these practices be stopped when it comes to your child. (These practices have become exceedingly common, even in special education classrooms.)

There are no hard and fast rules to determine if you can leave school out of the equation and still successfully reset your child's brain. Thus, unless it's very obvious that you need to do this, or it's relatively easy to arrange for school-based screen-time to be eliminated, I would advise you to try the electronic fast without addressing the school piece first, and then, if you don't see results, consider eliminating use related to school as well. That said, when I work with parents individually and we decide we need to eliminate school screen-time (either preemptively or as part of troubleshooting), I often accomplish this by writing a note to give to the teacher. Here is a template of what my note typically looks like:

Date _____
RE: Johnny Doe, Date of Birth: 1/2/03
To whom it may concern:

Because screen-time can overstimulate the nervous system and cause chronic hyperarousal (fight-or-flight), and thereby negatively affect attention, mood regulation, behavior, and/or sleep, Johnny is to be off all computers and any other electronic screen devices for the next ____ weeks, starting __ [date] and finishing __ [date]. Recommendations may be made regarding this issue thereafter, to be determined.

Sincerely,
_____, M.D. License#_____

I usually leave out the child's specific diagnoses, unless the parent wants the teacher or school administrator to know more in order to obtain accommodations, in which case it can be helpful to divulge more details. Also, I sometimes leave out the opening description of screen-time effects and simply write that "for medical reasons" the child's computer use at school must be restricted.

At any rate, if a doctor's note is needed, you can bring in a template like this to your child's pediatrician (or child psychiatrist, if you have one) and ask him or her to consider signing it (or to write their own version, if preferred) to support your effort to try the Reset Program. Visit www.Reset YourChildsBrain.com to obtain a downloadable form (use password "reset docs"). Regardless of how much your child's health practitioner knows about how screen-time affects mental health, I doubt most clinicians will mind supporting you in *trying* something like this, especially if he or she knows your child is struggling; after all, it's risk-free. Most physicians will be aware of the American Academy of Pediatrics' current media or screen-time recommendation that children watch no more than one to two hours a day, and they will also be aware that most children are many times over that limit.

Depending on the school, the teacher, and whether your child has any accommodations already in place at school, it may be enough to simply put your request in writing by emailing the teacher and copying other relevant school staff on the email. If you want to incorporate school into the Reset, see also chapter 11, which provides more guidance on how to work with your child's school effectively.

Preparation Checklist

Did you . . .

- ❏ List three target areas and three goals?
- ❏ Tell everyone who is relevant to the plan's success?
- ❏ Structure your child's schedule to minimize downtime?
- ❏ Gather replacement toys and activities?
- ❏ Create and post an activity calendar for everyone to see?
- ❏ Perform a thorough "screen sweep"?
- ❏ Schedule breaks or treats for yourself?
- ❏ Establish clear television rules (if you're allowing it)?
- ❏ Arrange a stationary computer workstation in a common area for homework, if needed?

Chapter 5 Take-Home Points

- Preparing for the electronic fast by following the ten steps is essential for a successful Reset.
- Use a Reset-designated notebook for the exercises and a four-week calendar for planning and scheduling activities.
- To help track symptom progression and to focus your efforts, choose specific problems to address and goals for your child.
- Get others on board for support and to limit opportunities for "sneaking" screens.
- Replace screen activities with physical, creative, and parent-child activities, which supports whole-brain integration and self-esteem.
- If possible, have another parent do the Reset with you, for psychological and logistical support.
- If you allow some television watching during the fast, maintain restrictions on time and content.
- Eliminate as much school-related screen-time as is feasible.

WEEKS 2–4: THE ELECTRONIC FAST

Unplug, Rejuvenate, and Reset the Nervous System

Set your course by the stars,
not by the lights of every passing ship.

— Omar Bradley

Once you've finished your preparations for your child's three-week electronic fast, it's time to put the Reset in motion. Remember, the Reset is the first leg in a bigger journey: improving your child's quality of life by helping your child develop a more rested, balanced, integrated, and organized brain. In the coming weeks, between the changes the fast requires and the chaos of life itself, it's easy to become distracted from the task at hand. *Stay the course.*

This chapter gives an overview of the electronic fast itself so you know what to expect, and it provides action plans for each week. Ideally, read (or briefly review) all the chapters in part 2 before you actually begin. All the Reset Program chapters are companions to one another, and chapters 7, 8, and 9 look more closely at critical aspects of the fast, like the importance of tracking progress, dealing with uncertainty in yourself and resistance from others, troubleshooting problems, and planning for what's next. However, *it's of the utmost importance that you don't lose momentum or motivation*, so if you're ready to start the fast before you've finished reading, do so, and then complete your reading during the fast.

That said, when you're ready to start, the first question is when to tell your child. Per the sample calendar in chapter 5 (see page 140), I suggest announcing the fast on the Saturday before a Monday start (or two days ahead) and then doing the screen sweep the day before you start. It can be too abrupt to announce the electronic fast and immediately take away all devices, but waiting longer than a day or two only makes the start more difficult. In addition, children always ask if they can use screens up until the clock starts, so to speak, and I usually don't mind this "last hurrah." However, you know your own child best, so adjust the timing and presentation of the announcement in whatever way will cause the fewest problems.

Starting the Reset: Your Child's Reactions

Knowing what to expect when you inform your child of the Reset will help you feel empowered. Nearly all children will have a negative emotional or behavioral reaction when they hear their beloved devices will be gone, but know that if other parents have survived it, you can too.

In general, when informing your child of your decision to do the Reset, be matter-of-fact but compassionate. In your manner as much as your words, communicate that the intention of the fast is to help everyone; it's not a punishment. Be sympathetic and understanding with whatever your child's emotional reaction is, but at the same time, be firm and clear that the fast is not up for negotiation. In other words, you want to balance two messages: that you love your child and empathize with what he or she is feeling, but that you're not going to give in or backpedal on the terms.

Children's reaction to hearing the news varies. Some will take it hard, and some will take it better than you dared hope. But all children inevitably ask the same two questions: Why? And what happens afterward?

Answering the Hardest Questions

There are a couple of traps to avoid when answering the very valid question about why you are doing this. The first trap is that you aren't likely to convince your child, who isn't likely to agree with your explanation (even if he or she secretly senses that you are right), no matter how artfully you present your reasons. It's very easy to get caught up arguing and debating whether there's a problem and whether this is the right solution — which is exactly what you don't want. Children will always have more energy than you, so it's to their advantage to keep you engaged. It's to yours to keep it short!

The second trap is allowing guilt to influence your actions. Children will complain that what you're proposing is unfair or insist that you're "being mean." In this case, if you get into a debate about why a fast is necessary, it just gives children the chance to try to prove that you *are* being unfair and insensitive. These accusations sting. Sometimes parents report that their hearts break when their child expresses how awful it'll be when everyone else is still playing, texting, and so on, and they're not. With some children, these feelings are expressed without an ounce of manipulation, purely out of despair, which can make a parent feel even more tempted to console by making concessions. In other cases, children can become downright spiteful, and the discussion becomes so toxic that it becomes intolerable for the parent. Indeed, some parents admit that anxiety over feeling like their child "hates" them is what makes them reluctant to do the fast in the first place. But a child who senses this will exploit this vulnerability to high heaven, so if this is one of your concerns, be extra prepared to keep the conversation brief.

So, the first thing I advise parents to say when kids ask why is that it's "an experiment," which is the truth. You're trying this out for a short time to see if everyone feels better when they have less screen-time. Remind your child that it won't be forever, and console yourself with the knowledge that your child is reacting to whatever he or she *imagines* is going to happen, which is far worse than what the reality will be. This answer also sidesteps many of the traps described above because it doesn't provide much to argue against.

If you feel obligated to offer an explanation in terms of brain health or functioning, keep it simple. You might say something like, "Doctors are finding that video games and screen-time can sometimes be bad for our brains, particularly children's brains, which are still growing. So we're going to give up electronics for three weeks to see if we feel better."

If you've already been working on specific issues, like meltdowns or falling behind in school, you could mention that and use a computer analogy. Something like: "You know how we've been dealing with [name the symptom]? Some doctors think what may be happening is similar to when a computer freezes or slows down because too many programs are running. There's too much information being processed at once and the computer gets overloaded. The same thing might happen in our brains when we use electronics too much, so we're going to give them up for a while and see what happens." Be sure to frame what you're aiming for in a positive way that doesn't make the child feel shamed or defensive. Say something like: "This might be a way to help you feel more in control [or less stressed, or do better in school]."

With older teens and young adults, you might choose to be more forthcoming about specific reasons based on what you've learned about screen-time's impact on the brain, but share only to the extent that it helps them to understand, and stop when you sense they are using the discussion as a tool to negotiate. The same questions may come up periodically during the fast and afterward, and the child's receptiveness may evolve as they become less defensive.

Of course, once you've dealt with why, children immediately want to know what will happen once the fast is over. *I'll get everything back then, right?* You may be tempted to discuss which devices will be returned or what activities will be allowed, but these are promises you might not be able to keep. The truth is, you don't know what sort of limits you'll want or need to continue after the fast. That depends on how your child responds and on your child's underlying vulnerabilities, as well as on other factors that are the subject of chapter 9.

So, reassure your child that this won't be "forever," but don't commit to specifics about what happens next. Say, "We'll see. We're not sure yet exactly what will happen afterward. For now, this is what we need to do, so let's focus on getting through the next few weeks."

Grade-School Age and Younger Children

Young children will typically have a bit of a panicky reaction upon hearing the news that all screen devices will be taken away. The child typically starts to cry, attempts to negotiate, or tells the parents why they think the plan isn't a good idea. Sometimes the child may seem okay with it at first, but as the conversation continues and the news hits them, the tears begin to flow. Expect this, and expect a fair amount of arguing. Children may also become angry or agitated. Whatever the reaction, empathize with how the child feels, acknowledge that you know it feels like it'll be hard, but that you're going to help them through it. Remember, from their perspective, something significant and substantial is being taken from their lives, and children have no idea how they'll fill the void, so it's appropriate to comfort them around this.

Once you've explained the fast and empathized with your child's reactions, you can try to shift the conversation to how you plan to make up for it.

For some children, talking about what you'll do instead (the special activities or treats you've planned) can be a source of comfort, while others will refuse to entertain such thoughts until they've accepted that the fast is really going to happen, in which case you should revisit this task and brainstorm with your child when he or she has calmed down.

Tweens and Teens

Adolescents may cry, too — but they're also more likely to get mad. I've had teens storm out and slam doors in my office — once hard enough to knock a picture off a wall. Other teens will sit and stew during the initial discussion, only to boil over and become explosive once home. Not uncommonly, teens will make threats — sometimes out of desperation to get you to change your mind, and sometimes out of an intense fear of feeling lost or unanchored. If violent behavior or extreme depressive states are a concern for your child in general, a safety plan may be in order (see below).

When you discuss why you are doing the fast, be careful not to use the term *addicted* or *addiction*, as the term tends to engender defensiveness. Teens often feel no one understands their inner world, so be sure to empathize by mirroring back whatever they say about how they are feeling, but don't waver in your commitment. For example, if a teen reacts with, "What?! Why? Video games are the only thing that makes me happy!" You might respond: "I know this is upsetting, and I realize video games are something you really enjoy. But we plan on doing other things to help make up for it."

With teens, another huge concern is social media and texting, both in terms of communication and the so-called "fear of missing out." Again, it's appropriate to offer comfort about this, since losing their devices will impact how they interact with their friends. If your teen cries, "Hell-*oh!* How am I supposed to talk to anyone or know what's going on?!" You could respond with something like: "I know it feels like you're going to be cut off from everyone, but you'll still see your friends in person and you can talk to them on the landline."

Older Teens and Young Adults

Young people in this age group can exhibit anxiety or anger, too, or alternatively they may become subdued and depressed. Youths may withdraw from the conversation and display a very "flat" or apathetic mood, or they may appear to think and speak more slowly, deflating like the last bit of air being let out of a balloon.

On the other hand, the older children are, the greater their potential ability to self-reflect. They're better able to examine what's not going right in their lives and may be able to identify future goals, which can open a doorway to aligning their goals with yours. When Emma came to see me, she was a nineteen-year-old college student on a scholarship who spent countless hours a day on the computer. Emma informed me that she was about to get "kicked out" of her scholarship program for failing grades. She expressed that she wanted "to be normal" and "go to school like everyone else my age," but that she couldn't keep up or stay focused. Emma could sense she was at a crossroads in her life: if she messed up another semester, it would drastically limit her choices and resources, and she'd be forced to get a full-time job. Our initial conversation about doing the Reset went smoothly, but she suddenly began crying after we'd moved on to another topic. Emma then admitted she felt worried she "wouldn't survive" without her laptop, even though we'd already problem-solved how to get her schoolwork done without it.

We circled back to her original reason for coming in. I quoted back to her what she'd said about what she wanted, and that the reason to do the Reset was not because anyone was "making" her do anything, but because her goal was to be successful in school, and in order to do that she needed to improve her attention and time management. If the Reset could help her do that, then it could help her get back on track to achieving this goal. As we talked, her demeanor changed as she shifted from feeling despondent about losing her laptop to being empowered about taking charge of her own future. Because she had the capacity to think about how her current circumstances were at odds with how she saw her future, she was able to be motivated in a way a younger person might not be.

Relief

A sizeable minority of children and teens who are dysregulated from ESS will have a sense that video games, their smartphone, or an iPad has taken them hostage. In these circumstances, upon being informed of the fast, the child might become upset but at the same time experience a release. Parents will sometimes tell me, "My son cried, but he also seemed a bit relieved, like he knows at some level that video games are bad for him." Following the fast, maybe a quarter of all children will start to become self-aware of the negative effect that electronics has on them. Particularly when children have been off of them for a few months, they may notice a difference in how they feel or will be able to identify the negative effects from screen-time in their friends.

Withdrawal Reactions

The term *withdrawal* is often associated with addiction, but really it is simply a reaction to a sudden reduction of an influence in the brain's environment. With screen-time, withdrawal can occur because of both psychological and physiological changes as the brain adjusts to a relative reduction in stimulation. True withdrawal reactions that resemble stimulant withdrawal can and do occur, and these include agitation, exhaustion, sleep disturbances ("crashing"), depressed or irritable mood, apathy, and lack of motivation. Severity of the symptoms depends on the total amount of cumulative and recent screen-time, how desensitized the dopamine-reward pathways have become, and on the resiliency of the individual. Certain biological factors may predispose some children to be more prone to experience more intense withdrawal, such as depression, autism, or a genetic predisposition for addiction. Meanwhile, having a strong social network is protective. That said, in my clinic I've only seen a handful of cases in which the withdrawal symptoms lasted several weeks before improvements were seen. Most typically, symptoms last a couple of days to about a week. Here are some rules of thumb about "withdrawal" reactions:

- Younger children bounce back more quickly (usually in one to three days).
- Adolescents typically take about a week or so to bounce back, and they may initially be more rageful, emotionally inconsistent (angry one minute, sobbing the next), or depressed, especially during the first few days.
- The most severe reactions are typically with older adolescents and young adults with years of extensive screen-time use.
- Children who use electronics as an "escape" from intolerable social lives may have an extreme reaction out of distress.
- Children who express sentiments such as "it's the only thing that makes me happy" may show signs of depression.

A Safety Plan: Handling Rage, Threats, and Depression

This section is not meant to alarm parents who don't expect their child to have an extreme emotional reaction to doing the Reset and who don't consider safety to be an issue in general. Rather, parents who need or will benefit from a safety plan typically already "know who they are," so to speak, because they've experienced threats or destructive behavior in the past when screen-time limits (or other limits) were set. Regardless, it is not uncommon for parents to worry that their child will become uncontrollably aggressive or hurt themselves in conjunction with the Reset. If you're concerned about your child hurting themselves, damaging property, or hurting others (including you), a safety plan should be put in place. Do this whether or not you feel your child's threats or behavior are purely manipulative — in other words, whether you think the behavior is a choice or is out of the child's control. Safety plans are powerful: they shift a parent from being paralyzed with fear to being mobilized and in charge.

Threats and destructive behavior tend to occur in children who are severely dysregulated, whether from ESS, full-blown tech addiction, other addictions, or psychiatric disorders. Often, the dysregulation itself can turn the hierarchy of power in the home upside down, with the child "running the show," which further exacerbates the situation. Whatever the cause, safety plans can help. Safety plans range from simply preparing mentally for how you'll handle your particular situation to formalizing a plan in writing, and it may or may not involve mental health professionals.

First, a word on boundaries. Safety is all about boundaries. An interesting but unfortunate aspect of screen-time is the quality of "boundarylessness"; cyberspace and some video games, for example, go on virtually forever. Needless to say, in addition to all the other effects we've discussed, this quality works against what children need. Boundaries are what make children feel safe. Conversely, when a child feels out of control, the child will push boundaries in order to *force* some containment because it's uncomfortable and unsettling to be without them. Thus, we want to help children feel a sense of firm boundaries without them having to force our hand. Two ways to promote this sense of safety and containment in children who feel out of control are 1) to have a plan that will keep everyone safe no matter what, and 2) to have adults who are in charge and who are communicating with each other. In this way, the plan *itself*— above and beyond what's actually *in* the plan — helps accomplish a sense of containment because the child knows they'll be safe, and because the parents feel more empowered and confident. That doesn't mean the child won't test the new boundaries, but it does remind you that safety plans work.

ANTICIPATING DESPAIR

For concerns about depression or a child hurting themselves in relation to the Reset, the safety plan's main focus is to ensure that there is no time during which the child is left unmonitored by an adult until the child's feeling better as well as safe. Worsening depression and intense anxiety are most likely to occur upon separation from devices, and at night if a child is accustomed to the "company" of a device before bedtime, so focusing on the time between informing the child and the end of the first week of the fast is most crucial. One mother I worked with slept in her thirteen-year-old daughter's room the first four nights. The mother reported: "She was furious at me but I could tell she liked that I was there." Indeed, the fear of being isolated and alone is part of what prompts a child's despair, so close monitoring and "being there" during this period can help provide a sense of grounding and connectedness — even if the child acts as though he or she doesn't want you there.

Remember that screen-time and light-at-night worsens depression and suicidality, so the risk of *not* removing devices is much greater than removing them. It may be reassuring to know that I've worked with children who have threatened to hurt themselves if screens are taken away, and I've seen children go through some depression or anxiety during the initial stages of the fast, but I've never had a child commit an act of self-harm in relation to this program. In fact, children with a history of self-injurious behaviors tend to get better, not worse.

CONTAINING AGGRESSION AND EXPLOSIVE BEHAVIORS

When you are concerned about the risk of aggression toward others, on the other hand, the safety plan should address specific high-risk times, such as when the child is informed of the fast and when devices are first removed. To reduce the chances of escalation during these moments, avoid informing your child about the Reset when he or she is using or has just been using a device, have at least two adults present when informing your child, and perform the screen sweep when your child is not home, such as while he or she is at school. If you're concerned that the child will explode upon coming home to find devices have been removed, you'll need another adult with you at this time as well.

Aside from the specifics of the Reset, however, the safety plan should convey to the child that you and other adults are in charge. If your child has a history of explosive behavior — in regard to screens or anything else — I recommend putting a safety plan in place and going over it with your child *prior to* discussing the Reset. This prevents your child from feeling blindsided when screen-time boundaries are set, and it shows your child that safety comes first and applies to everything, not just screen-time. It also gives you a chance to go over what behaviors are and are not acceptable. For example, getting mad and yelling are okay, but hitting, shoving, and throwing things are not.

When managing explosive or threatening behavior, it's important that both child and parent feel a sense of containment. Thus, if you feel you can't comfortably handle safety issues on your own or with other friends and family, enlist mental health professionals to help make the plan, be a part of the plan, and enforce the plan. In cases of aggression, the more adults who are involved in forming a "united front" and the more solid the plan, the safer the child will feel (despite protests to the contrary). Often though, in regard to the Reset, situations can be contained simply by having both parents present while informing the child, or by having another adult present that the child knows and respects, as in Lily's story, which we'll get to shortly (page 174).

A Safety Plan for Aggression

What does a safety plan for explosive behavior look like? In general, it should include coping strategies to lower the child's arousal levels, either through redirecting energy or giving the child time and space to calm down. Coping strategies or skills should be put in writing on the plan, and they can be changed as you figure out what works best. The plan should also include what you'll do to maintain safety. With this, what your own response will be depends not just on the child's behavior but on how safe you feel, or on how confident you feel that the behavior can be contained. In other words, if you feel you can handle an hour-long rage as long as no one gets hurt, so be it, but if a five-minute rage makes you feel that things are spiraling out of your control, then you'll need to take additional steps more quickly to contain the situation.

With bigger children, teens, and young adults who have been explosive in the past, I suggest including in the plan as a last resort "call 911." Adding this can make some parents feel uncomfortable, but the message to the child is that he or she will be contained *no matter what*. Truly, if someone is being injured or the child is hurling objects and smashing property, this is what needs to be done. When parents do call 911, either the police or a psychiatric emergency team (PET) comes to the home, and they'll de-escalate the situation if it hasn't been defused already. Often, when parents follow through with this step, the child is so shocked that episodes never rise to this level again.

The safety plan should be gone over verbally, read, and signed by the child and all adults involved (including any therapists). Here's an example we used for a fourteen-year-old boy, Harley, who was prone to rages:

HARLEY'S SAFETY PLAN

- If Harley is beginning to escalate, parent(s) will attempt to calm him by giving a time out or by redirecting him with coping skills (tearing up phone books, punching a pillow, playing basketball in the driveway, doing pushups, or calling Aunt Theresa to vent).
- If Harley continues to be unsafe or is escalating further, parent(s) will call Joe (next-door neighbor).
- If the above interventions aren't possible or don't work, and there is concern for danger to self or others, Harley will be warned that if he can't be safe, parent(s) will call 911.
- Timer will be set for ___ minutes. Harley will be given a warning that he has ___ minutes to calm down and be safe, or parents will call 911.
- When the timer "goes off," parents will determine whether Harley is being safe or is containable.
- If Harley continues to be unsafe, parents call 911.

I often add the timer step because the timer itself is a boundary, and it gives the child a chance to cool down. Obviously, if someone is being injured, you needn't wait for the timer to go off. I suggest setting the timer for somewhere between two and ten minutes, depending on how acute the situation is. Some final advice regarding dealing with a raging child: keep your voice calm and even; don't react or respond to verbal abuse (such as name-calling); don't attempt to reason or lecture (which tends to escalate a child further); and lower the stimulation in the room (turn down lights, turn off the TV and any music or radio, and so on).

Regardless of what you use the safety plan for, remember it can empower you to put the Reset plan in place, and realize that the Reset itself will further reduce these behaviors.

LILY: MOM TAKES CHARGE

In chapter 3, I told the story of Lily (see page 64), a sixteen-year-old girl with bipolar disorder who had been expelled from school because of her rages and erratic behavior. There, I described Lily's history during and after the Reset; here I'd like to share more about how we first set the wheels in motion. When I met Lily and her mother, they'd just begun homeschooling, but it wasn't going well. Lily was on the computer for more hours than ever, and when Lily's mom once tried to enforce a screen-time limit on her own, Lily had flown into a rage.

When I suggested that Lily do an electronic fast, Lily's mom expressed worry about how Lily would react. "She's bigger than me," her mom said, "and my husband works late and sometimes travels. I don't know if I can contain her if she flips out when I tell her what we're going to do."

So Lily's mom and I came up with a safety plan.

First, we spoke with Lily's dad and made sure both parents agreed with the approach and supported the plan. Since Lily's father couldn't be physically home most of the time, Lily's mom enlisted a trusted neighbor for support. The neighbor was with Lily's mom when she informed Lily of the plan and also when Lily's phone and computer were removed from the house. In both these moments, Lily flew into a rage, as expected. If the situation got out of hand, the safety plan included calling 911, but thankfully it never got that far. Mom held her ground, and though it took several more days, Lily's rages eventually subsided. By the end of the second week, there was a dramatic decrease in her symptoms, and Lily successfully completed the fast.

The Electronic Fast: Week by Week

While resetting or rebooting a computer may take a matter of minutes, the brain is immensely more complicated and thus needs more time to rest and turn things around. These three weeks allow your child's brain the chance to rejuvenate by obtaining the deep rest it needs to reset out-of-balance systems and redirect energy, blood flow, and nutrients to the brain's frontal lobe.

Week 1: Unplug in Order to Reset

The first week your child may or may not be in the throes of a true withdrawal syndrome. With school-age children, during the first one to three days they might mope around, complain, and not know what to do with themselves, but they quickly adapt — faster than you might think. Younger children also tend to "forget" about playing video games or using the computer sooner than older children do.

The removal of electronic screen devices immediately sets into motion a healthy chain of events. Removing the bright screen helps initiate a resynchronization of the circadian rhythms, allowing melatonin (the sleep hormone) to be secreted earlier in the evening and in larger amounts. In addition to being a sleep aid, melatonin is a powerful antioxidant in the nervous system — one of the *most* potent, actually — helping mitigate chronic stress-related damage caused by inflammation. Melatonin is also the precursor to the brain chemical serotonin, which keeps us calm and happy. A lesser known role of melatonin is that it influences the sex hormones. Melatonin exists in much higher levels in children, and suppression of it is speculated to be a cause of early puberty, which has become increasingly common in girls.[1]

Thus, brain chemistry and hormones enjoy an immediate shift toward normalization once melatonin is no longer suppressed. Likewise, dopamine is no longer forced into a "surge and deplete" pattern, which serves to improve mood and attention span. Upon the removal of unnatural and intense sensory and psychological stimulation, the nervous system will seek out more balanced stimulation through physical interactions with the environment. The brain has taken shelter from the storm, and instead of being in a protective state of reacting and defending, it shifts to a proactive mode and begins to self-organize.

What does this mean for your child? In Week 1, you can expect the following:

- A return to healthier, more imaginative, and more physical forms of play as creative energy returns
- Improved mood and less-extreme or less-frequent meltdowns as dopamine and serotonin regulation begin to normalize
- Improved compliance and less oppositional-defiant behaviors as the brain moves away from protective-defensive mode

As for parents, they often feel a lingering ambivalence about whether they can get through the whole three-week fast. They feel worried about "what it will take." If your child's meltdowns are worse during this week, you may start to have doubts. Hang tight!

WEEK 1 ACTION PLAN

1. Start tracking the problem areas you identified in chapter 5 ("Step 1: Define Problem Areas and Target Goals," page 130), which you already counted, measured, or rated the previous week to establish a baseline (see chapter 7 for more on tracking). At the end of each day, write down whatever information you've collected in regard to meltdowns, sleep reports from the previous night, missed homework, or whatever it is you've chosen to monitor. Keep a notebook at your bedside to remind yourself.

2. Make sure you review with your child the "Accountability Act" (see chapter 5, "Parental Screen-Time and Accountability," page 147) to go over whatever you (the parent) agreed to do in terms of activities and screen-time limits for yourself.

3. Fill in any schedule gaps for the coming weeks, such as unstructured time, access to electronics missed during the initial screen sweep, or unreliable caregivers. Take whatever steps you need to get rid of potential "holes."

4. At the end of the week, check in with your spouse and any other Reset support members and go over what is working and what isn't. If you're doing this on your own, schedule a time to journal about your assessment of the week, and add any ideas you've had that

might make things easier. If another parent-child team is doing the Reset with you, compare notes with them.

5. Mark the days off on the calendar and pat yourself on the back. Week 1 is the hardest!

Week 2: Allow Your Child's Brain Deep Rest

By the second week, your child's brain chemistry and biorhythms are a lot closer to normalizing, thanks to deeper sleep and reduced exposure to unnatural stimulation. Brain waves become more coherent and less erratic, and stress hormones diminish. Fight-or-flight symptoms or reactions may still be present, but these should start to ebb. On the other hand, underlying factors such as concurrent psychiatric or neurological disorders, or ongoing psychological stress, may continue to play a role, and their severity may affect how long it takes the brain and body to return to calmness.

As circadian rhythms resynchronize, serotonin levels rise. As the heart and the rest of the cardiovascular system experience less stress and more calm, a rhythm known as *heart rate variability* (HRV) becomes more coherent. Interestingly, coherent HRV patterns in turn induce coherent and more synchronized brain waves, implying that reduced cardiovascular stress improves brain integration.[2] Since HRV, blood pressure, and heart rate are negatively impacted by interactive screen-time, these markers should improve as the electronic fast progresses.

The things you can expect for your child in Week 2 include:

- Deeper and more restful sleep — although it may not be completely restorative yet
- Earlier bedtime or less resistance to bedtime and more energy upon awakening
- Continued improvement in mood swings and meltdowns
- Better organized behavior (child gets ready for school more easily, keeps better track of belongings or schedule)
- Improved impulse control, "cause-and-effect" thinking, and attention due to improved frontal lobe function
- Less arguing and negotiating about returning screen devices
- Increased spontaneous play and use of imagination

As parents start to see signs of improved mental health, they feel a mix of hope, relief, and increased motivation. During Week 2, there is typically less concern about one's ability to complete the fast.

WEEK 2 ACTION PLAN

1. Check in with your child about the "Accountability Act." Is there anything you missed or haven't followed through with? If so, did you pay the "tax"?
2. Ask your child how he or she has been sleeping, and take into account your own impression as well. Is your child still having trouble falling or staying asleep?
3. Double check that there are no handheld devices being sneaked under the covers at night or stashed in a backpack. If you didn't take your child's phone away, even if it's a flip phone, have your child turn it in as soon as he or she walks in the door, and make sure it's still checked in before you go to bed.
4. Continue to examine and fill the schedule. Do you have too much unstructured time? Are there are any upcoming activities that might provide opportunities for using electronics? Do whatever it takes to eliminate those risks. Take it seriously — you've put in a lot of effort already not to let something slip in.
5. Continue to collect data and document it nightly or as often as you can.
6. At the end of Week 2, check in with your spouse and any Reset partners. Is everyone getting enough support? Is the program creating more work for one parent than the other? Do the breaks and work load need to be rebalanced? If you're a single parent, do you need friends or family members to help you carve out more breaks?

Week 3: Healing and Reclaiming the Brain

Be careful not to get lax during Week 3. If your child's most extreme symptoms are dissipating or disappearing, you may feel tempted to start bending the rules a little. But now's not the time get sloppy — your child's brain is still healing. By now, biorhythms and brain chemistry may be close to normalizing, and as healing continues, stress and sleep hormones rebalance and promote calmness rather than hyperarousal. From the cell to the entire brain, oxidative stress and inflammation lessen, due to reduced stress load, and hormones will start to rebalance. As your child moves out of a state of chronic stress, the brain's energy is freed up to do other things — like learning new concepts and processing emotions. In contrast to the survival state, which is inherently selfish, impulsive, and one-track-minded, your child is now on his or her way to becoming healthier in mood, thought, behavior, and relationships.

In the final week of the fast, your child may experience or display:

- Dampened stress response and improved coping due to ongoing deep rest
- Reduced signs of anxiety, like nail biting, nightmares, headaches, or stomachaches
- Heightened curiosity and improved retention of new information
- Better manners and more respectful attitude
- A "virtuous circle" of improvement, in which better rest begets better mood and attention, which begets improved self-image, which begets better sleep, and so on

As for yourself, the fast will likely feel much easier to manage at this point. Your own stress levels will likely be significantly lower in general. Particularly if you've reduced your own screen-time, you may feel an enhanced sense of being "in the moment" with your child.

WEEK 3 ACTION PLAN

1. Journal about your experiences during the fast: What's become easier, and where did you run into unexpected roadblocks? How has the fast affected you?
2. Continue collecting data. During the week, review your original list of problems and goals. Do you have a general sense of whether things have improved? Have other symptoms or issues improved as well? To explore this, see the next section below, "After the Fast: Assessments and Next Steps."
3. Notice and write down any positive new changes in your child. Is he or she picking up any new interests, showing more curiosity in

general, or being more sensitive and kind to others? These things may become more pronounced with time, but recognizing them can be a particularly poignant reminder of how screen-time has been hindering your child's development.

4. Make sure you continue to schedule breaks for yourself. If you tend to schedule them but not take them, break that habit this week. Just as your child's brain needs to rest, *you* need to rest.

5. Check in with your spouse and other partners. As before, review what's working and what isn't. Did you do anything different during this week that helped, like rebalancing workloads? Make a note so you don't slip back into old patterns.

6. Begin to develop a game plan for what you'll do next by doing the exercises in the next section and by reading chapter 9. Do you feel a complete fast should be continued, or will you start to reintroduce screen-time in small amounts, and if so, how? By week's end, you want to have a considered answer.

7. Appreciate that the rule of thumb for creating a new habit is twenty-one days. By the end of Week 3, you and your family should start to feel more matter-of-fact about living screen-free: "That's just the way it is now." Congratulate yourself for putting in enough solid time to make a healthy habit "stick"!

After the Fast: Assessments and Next Steps

At the end of the fast, take some extra time to assess how things have gone, what's changed, and what you want to do next. Parents have lots of questions at this point: What if the Reset didn't work? How do I know if I need to do the fast for longer than three weeks? How do I decide whether to reintroduce screen-time, what kinds, and how much? Answering these questions is the focus of chapter 9, but first let me share with you a couple of things I've learned from working with parents.

First, it is not uncommon for parents to decide to continue the electronic fast for longer than three weeks (or for me to persuade them to do so!). We've seen this in several of the case studies I've described so far, such as with Dan in chapter 3 (see page 60), who needed six weeks of abstention before his depression lifted, and who afterward could only handle limited amounts of computer use without triggering symptoms again. In other cases, parents decide to continue fasting for several months in order to get their child's symptoms under control, while still others choose to eliminate interactive screen-time on a more permanent basis because they've determined the risks are too high. Then again, many parents want to try reintroducing screen-time after the three-week fast, but in much smaller amounts. In any case, what to do next is not a casual decision.

This brings me to my second point, which is that, in all likelihood, some things will improve during the fast and some won't. Odds are high that you and your child will experience enough relief and benefits to make the fast clearly seem worthwhile. But if what remains still causes a lot of stress, it can be discouraging, which makes it easy to dismiss any gains: "Well, yes, a, b, and c improved, but we're still dealing with d, e, f, and g...." If this is the case, try to curtail this tendency, and during your assessment, focus on identifying and quantifying all the areas that have improved, rather than on what's still bothersome. Know that some children need more time than others, and recall from chapter 4 that benefits accumulate and build over time. *Stay the course.*

EXERCISE *Analyze Your Data*

Return to the two or three prioritized items you chose to track. Summarize all your notes during the three weeks and rerate or measure them now. If the data allows, chart whatever you decided to track, and compare baseline to endpoint measurements. Did each problem area improve, and by how much? How would you rate each item post-fast as compared to pre-fast?

For example, say you decided to track homework completion. Say you found that your child completed four of eight assignments in the two weeks prior to the fast — a 50 percent completion rate — and then you found that he or she completed four out of five assignments during Week 3 of the fast — an 80 percent completion rate. This would mean your child had increased his or her homework completion rate from 50 percent to 80 percent. Although it's still not perfect, that's a highly significant improvement. If you decided to measure meltdowns, say you noted that the severity remained about the same, but that the frequency decreased, perhaps from once or twice a day to once or twice a week. Even conservatively, that change represents a 70 percent decrease! Although each individual meltdown may make you want to tear your hair out, looking at raw data like that can be highly encouraging.

EXERCISE *Acknowledge Positive Changes*

Near the end of Week 3, write down *all* the improvements that you've noticed in your child, including those related to the problem areas that you tracked as well as any other positive changes you've noticed. Think in terms of behavior, mood, cognition, and physical well-being. Even if you're not sure each and every improvement is directly related to the fast, note them all; indirect changes count, too. Did mood or attention improve? Did your child listen better when asked to do something? Did a teacher or relative make a positive comment? Did you notice your child rediscovering toys or activities? What were they? Be as specific and detailed as possible.

Meditate on these improvements. Appreciate this "new normal" and consider how it relates to all the other changes you've made in the last three weeks (in addition to restricting screen-time). Keep these improvements in mind when you read chapter 9 and consider what to do next.

Chapter 6 Take-Home Points

- Be ready for your child's negative reaction when you inform him or her of the fast, prepare for common questions, and don't engage in arguing or negotiating.
- If your child becomes despondent or angry, validate the child's feelings and comfort him or her while standing firm; keep the conversation matter-of-fact and the expectations clear, and present the alternative activities and special treats that will replace screen-time.
- Safety plans can and should be made in the case of concern about a child hurting him- or herself or others.
- The first week of the fast is the hardest, but it immediately sets into motion a chain of positive events that influence circadian rhythms and brain chemistry, whether you see outward signs of improvement or not.
- The second and third weeks become easier, and improvements in symptoms and functioning become more evident, sometimes dramatically so.
- Near the end of the fast, consider next steps; children who show fewer improvements may need a longer fast.

CHAPTER 7

TRACKING AND TROUBLESHOOTING

Deciding What's Working and What's Not

Courage means to keep working a relationship,
to continue seeking solutions to a difficult problem,
and to stay focused during stressful times.

— Denis Waitley

This chapter discusses two separate but interrelated issues: tracking symptoms or dysfunction to document improvements, and troubleshooting what might be going wrong if improvements don't arise. Tracking is the most objective way to determine whether the fast has been effective, and if it hasn't, then I always ask parents to troubleshoot for common problems or mistakes that can happen when implementing the Reset.

Tracking Your Child's Progress

The vast majority of the time, the benefits of the fast will be obvious to you and to others. You will see major changes in your child and feel palpable relief. But sometimes, when whatever symptoms that still remain continue to be disruptive or stressful, improvements are not as obvious. It's for these cases that tracking becomes most critical. In an objective manner, tracking answers the all-important question: *Is the fast worth it?* When embarking on a lifestyle change like the Reset, everyday life can easily get in the way of maintaining objectivity about improvements, since even as some urgent problems subside, others move to center stage. This process can make a stressed parent feel like progress is not being made, when in fact it is marching right along.

Tips for Successful Tracking

Tracking boils down to obtaining objective baseline measurements of the problem areas you have identified, collecting data during the fast, and then assessing these areas again at the end of it. For example, if we picked "meltdowns," we could track frequency, severity, or both. Here is a breakdown of the process.

1. *Collect data daily:* Try to track daily or at least every few days so your memory of events is fresh. It is sometimes like pulling teeth to get parents to track, but it's helpful, and not just for the information: the ritual of writing down observations helps focus your intention and awareness. Parents who track stick to the fast better and have more success.

2. *Quantify as much as possible:* There are three main ways to quantify: *counting* (such as the number of meltdowns in a day), using a *rating scale* (such as the severity on a scale of 1–10), and *calculating a percentage or average* (such as the average amount of homework completed in a week). You could also use time, such as tracking what time your child goes to bed, or how long it takes to do homework.

3. *Write in a dedicated notebook:* In the "spirit" of screen liberation, track on paper in a dedicated notebook or journal, which you can leave out as a visual reminder. For example, putting the notebook on your bed each day can help you remember to do the journal exercises before hitting the hay.

4. *Define a larger mission:* Remember, tracking (and the Reset itself) is in service of your child's health and quality of life. Don't miss the forest for the trees. Create a mission statement (per chapter 5, "Step 10: Set Your Intention," page 155) that articulates the positive vision you're seeking. This helps you prioritize, stay on track, and be successful.

5. *Post your one-month Reset calendar:* Per chapter 5, "Step 3: Set a Date and Create a Schedule" (page 139), posting the calendar in a common area will provide a visual reminder to track every day, and it reminds you where you are in the process.

6. *Set a reminder to track endpoints at the completion of the fast:* The most important data points are your baseline (pre-fast) measurements and the endpoint (post-fast) measurements. So if you start out strong but forget to track during the middle of the fast, that's okay. Just make sure you get some measurements down from the end of Week 3. Put a reminder both on the Reset calendar and in your phone.

7. *Accept the true nature of change:* Progress naturally proceeds in fits and starts, and each situation and person is different. You may see dramatic positive changes and then sudden, unexpected pullbacks. Or, change may be very gradual and hard to notice at first. Track with an open mind, and remain committed for the full three weeks. Don't stop the fast halfway through or decide not to track just because you're not seeing the results you hoped for.

To see how tracking can make a meaningful difference in the interpretation of a Reset, let's look at two cases. Both families had adopted children who were struggling with attachment issues. The first involves a family who failed to track, which undermined their confidence in the effectiveness of the Reset, and the second involves a family who tracked successfully, which provided them with objective data with which to make decisions.

Misha: A Lack of Evidence

The Barringtons adopted their little girl, Misha, when she was three. Misha was from an orphanage in Russia, and like many adopted children who've suffered early neglect, Misha was prone to rages. I'd been seeing Misha with her parents since shortly after Misha's adoption. When Misha turned eleven, she received her first cell phone, a birthday gift from her parents. Misha began texting her friends throughout the day and also at night when she was supposed to be in bed asleep, and it didn't take long before her rages became worse — much worse. Because of her history, Misha had significant attachment issues, so when I mentioned that her rages had grown worse since she'd been given the phone, her parents were not at all convinced that the phone was any part of the problem. Finally, after months of urging, I convinced the family to take Misha's phone — her sole device — away for a month to see what would happen.

Per my usual practice, I'd been tracking the frequency of Misha's rages as reported by Misha's parents. Just prior to the Reset, Misha was averaging two to three rages a week that were severe enough to result in property damage. Just before they began the fast, I asked the parents to make the four-week calendar and to note two or three behaviors — including the rages — that they'd like to reduce, to rate the behaviors in terms of severity and frequency before the fast, and to do the same each week until I saw them again. When I saw them a month later, they admitted they'd forgotten to track, but they said they had indeed gone through with the "no phone" fast.

"It didn't seem to make much of a difference. Our lives are still a nightmare," Misha's mother declared about the Reset.

I asked her to estimate how many rages Misha had had over the last three weeks, and she said, "Misha had a major one last week, over nothing. It was unbelievable. She flew into a rage over me refusing to buy her this pair of shoes —"

"I'm sure that was frustrating," I said, interrupting her. "But let's nail down the frequency, and then we can get back to that. She had one rage last week. How about this week?"

"None this week, but the one she had last Monday in the store was a doozy..."

Misha's mother continued to focus on what had happened during that single incident, but the fact that Misha had experienced only one rage over the past two weeks was not lost on me. Previously, Misha was experiencing four to six times that many meltdowns in the same period. When I pointed this out, Misha's mother replied, "Yeah, but how do we know it had anything to do with the phone restriction? I mean, it could have been anything."

"We don't know for sure," I admitted, "but the whole point of tracking is to give you objective evidence about whether the rages or other behaviors have improved. Let me show you what I wrote in her chart from your last visit."

I showed Misha's mother my notes from the month before, but Misha's mother said she was still "not convinced" that it was the phone that had made the difference. "Besides," she said, "I like her to have the phone so I know where she is." Lacking additional hard evidence, I couldn't convince Misha's mother that electronic stimulation and light-at-night were contributing to the very behaviors she was complaining about. She was "stuck" on the severity of the rages themselves as well as on the convenience of the phone, and her subjective sense was that nothing had really changed. Thus it was difficult for me to help her see that it might be a worthwhile intervention to continue.

This is why tracking is important: it gives you concrete data about what, if anything, is improving so that you can make informed choices, which is particularly important when you're stressed and everything seems like one more demand. Tracking can also reinforce your subjective impressions, which strengthens conviction. Banning a phone wasn't going to solve all of Misha's problems, but it certainly might have made things easier.

Melody: Signs of Improvement

The Rodriguez family adopted their little girl, Melody, also when she was three, and they adopted her three older brothers shortly thereafter. When Melody was in fifth grade, she began stealing compulsively, and after about a year of this behavior, the family came to me for help. With four children, they were a busy and stressed family, and the parents weren't thrilled by the prospect of doing a Reset. But they agreed, and for the three-week fast, we decided Melody would use no electronics at home — no computer, no phone, and no social media — but she would be allowed to use a computer at school. Mrs. Rodriguez agreed to track the stealing incidents plus two other problematic behaviors. She then had the foresight to propose an idea that proved quite useful: "If this Reset plan does make a difference, and we need to minimize computer use at school as well, it would be good to show the teacher some hard data."

The three problem areas Melody's parents picked were stealing (which was being exhibited at home and at school), insomnia, and not turning in homework assignments. Prior to beginning the fast, Melody's parents noted the following, which they used as a baseline: stealing was occurring on a daily basis at home and at school, Melody was falling asleep at around 1 a.m. on average, and her homework score was "pretty much zero."

When I met with Melody's parents at the conclusion of the fast, they reported that by the third week, Melody had stolen at school only twice (that they knew of), but that at home she was still stealing on a daily basis. She was now going to bed by 10 p.m. on most nights without much of a fight, and she was asleep by 11 p.m. on five of the last seven nights. Lastly, she had turned in three homework assignments that week, compared to virtually none at baseline.

"Obviously, she still has miles to go," her mother said, "but at least we're seeing some seedlings of change. We have decided to continue to hold computer, phone, and social media and see how it goes. We also showed the teacher our tracking results and talked about how screen-time can increase compulsive behaviors. She was impressed enough to try 'no computer' at school, too, to see if it would help."

Over the following year, Melody's parents continued to uphold these restrictions, and Melody gradually ceased stealing altogether. She continued to sleep better, and she became more conscientious about turning in her schoolwork.

There are a couple of important points that Melody's story illustrates. One is that if Melody's parents hadn't actually tracked the stealing as a problematic behavior, the symptom might have "felt" unchanged, since Melody was still stealing nearly every day at home. Part of the difficulty in addressing behaviors that are upsetting, embarrassing, or difficult to relate to is that it's hard to praise a child for doing "less" of them: "But she just stole yesterday. Am I supposed to praise her for stealing *less*?" Yet that's exactly what needs to happen. By measuring stealing incidents at school and looking at other markers as well, Melody's parents could objectively see a difference and be proud of their daughter's improvements, which reinforced her progress. The second is that tracking can provide clear evidence that can convince others, such as mental health clinicians and teachers, to support screen-time limits as part of an ongoing intervention. In the case of school, where teachers and the principle have to devote much of their energy to the most disruptive children, data like this might be particularly compelling.

Did going screen-free help Melody to be less impulsive because of improved frontal lobe function? Was better dopamine regulation mitigating her compulsive behaviors? Or was she simply spending more quality bonding time with her family and felt better about herself? In truth, we don't know for sure that it was the reduction of screen-time that helped, much less the weight of individual components. But we do know that tracking allowed these parents to "see" small but positive changes, which gave them hope and helped them shift their focus onto the most important goal: helping their daughter feel secure and loved.

Troubleshooting Reset Problems

What happens if you track diligently and complete the three-week fast, but don't see any results? Before you decide that screen-time is not impacting your child, take a closer look at some of the following issues that can undermine a Reset. If you troubleshoot these and try again, odds are good that you'll get a better result. You've got nothing to lose and potentially much to gain.

Issue #1: Overlooked Devices and Opportunities

Did you miss something? If a child exhibits classic signs of Electronic Screen Syndrome and is receiving interactive screen-time on a daily basis, then a properly executed electronic fast will almost always effect some type of positive change — even if there are *multiple* other variables going on. Why? One reason is that better sleep tends to improve psychiatric symptoms across the board, and as you now know, removing electronics improves sleep. So, in cases like these — involving a child with classic ESS symptoms plus confirmed screen-time exposure — if parents tell me the fast "didn't work," I am almost certain something was overlooked.

Here are some cases that demonstrate how easy it is to miss something.

GEORGIA: OVERLOOKED DEVICES

When I started working with Georgia, she was sixteen and struggling with ADHD. Georgia continually fell behind in school, even after we arranged for accommodations at school to help keep her on track. Georgia had two younger siblings at home who were toddlers, and she often complained she couldn't concentrate enough to get her work done when the kids were around. So we problem-solved that issue, but even after Georgia was able to work quietly without distractions, she continued to struggle. She also felt depressed and lonely, and her parents complained that she rarely got her chores done. We repeatedly discussed setting screen-time limits during family meetings, but Georgia's parents had their hands full with the two little ones, and so they were fairly lax about enforcement.

By her junior year, Georgia was so far behind that the school warned the family that Georgia might not graduate on time. At this, Georgia's parents decided to take action and began the electronic fast. Within several days, Georgia began dedicating more time and effort to her schoolwork, but she had quite a bit of catching up to do.

Three weeks into the fast, Georgia came to my office by herself for a visit and sobbed uncontrollably about not having her phone. Her level of despair made me suspicious that she was still dysregulated, but she denied using any other screen devices. The next day, however, her mother emailed me and said they'd discovered a touchscreen Kindle in Georgia's room that they'd forgotten to remove, and that Georgia had admitted she'd been playing games on it in bed each night. Shortly after that discovery, Georgia got caught using an old cell phone that had been stored in a junk drawer. After performing another screen sweep for good measure, Georgia's father took the devices to work — at which point the *real* Reset began.

With no electronics to distract her, Georgia managed to catch up on a massive number of missed assignments. She began engaging in more face-to-face social activities, and with continued strict screen management, her loneliness and depression lifted. Meanwhile, her reinvigorated social life gave her parents newfound leverage over getting her chores done. Over the following months, Georgia wound up making tremendous strides in multiple realms — but it might never have happened if her parents hadn't uncovered those overlooked devices.

JT: Overlooked Opportunities

In this case, an eight-year-old boy named JT displayed significant improvements in mood within the first week of the fast. During the second week, however, his parents became dismayed when his tantrums and explosive behaviors returned. After some sleuthing, they discovered that one of JT's friends was letting JT play a handheld game during the half-hour bus ride to and from school each day. To solve this problem, JT's father drove him to school for a few weeks, and sure enough, JT's mood improved again. After deciding to continue elimination of video games for several more months, JT's mother spoke to both the bus driver and to the friend's parents, who agreed to help with the restrictions. As it turned out, JT much preferred riding the bus with his friends, and he stayed compliant with the fast rather than risk having to ride to school again with dear old Dad.

Jackson: False Promises

When Jackson began seeing me, he was twenty years old. He had mild attention issues but was otherwise quite bright. Still, he repeatedly fell behind in his college classes and wound up dropping out of them every semester. After months of insisting that his video game habits weren't affecting him,

Jackson finally admitted how much time they took up and how they affected his motivation. Since Jackson lived at home, he and his mother agreed that she would physically remove the video games from the home so that Jackson could focus on school.

Upon returning home from my office, however, Jackson changed his mind and told his mother to leave the console in his room. He promised that he simply wouldn't play, but of course he continued playing just as before. So Jackson's mother made him a deal: she'd buy him a ski pass if he handed over the game controllers. They shook on it, and upon taking possession of the controllers, she bought the pass. When I later asked his mom why she hadn't removed the whole unit, she replied, "It was too much of a pain." When I asked if the controllers were out of the house, she said she'd hidden them in the closet.

Needless to say, Jackson found the controllers. At first he hid them under his bed and played when no one was around, but eventually he returned to playing openly, since the ski pass had already been paid for and given to him.

At that point, I continued to see Jackson but dropped the subject, since it seemed the family was not ready to follow through. About a year later, Jackson marched into my office and announced he'd taken the entire gaming system out of his room and handed it over to his mom. He told me, "I thought I could handle it and just play once in a while, but I can't. The only way for me to *not* play is to not have it available." Jackson began earning As and Bs in school, he stopped dropping classes, and he wound up losing twenty pounds.

When faced with the prospect of an electronic fast, children will promise not to play games or to use their devices anymore — so long as you don't take them away. Many times this is simply manipulation, but even when children truly mean it and believe it, we don't do children favors by "trusting" them in this regard. Leaving devices available is simply too tempting. I've *never* seen a child with screen-related issues be able to voluntarily give up using them for more than a few days when devices remain accessible. Devices must be physically removed from the house, not just hidden in a closet or unplugged. As I discuss below, kids are smart, and where there's a will, there's a way!

Don't Underestimate Your Child's Determination

When you do a screen sweep, the purpose is to eliminate any and all temptations. Often, parents remove their children's devices but leave their own lying around the house "locked" with a password or some other blocking application. This is a mistake. If there's a workaround, kids will find it faster than your company's IT guy. And don't think removing the battery from a phone will prevent a determined child from using it, either — they'll find another.

So, if you suspect something is being missed, consider the following:

- Review your child's schedule, hour by hour, day by day. Don't forget about time spent riding the bus, carpools, recess, and downtime during sports practice as potential screen-time opportunities.
- Make a list of devices, old and new, even if you think your child isn't interested in them anymore. An old handheld game becomes enticing if the current ones aren't available.
- Don't forget about old phones. Most have games on them, and your child will notice and find them if they are simply stashed in a junk drawer.
- Consider every place your child goes: to an ex-spouse's house, to daycare, to after-school care. Children may also lie to other caregivers and tell them they're "allowed to play now." Make sure you remind everyone involved. Sometimes grandparents don't realize that older phones might have games installed on them, and hand one over, thinking it's harmless.
- Finally, don't allow a device to be kept simply because it was a gift or because "she bought it with her own money." Smartphones and other devices are often inexpensive or even free these days, leading them to be given as gifts like never before — but that doesn't mean children should have them.

Issue #2: Insufficient Fast Length

Although the majority of children and teens can reset with a three-week fast, sometimes three weeks is not long enough. Most often this occurs in older teens and young adults who are either physically addicted or who spend upward of ten to twelve hours daily on a screen (which is more common than you might think). When the need for a longer fast occurs in a school-age or younger child, it's typically because of complicating factors like autism, sensory issues, or an underlying mood disorder, and it may be a sign that the child simply can't tolerate much — if any — electronics use at all.

Chapter 9 discusses this in more detail, but simply put: if you're not sure why you haven't seen improvement, *you can't go wrong by extending the fast.* Parents seem to have an intuitive sense about this; if you find yourself wondering if you should go longer, just do it.

Issue #3: Relaxing the Rules

There are two main reasons why a strict fast can become progressively less strict, and therefore less effective, over time. The first is fatigue. Maintaining a strict fast without adequate support may feel too difficult, so parents start letting things slide and don't monitor things as closely. Aside from not getting enough breaks or having enough help with child care, fatigue can occur when parents experience a lot of resistance about the fast or about screen-time issues from others, such as relatives, clinicians, caregivers, and so on. Parents can grow tired of explaining and justifying their position, and start giving in. This issue, and how to handle it, is discussed in chapter 8.

The second main reason rules get loosened is early success. When parents see some positive results fairly quickly, say during the first week, they might knowingly or unknowingly become lax about the rules during subsequent weeks. When their child's behavior worsens again, the parent thinks, "I tried, but it's not working!" So be honest with yourself: Did you become lax with the rules — for whatever reason? Did the "fast" become something less? Did screen-time creep in? Remember that it really does take three weeks or longer for the brain to be adequately rested and rejuvenated — not one week. You have every reason to celebrate early improvements, but that isn't a reason to loosen the reins. If you realize this may have been what happened, then do the Reset again as soon as you can, and double down on your commitment to stick to it.

Issue #4: Too Much Resistance or Too Little Support

Lack of support, or too much resistance from others, can doom a Reset before it begins. Virtually every parent has to cope with doubt and skepticism about ESS from others, as well as varying degrees of cooperation with an electronic fast. It could be that the fast didn't *become* more relaxed over time; it simply was never strict enough to begin with because of a lack of help. This is such a huge, critical issue that I've dedicated the second half of chapter 8 to it.

Issue #5: School-Related Screen-Time

If your child is exposed to too much screen-time either during the school day or during homework time, or if your child is particularly sensitive to becoming dysregulated, you may need to eliminate school-based screen sources for the brain to adequately rest and reset. In some cases, it's only necessary to eliminate school-related screen-time during the fast, and in other cases it may be important to restrict or eliminate it long term. Revisit chapter 5, "Reset Planning and School" (page 158), for information about requesting that screen-time be eliminated during the fast, including a template for a doctor's note, and read chapter 11, particularly "Working with Your Child's School: Effective Attitudes and Approaches" (page 276).

Issue #6: Other Electronic-Related Instigators

Finally, if you're sure you haven't missed any unwanted screen devices or opportunities, consider whether other electronic-related impacts might be causing dysregulation and preventing your child's nervous system from healing. The three major ones are EMFs, television, and unhealthy lighting.

RADIATION FROM ELECTROMAGNETIC FIELDS (EMFs)

EMFs are everywhere, and individuals vary in their sensitivity to them. All wireless communication from WiFi and mobile phones emit them, and there is a growing body of evidence that suggests manmade EMFs produce stress-related changes that may contribute to hyperarousal symptoms, at least in some. Certain conditions may predispose one to EMF sensitivity, including autism, autoimmune disorders, allergies, and some cases of ADHD. In turn, EMFs may worsen or accelerate these conditions.

Since WiFi is a continuous source of radiofrequency EMFs whether you're using the Internet or not, to troubleshoot the Reset, turn your home's WiFi connection off for a month and use wired (cabled) Internet access instead. For a fuller discussion on possible effects, see appendix B, "Electromagnetic Fields (EMFs) and Health: A 'Charged' Issue."

(See also chapter 11 regarding school-related WiFi.)

LOSE THE TV

As I discuss in chapter 5 ("Television Viewing During the Reset," page 156), I do typically permit some television or movie time during the Reset, but sometimes this allowance backfires. Why? Sometimes families don't follow the TV guidelines: either the child is allowed to watch fast-paced cartoons and children's shows on a mega-screen TV, sitting right in front of the set; or the family leaves the television on all the time, even when no one's watching it. As I discuss in chapter 3, studies show that even background television can be harmful to attention and it reduces the amount and quality of parent-child interaction. Meanwhile, television viewing is linked to learning, reading, and behavioral difficulties. Whether you've followed the Reset's TV rules or not, if your child struggles during the Reset and you've troubleshot all the other issues, consider giving up television, too.

UNHEALTHY LIGHTING

Research suggests that several factors related to the light quality emitted by energy-efficient lighting can contribute to hyperarousal, including studies demonstrating fight-or-flight stress reactions and more shallow sleep.[1] Because of this, one suggestion I make when other electronic causes seem accounted for is to switch all compact fluorescent lights (CFLs) and LEDs in the home to light that is less blue-toned and fuller in spectrum. If this isn't possible, at least switch out the lights in your child's bedroom. Incandescent bulbs are the healthiest, since they emit full spectrum light and in a continuous manner that's easy for the eye and brain to process, but these are hard to come by these days. Next best are halogen bulbs, which don't have as perfect a spectrum balance as incandescent, but it's close. In contrast, both CFLs and LEDs have strong blue and white tones, and they emit light in "bursts" rather than in a continuous manner, creating a less soothing light.[2] Between the two, fluorescent light looks and feels more irritating, and it also emits more radiation.

One of the reasons we know that fluorescent light can be a visual and nervous system irritant is because in certain sensitive individuals, such as those with autoimmune disorders, migraines, seizures, or tics, fluorescent lights can precipitate a reaction (such as a rash, headache, seizure, tic, and so on). Conversely, studies show people report a greater sense of well-being when under incandescent versus CFL lighting.[3] There's a reason we call it "mood lighting"!

Changing out bulbs is a relatively easy thing to do. Even if you don't see a difference right away, reducing the stressful influence of energy-efficient lighting may prove to pay benefits over time.

Chapter 7 Take-Home Points

- Lack of objective tracking can sometimes lead a parent to feel like the Reset didn't help when in fact it did.
- Proper tracking can help you prioritize the most pressing problem areas, establish clear goals, and maintain fast strictness when dysfunction is occurring in multiple areas.
- If the Reset appears to have been ineffective, troubleshoot possible reasons why before deciding screen-time has no impact.
- Common troubleshooting issues include missed screen devices or opportunities, insufficient fast length, a "loosening" of the Reset rules, lack of proper planning or support, school-related screen-time, and other electronic-related instigators.
- In some children, television viewing may need to be reduced further or even eliminated for the nervous system to properly reset.
- EMF exposure may cause many of the same stress reactions as interactive screen-time, so minimizing manmade EMFs by turning off WiFi may boost the Reset's effectiveness, especially in sensitive children.

CHAPTER 8

DEALING WITH DOUBT
AND SHORING UP SUPPORT

All truth passes through three stages. First, it is ridiculed.
Second, it is violently opposed.
Third, it is accepted as being self-evident.

— Arthur Schopenhauer

The very subject of screen-time touches a collective nerve. It triggers anxiety about parenting practices, guilt over allowing screen-time to cause negative effects in our children, and defensiveness regarding one's own screen-time habits. Parents feel helpless and angry when schools make sweeping changes that leave them without a choice, and they feel alarm when they hear their children's data is being mined and sold. Some resent that the medical community hasn't been forceful enough regarding screen-time warnings, while others resent being told how to live, how to parent. At the same time, innovation in general is often tied to screen-based technology, and we're told so often that technology holds such promise that questioning its role in any arena feels almost unpatriotic. All these conflicting feelings — felt at both the individual and societal levels — produce burning questions for parents: Is screen-time truly dangerous or are fears overblown? Does it affect all children or just a few? Does it help learning or hinder it? What options do I have if it's affecting *my* child? Meanwhile, screens are everywhere. We use and rely on them more every day, and the idea of limiting screen-time — much less following a strict fast — can seem like folly.

Doubt and uncertainty about screen-time is such a universal issue, and it can be such a critical roadblock to a successful Reset, that it deserves its own chapter. If you are uncertain about ESS and about whether ESS is affecting your child, know that you are not alone. Almost every parent who does the Reset Program wrestles with doubts. Many times it is only by persevering and following a strict fast that parents see for themselves how screen-time is impacting their child.

On the other hand, all parents without exception must deal with the doubts and skepticism of others. This can create quite a challenge at times because it is impossible to do a Reset without help, cooperation, and support. So in addition to addressing the doubts that parents might have, this chapter addresses how parents can work with others and enlist help — no matter what people think about ESS or what they believe about screen-time's effects.

That said, not every parent I work with has doubts. Some, in fact, feel validated when I discuss ESS, for it confirms what they've witnessed in their own lives, with their own children, and with others. These parents are eager to do the Reset, for they are already convinced it will help. But even those readers will benefit from this chapter as they build support with a range of helpers who may not all share that conviction.

Personal Doubts and Uncertainty

When I work with families on screen-related issues, one of my most important tasks is to address parental doubts and uncertainty about the Reset Program. It's crucial to figure out what's *behind* any doubts or reluctance, since a lack of commitment can easily undermine a Reset. Essentially, I find this boils down to two areas: 1) doubt or disbelief regarding the adverse effects of screen-time (and thus the effectiveness of the Reset), and 2) doubting one's ability to carry out the Reset Program.

It's impossible to address in this book all the doubts that a parent might have. The first three chapters explain ESS and provide a wealth of scientific and research support for the negative effects of screen-time. When parents want the "evidence" for my claims about screen-time's propensity to dysregulate a child's brain, I share with them this research, as well as my firsthand experience treating others. Chapter 4, meanwhile, summarizes what I've found to be the benefits of the Reset Program. However, none of this answers the real question: Is screen-time having a negative effect on *your child*, and what benefits would *your child* get from a Reset?

In truth, no parent knows either of these things with absolute certainty before attempting an electronic fast. Every parent must do the Reset despite any doubts they have about whether ESS is affecting their child and what benefits a fast will bring. Some cases are clearer than others, some parents more willing than others, and some kids more amenable than others. But it's only in retrospect, once the fast is complete, that you can say with certainty what impacts screen-time is having and what improvements removing it will bring. As we've seen, impacts and benefits are both direct and indirect and depend as much on what naturally replaces the missing screen-time as on removing screens themselves.

Is it worth it to do the Reset when you aren't sure what the results will be? That's really up to you to decide, but when parents are uncertain, I ask them to do what is essentially a cost-benefit analysis. I ask parents to list what they think will be the "costs," or negative impacts, of doing the Reset against what they think the potential short- and long-term benefits could be. In many ways, this is a companion exercise to the one in chapter 5, in which parents identify which of their child's problematic behaviors they want to address and what goals they want to aim for. Each of these steps helps parents clarify their goals, purpose, and mission.

EXERCISE *Reset Cost-Benefit Analysis: Tallying the Costs*

As with any cost-benefit analysis, this exercise consists of making two lists, comparing them, and then making your decision to do the Reset based on whether the costs outweigh the benefits or whether the potential benefits justify the costs. Unlike a financial cost-benefit analysis, there is no set or predetermined value for any item. You must decide how much things are worth, both to yourself and your child.

In any case, simply the act of defining these things is helpful. In their anxiety over how much trouble they imagine the Reset to be, some parents resist without really examining what they are afraid of. Nor do they really balance this against what success (in their terms) would bring if the Reset works. In fact, some of the typical "costs," particularly the fear that the child will be extremely upset and angry, are indications that a Reset is needed and indeed would be effective, since this reaction in itself indicates a level of attachment and dependence that is associated with other negative impacts. Often the feared "costs" are the flip side of what the program may in fact get rid of.

To begin this exercise, write a list of the costs you anticipate during the one-month Reset; for now, put aside concerns over continuing screen-time limits into the future. When tallying costs, be as specific and detailed as possible. Perhaps also rate each item's "value" on a scale of one to ten in relation to its real or imagined impact. This list also functions as a survey of all the areas of difficulty where you might want to seek help and support from others. Here is a list of possible items or areas that parents often mention:

- My child's reaction may be intensely negative, provoking rage, depression, or aggression.
- My child may blame or "hate" me for taking electronics away.
- I will lose a necessary or often used "electronic babysitter" for peace and quiet or to get work done.
- I will lose bonding time with my child, since "game time" is shared or done together.
- Losing electronics may separate, isolate, or single out my child from peers who use electronics.
- A strict fast seems too hard to accomplish, since electronics are so pervasive in the home and elsewhere.
- It's too inconvenient to have my child do computer-related homework in a common area.
- My child may "drive me crazy" because he or she doesn't know how to entertain him- or herself.
- I don't want to cut back or change on my own media use and screen-time.
- Convincing my spouse and other vital caregivers to agree and cooperate may be difficult.
- Replacing screen-time with other activities may mean more work than I have time or energy for.
- I may feel even more stressed and exhausted than I do now.

As I suggest, when listing costs, be as specific as possible. For instance, if you're concerned over lessening your own screen-time at home, distinguish how much of this screen-time is convenience and personal pleasure, how much is practical and necessary, and how much is related to making yourself available to others for work purposes. By making this distinction, I don't mean to dismiss the "convenience factor" as a cost; this cost is real and should be accounted for. However, while convenience is often the first cost many parents think of, it's often given more value than it deserves, and it's rarely the most important issue at the end of the day.

EXERCISE *Reset Cost-Benefit Analysis: Specifying Potential Benefits*

Tallying the costs may make you groan, but it's better to go forward with eyes wide open so that you anticipate and plan for difficulties. Facing fears or acknowledging risks has a way of loosening their hold on you.

Next, think about and list all the potential benefits, both short-term and long-term, that the Reset might provide. Again, be as specific as possible. Obviously, you don't know what the benefits will actually be until after you do the Reset, but list those things you feel you can reasonably expect and hope for, based on what you've read in the book so far. Table 3 below lists some potential short-term benefits, along with how these can translate into long-term gains over time.

POTENTIAL SHORT-TERM GAINS	POTENTIAL LONG-TERM GAINS
Improved frontal lobe function • Mood: happier, more even-keeled, less irritable • Cognition: better focus, more organized, improved stress tolerance, more creative • Behavior/Social: less impulsive, more "in tune," more compliant	Improved frontal lobe development • Better mood regulation and stress management • Optimization of academic, career, and/ or creative potential • Deeper thinking • Responsible, empathic • Richer relationships, enhanced self-esteem • Lower risk of drug use and delinquency
Better rested and more physically active	Balanced hormones and immune system Healthy weight and heart
Avoid or minimize medication use	Avoid or minimize long-term medication risks
Save money and resources (spent on tutors, therapists, and so on)	Save money for future
Less household stress, more bonding	Less strain on parents' marriage, stronger sibling ties

Table 3. Potential benefits of Reset and ongoing screen management

Below is an example of an actual cost-benefit analysis that one mother, Shauna, came up with regarding her son, Steven, after we'd discussed screen-time's effects, ESS, and my experience in working with children similar to her son. Hopefully, table 4 helps you see how the general items in table 3 might apply or be expressed in a real situation:

RESET COSTS	POTENTIAL SHORT-TERM GAINS	POTENTIAL LONG-TERM GAINS
Energy to convince others (esp. my husband) Time/energy/money to replace activities It's inconvenient! Dealing with Steven's reaction Losing the breaks it gives me (e.g., to get dinner on the table, quiet time)	Tics might get better More interest in playing outside Better sleep, fewer nightmares More compliant (does what I ask) Easier time getting ready (for bed or school) Happier, less cranky Get more homework done, with less of a headache (me) Could go places without worrying he'll have a meltdown (me) Relief or less stress if behaviors reduce	Better sense of himself and his identity Richer relationships with friends and future girlfriends Help him go further in school and reach his potential More mature and respectful of adults More responsible and more likely to get (and keep) a good job Broader interests Better grades Avoid use of medication Tics could continue to get better, would be less "reinforced" (me) Less stress on my marriage (me) I'd be better able to pursue my own wants/needs/interests

Table 4. Shauna's cost-benefit analysis of the Reset for Steven

The Reset Program is literally an investment in your child's health. All worthwhile goals cost work or energy — there is no such thing as a free lunch. In the end, if the Reset isn't very effective with your child's symptoms, or isn't worth the cost, then you move on and try something else. Yet if the Reset works and you realize many of the most important benefits, then the anticipated costs often pale in comparison. If you're worried that the Reset will be too hard, I strongly encourage you to evaluate very closely the benefits you might be giving up. Particularly if you treat the fast as a three-week "experiment," you limit your costs as you confirm the benefits for your child, making it one of the cheapest investments with one of the longest running potential returns you might ever make.

Convenience and the Electronic Babysitter

While I don't use the term *electronic babysitter* in practice because it carries a negative connotation, it is a term that everyone's heard of and understands. Even in a two-parent household, the pressure to let children use electronics so you can hear yourself think is tremendous. If you admit to using video games or other screen media to have some peace and quiet or to get things done, kudos for being honest.

But when parents feel they *need* electronics for "babysitting," what this often implies is that there is a support issue: there is not enough child-care help, too much day-to-day stress, or not enough peaceful downtime or enjoyable moments during caregiving. If you had more breaks, would you still need to use electronics for respite? If the baseline level of stress in the home was lower and your batteries were recharged, wouldn't that work just as well?

Remember: if the Reset is successful, your child will be more capable of engaging for extended periods in healthier solitary or joint play peacefully. What if you could get the same kinds of breaks each day at home by handing children a book, a crafts project, or a game that they could play on their own? This isn't a fantasy. As I've described, the Reset Program improves frontal lobe functioning, which enhances the ability to self-initiate activities, tolerate frustration, lose oneself in imaginary play, read quietly, daydream, cooperate with siblings, and find wonder in nature. Don't get overwhelmed by imagining a life of parenting without screens. Focus on the fast, and if it works, many of the inconveniences that seem so daunting right now may resolve themselves naturally.

Building a Circle of Support

Implementing an electronic fast requires effort and dedication, and thus the Reset is much more likely to be successful if adequate support exists or is created. Conversely, inadequate support is one of the most common reasons for the Reset to fall apart. Think of your support circle as having two arms — one to support the electronic fast (both in spirit and logistically), and the other to promote your own self-care.

If you're married or living with your partner, an important source of support is your spouse. I discuss getting your spouse on board in chapter 5. Even if one parent remains skeptical or doubtful that the Reset will help your child, having that person's cooperation and help with the fast anyway can make a world of difference. As with any parenting issue, if parents aren't on the same page, children get mixed signals, and they will likely exploit these differences to avoid screen-time restrictions and limits. Conversely, because spouses share a mutual goal of supporting the child's well-being, supporting each other during the Reset can create a bonding experience.

But whether there are one or two dedicated parents on board, there is work to be done: legwork to talk to the relevant people involved, organizing schedules and activities, carving out time to spend with your child, and so on. If you start to do all the extra work without allowing for self-care, you are more likely to throw up your hands and "give in" on the days that you're tired. The need to plan for breaks is particularly important for mothers, who tend to take care of others' needs first and then forget about their own. Remember, this is a recipe for burnout. On the other hand, if you can say to yourself, "Hey, I'm utterly exhausted, but Thursday night is my dinner out with friends," it'll be easier to stick to the program because you know a break is on the horizon. If you're that breed of parent who feels guilty when you do something for yourself — and many parents are — remember that "honoring the self" models good self-care for your child.

EXERCISE   *Identify Gaps in Your Support System*

To build your support circle, think of those closest to you and work your way outward. Make a list of all the people you can think of who already help you, the roles they currently play in your life, and what "extra" things you might need or want to ask of them during the three-week fast.

Then start approaching people and determine their willingness to support you. When you tell each person about the Reset Program and ESS, how do they react? Are they skeptical or open? Aside from your spouse and key indispensable caregivers, don't spend too much energy convincing others. All you need is cooperation with the fast, not agreement that this treatment is worthwhile or effective. Figure out quickly who in this process is crucial to get on board, who supports you and who doesn't, and work from there.

As you do this, continually evaluate: Where is support lacking? Where are there gaps, weak spots, or places where electronics might sneak in during the fast? Is it at school, with certain friends, or at your ex-spouse's house? Where is support strongest, and can these people or situations help make up for areas of weakness?

Keep updating your support list on an ongoing basis during your preparation week, and devise measures to make sure nothing — including your sanity — falls through the cracks. Figure out logistically when and how you'll get breaks. Married spouses should help each other with screen-free activities *and* child care, so that each spouse can take breaks. Allowing each parent one night "off" every week is helpful. If it can be the same night each week, even better, because then you'll know exactly when that next break is coming.

Sam: The Single Mom and the Electronic Babysitter

As I've said, sometimes screen-time becomes a problem precisely because parents lack support and rely on electronics too much. In fact, some parents may need to build more support before they can even contemplate a fast. This was the case with Sam's mother, a single parent who allowed her son to play video games after school each day before starting homework. Sam's teachers were complaining that Sam was disruptive and falling behind in reading and math, and his mother was at her wit's end.

"When he comes home from school, he's a mess," his mother told me. "At first he was getting game time only if he had a decent day at school, but to be honest, I need the break it gives me. So now he pretty much gets it every day. It allows me to get dinner started, and it keeps him quiet. It seems to be something that's working right now."

Sam was then in second grade. I explained to his mother the vicious circle the daily gaming habit was creating: how, after the intense stimulation and excitement of playing, his brain would go through a dopamine "withdrawal," and he would become irritable and have trouble concentrating, then he'd be unable to get his homework done and would have difficulty falling sleep, and the cycle would repeat. I told her, "He won't be able to move forward academically without eliminating the video games."

"Yeah, I see what you're saying," she replied, "but I'm a single parent and sometimes it's all I can do to get through the day. I have no one to help me. And for him, I really think it calms him down, at least while he's playing. And I need the break, too, because I know the rest of the evening is going to be hell trying to get his homework done."

Sam's mother clearly needed more support before she could attempt a fast. She couldn't contemplate how life would be without the break screen-time allowed, so we tried to solve that problem first. Sam loved playing outside, but up until then, his mother had been restricting this because he'd fallen so behind in school. So the first move was to allow Sam to play outside for forty-five minutes to an hour after school each day, no matter what. Next, we worked with the teacher to get rid of all homework until further notice, to allow more "brain rest" time, and to make the evenings less draining for Sam's mother. Once we did this, Sam's mother was ready to try the Reset.

Now, with the dreaded hassle of homework gone, Sam's mother had more energy to plan healthy play activities. She also started teaching Sam how to help out around the house, for example, by having Sam help prepare dinner and set the table. She'd ask him to fold the napkins in different shapes each night, a simple but entertaining and creative task for him. Over the next several weeks, between the extra physical time outdoors, the healing of his brain from the fast, and the bonding time with Mom, Sam's concentration and self-esteem improved — and learning became fun again. Once the Reset was finished, we arranged to have 90 percent of Sam's homework completed at school with an aide, and he continued the outdoor play when he got home along with no gaming during the school week. Sam still had his challenges, but his math and reading scores improved, his behavior became more respectful and helpful, and his mother was able to enjoy spending time with him in the evenings again. It's worth noting that this single mother made all these things happen without extra child care — and without spending an extra dime.

The Permission Phenomenon

The *permission phenomenon* is a dynamic that occurs when someone confirms an internal belief we have that goes against societal norms or beliefs, and the confirmation or validation gives us "permission" to act on that belief. With screen-time, the permission phenomenon arises when someone suspects that there is something inherently wrong with screen-time in general or perhaps with certain screen habits, like daily gaming, nonstop texting, or being obsessed with social media. The person senses that their views are in the minority and thus won't be heard, but upon hearing an explanation regarding the nature of screen-time that resonates with what they silently believe, he or she suddenly feels free to act.

Often, this individual will have a frustrating story to tell when the subject of dysregulation from screen-time comes up: "I can totally see that. My niece is out of control, and I've always wondered if it was because she's on her phone 24/7." Or, "I've been trying to tell my husband that I can tell video games aren't good for our son, but he just tells me that research shows it improves attention." Similarly, when I receive emails from parents who've read an article of mine, they often tell me that other clinicians and professionals have shot down their suspicions that screen-time was having negative effects: "I told my doctor I felt like gaming was affecting my younger son's ADHD, but he said my son's disorder is genetic, and that I shouldn't punish him by taking games away." Or, "I told the teacher that my son needed to be playing outside during recess — and not playing video games — but the teacher insisted that the games are educational."

When you approach others for support with a fast and the permission phenomenon occurs, the person listens intently to what you're proposing (and to the reasons why), and conveys little resistance to doing what it takes to help your child. You'll feel the resonance because you're on the same wavelength; it's as though you're suddenly on the same team. By introducing the rationale behind screen-related symptoms and the fast, you're offering validation regarding something this person has already intuited, plus offering a chance to help a child — yours and perhaps theirs, too — an appealing combination. Even parents of children who use electronics all the time may be more open than you think; sometimes parents simply work a lot and feel helpless (or too busy) to orchestrate healthier activities. Herein lies the "permission" — you're providing information that allows them to act according to what they already believe. It can be highly satisfying to connect with someone in this way, as it is for me when I talk to or hear from parents, grandparents, teachers, and therapists from around the globe who acted on their beliefs after resonating with something I've shared in an article. So be brave, open the door to conversation, and see who might join you.

Parents of Playmates

As you build your support network, you need to take inventory of who your child will be spending time with during the fast — beyond the caregivers who supervise your child on a daily basis. In particular, you should reach out to the parents of your child's friends, tell them what you're doing, and ask if they will abide by the "no-screen" rules when your child is at their house. If any of these parents do not agree, or you aren't quite sure they'll follow through, your child cannot play at their house — it's that simple.

If you're not close to a particular set of parents, you may wish to preserve your own or your child's privacy, and so you may not want to divulge all the issues your child is dealing with or the reasons you're doing the Reset. Even with family, parents sometimes prefer to remain private about a child's behavior issues, sometimes out of embarrassment and sometimes because they don't want to burden others. One vague but still truthful explanation for the Reset is that your child is under "doctor's orders" to have a break from video games to improve his or her sleep. Most people will have heard of the link between sleep and electronics use, and citing a doctor's authority takes the burden off of you. Emphasize the importance of strictness: explain that these are similar precautions to an elimination diet when assessing food sensitivities. The assessment won't be accurate without a complete ban for a prescribed period of time.

That said, as I mention in the sidebar "The Permission Phenomenon" (page 209), you're likely to be surprised by the openness of at least some of these parents. Don't assume that just because another parent seems very permissive or blasé that they don't share your concerns. Busy parents may *want* to be more involved, and permissive parents may *want* to instill healthier habits in their child, especially if they can do it with someone who offers mutual support. If you share information about ESS with these parents, you may get more than a parent willing to enforce the fast whenever your child is over — you may get a partner for the fast itself. Your own involvement might be just the support someone else needs to give it a try, at which point you can coordinate mutual accountability and taking turns orchestrating activities, thus providing one another with precious breaks.

Anna was a single mother of a fifteen-year-old girl, Kayla, whom I was seeing for depression. Kayla was posting sexually provocative pictures on her Instagram account, exhibiting rages, and failing in school. Concerned about the potential repercussions of her actions and the severity of her irritability, I prescribed a strict fast and advised she not be allowed any social media access, even after the fast. Kayla's best friend, Breanna, was a couple of years older and had a single mother as well. Breanna herself used social media obsessively and had unrestricted access to various electronic devices at home. When Anna informed Breanna's mother that Kayla wouldn't be allowed to spend time at Breanna's house for several weeks because of the fast, Breanna's mother unexpectedly expressed that she thought the fast was a great idea. In fact, she placed *her* daughter — who was extremely oppositional — on the fast as well.

This move helped both mothers, in terms of reining in out-of-control behaviors. For Kayla's mother, the additional support from another parent also allowed her to tackle Kayla's other serious issues more effectively, without the added burden of restricting where Kayla spent much of her time.

Friends and Relatives

When building support, don't think only of the people your child will be involved with during the fast. Think of anyone who might assist you with your own self-care. Ask friends to join you for an evening out, or ask a close relative to call you and check in regularly — someone you feel safe venting to and who could hold you accountable.

I like to enlist grandparents for this role because they appreciate getting back to the basics, are often quite reliable, and can be extra motivated to support their own children as well as their grandchildren. But sometimes parents forget to let grandparents know what's going on with the fast. For one thing, it doesn't occur to parents that someone from an older generation might encourage electronics usage and constitute a "crack" in the plan. Grandparents *love* to indulge their grandchildren, and they often marvel at how adept kids are with technology. In addition, usually as part of a larger family dynamic, grandparents sometimes undermine their own children's parenting. More commonly, though, grandparents can be a huge asset in terms of both psychological and logistical support. Just be sure to get them in your corner and be explicit with the rules.

A rather dramatic example of unexpected support involves a family I worked with in which the maternal grandmother, Elaine, was the primary caregiver. According to Elaine, each time Casey, her seven-year-old grandson, would go to his dad's for his twice-monthly visit on the weekends, Casey would sit around playing video games all day, then come home "spun out" on Sunday night and take several days to recover. Casey had ADHD, could only tolerate low doses of medication, and was failing in school. As such, we had a pressing need to do the fast, but we needed Casey's father on board. Unfortunately, Casey's father didn't seem particularly concerned with Casey's welfare in general. For example, though Casey suffered from asthma, his father smoked inside the house during his son's visits, and he even smoked while they were together in the car. So, as we discussed what to do, Elaine and I figured there was *no way* Casey's father would agree to no video games for a month. "The only chance he'll do it is if he hears it from you," Elaine said. After my attempts to reach the father by phone failed, I wrote a doctor's order for Elaine to give to Casey's father.

Shockingly, Casey's father obliged. Neither Elaine nor I could believe it. He began taking Casey fishing — something he'd apparently done with his own father — and Casey started coming back to his grandmother's tired, but happy and relaxed. And because his dad was enjoying himself, too, he kept up their new routine. With the extended gaming sessions out of the way, Casey started to catch up in school. His teacher reported a much improved attitude, and Casey was happy that his dad was spending more time with him.

This was an avenue we could have easily just written off, if we hadn't given Casey's dad the benefit of the doubt — and the payoff was huge.

Parenting Communities

Are you part of an already-established parents' group you could utilize during the Reset? Even if these parents don't join you in the Reset, they may gladly help you accomplish it.

One group of mothers I worked with decided to do the Reset together because they'd done community homeschooling a few years before. These mothers were accustomed to shuffling the kids between various houses on particular days, and their system was very organized. Because each mother only had to have the children once a week (or even less), they were willing to organize healthy screen-free activities as well as whole-food snacks on the days they "hosted." The mothers who couldn't host because of working or other obligations paid in some other way, either by providing food, cash, supplies, or activities on the weekends.

Granted, working with a group like this takes a lot of organization up front, but once it is set up, it gives all the parents a win-win situation — one ripe with breaks, at that. Because of the relative ease with which these moms were able to pull off being screen-free, combined with the benefits they observed, these families ultimately decided to keep their children completely video game–free, and they only allowed small amounts of computer use for school once a week. For more on Reset communities and movements, see chapter 12.

Teachers and Coaches

Teachers rule the roost for a large part of your child's day, and coaches can be extremely influential, especially with boys.

To specifically address eliminating school-related screen-time during the fast, see chapter 5, "Reset Planning and School" (page 158). As I discuss there, in my experience, many teachers are open to screen-time concerns and are willing to help, but some are not. Approach teachers about whatever support you might need, and share information as you see fit. Become informed about school policies regarding phone use, texting, device use during breaks, and ask how they're enforced. Others within the school to consider talking to are the school psychologist, nurse, occupational therapist, resource teachers and special education staff, and the vice principal and principal. Many in these occupations are becoming alarmed at the amount of technology in school and welcome research-based evidence pointing to it being problematic. Indeed, technology in the classroom constitutes its own set of problems, which are discussed in chapter 11; see also "Working with Your Child's School: Effective Attitudes and Approaches" (page 276).

Having coaches on board with the Reset and with screen management in general can be extremely helpful. Coaches are often big believers in natural health, they can be instrumental in motivating a child to keep up his or her grades, and they can serve as role models or mentors to children. Additionally, coaches — like teachers — are often all too aware of the impact of screens on attention span, and some will even recommend to children that they give up gaming to improve grades and to sharpen focus during games. Kids listen to coaches. Recall the story of my nephew in chapter 3 (see page 82). Shy and inattentive when he was younger, my nephew attributes his becoming more confident, interested, and involved in class discussions to an instruction given by his high school football coach to give up gaming. After cutting down and then eventually quitting, my nephew describes how he actually felt a shift in how his brain was working. The change was clearly noticeable to others, too. He went on to be chosen for a leadership workshop in Washington, DC, after several teachers became impressed by his newfound impassioned involvement in class discussions.

Would this young man have blossomed in this way without the intervention of a coach insisting that his players be video game–free? Perhaps. He obviously had other things going for him. But I'd argue that this football coach liberated my nephew's brain — literally — and helped spur his development.

Doctors, Therapists, and Behavior Specialists

Medical and mental health professionals vary considerably in how well they understand screen-time's impact on mental health and in how willing they are to acknowledge a connection. For a Reset, since you won't necessarily need cooperation from every person involved in your child's medical or mental health care, focus your efforts initially on those providers who can either assist you in some concrete kind of way or potentially undermine your plan. Regarding the former, examples include talking to your child's doctor or therapist about providing a letter if you decide you need to eliminate school-based screen-time and working with a treatment team to construct a safety plan if you're concerned about aggression. Regarding the latter, typical scenarios that can undermine the Reset include behavior specialists or therapists using video games or computer time as rewards, speech specialists utilizing iPads for communication applications, and therapists who use video games or software programs to teach social skills. Since a parent isn't always in the same room when a child is receiving a therapy or service, make sure your wishes are known to anyone who sees your child. Ultimately, *you* are in charge of what goes on in your child's life, not anyone else, so you call the shots.

To illustrate how parents can help get practitioners on the same page, as well as how differing opinions from others can mirror conflicting feelings occurring internally, let's return to Michael, a little boy with autism whom I mentioned briefly in chapter 1.

Michael: Conflicting Opinions

When I first met Michael, he was six years old, and he was receiving formalized in-home behavioral services, a type of therapy known as applied behavioral analysis (ABA) that's commonly used to reduce autistic behaviors. Michael's treatment team contacted me for a consult when Michael's compulsive and repetitive behaviors suddenly became worse and seemed immune to ABA treatment. When I learned that Michael had been earning video game play throughout the day as part of his formalized behavioral plan, I immediately suggested that they lose the video games as a reinforcer.

The behavior team initially met this idea with much resistance. They hadn't come to me to adjust the behavioral plan, but to see what medication might help Michael. I was now in an awkward position: I didn't want to undermine the behavior team, but I also wasn't going to consider medication options until Michael had first tried an electronic fast. I discussed my thoughts with the parents and explained how gaming dysregulated the nervous system. I acknowledged that it must be unsettling to hear conflicting advice, but that ultimately, not only could the gaming be directly contributing to Michael's obsessive-compulsive behaviors, but it could also exacerbate the social dysfunction characteristic of autism as well — the very symptoms ABA was intended to reduce. Complicating the issue was the fact that the parents had been pleased that Michael liked video games because it was something a "normal boy his age would do." Indeed, they had hoped it would help him socialize with his peers.

As they considered the Reset, the parents wrestled with painful mixed feelings. They wished for Michael to live like other little boys as much as possible, and they felt guilty about taking something away that he enjoyed, when he had a difficult enough life as it was. As we talked over the next few sessions, other uncomfortable issues came up. What if, by allowing the gaming, they had been inadvertently hurting their child? How could this have occurred with treatment providers who specialized in autism? Who were they to trust? These parents had dedicated their lives to giving their child the best life possible, and these were unpleasant thoughts to ponder.

We talked about how even mental health and behavior experts tend to underestimate the negative effects of video games, and that the ABA *process* was supported by research — not the use of video games as a reinforcer. Video games work well in the short term, but they inevitably will backfire. We also talked about how it doesn't help to dwell on what has already happened; they hadn't done anything differently with Michael than any parent might do. We went back to the basics and revisited their "big picture" goals — for Michael to be as happy, well-adjusted, and as high functioning as possible. When they looked at his life from that angle, trying to be "like other boys" by copying unhealthy habits did not match those priorities. We also discussed how if gaming was indeed contributing to or precipitating symptoms, then stopping gaming would likely reverse this.

Eventually, Michael's parents decided to try the Reset Program. They then took the lead and informed the behavior team that they wanted the team to try finding another reinforcer so we could ascertain whether the video games were contributing to the problem. With the parents now on board, the behavior team agreed, and we put the Reset in motion. Michael's obsessive-compulsive symptoms resolved almost abruptly, and over the next several weeks we started to see social improvements as well. When the team realized they could actually take Michael into crowded public places without him becoming overstimulated, they no longer doubted the capacity of electronics to dysregulate. This allowed the entire treatment team to work together more effectively and productively, and ABA continued to be a big asset for Michael and his family for years to come.

After-School Care Programs

One particular area that can be a liability or an asset is group daycare or after-school program settings. On the one hand, it may be difficult to get cooperation with screen-time rules for your child that might affect other children; for instance, if handheld video games are allowed, then directors or caregivers may not want or be able to monitor whether other kids "share" these devices with your child. On the other hand, this is an arena where the permission phenomenon can come into play, and I've known parents to successfully navigate these waters and garner unexpected support.

One mother discovered that her six-year-old child was playing violent video games and watching scary movies at his after-school program. Her son suffered from nightmares, so she was highly motivated to keep him away from anything too stimulating. Upon discovering what was happening, during her next pickup, the mother looked through the videos and video games, picked up the games and the movies she objected to, and brought them over to the program director. "I know the other kids might be able to tolerate these, but my son can't," she told the director. "If these are lying around loose when my son's here, I can't keep him here. He just can't handle it."

The director surprised the mother by saying, "I'll gladly get rid of those! Sometimes parents 'donate' things and we feel rude if we don't have them out for the kids to use, but really they're inappropriate. I think having video games around when they have all these toys and each other to play with is just dumb. I'll lock up the video games, and tell the other staff that they're off-limits from now on."

It's also possible that program staff won't want to lose your business, so they may be motivated to work with you. Of course, things don't always go as smoothly as they did for the mother above, but you won't know unless you ask!

Chapter 8 Take-Home Points

- When it comes to ESS and the Reset, nearly every parent will face some degree of doubt and uncertainty, both from within and from others, but these barriers are surmountable.
- When considering the Reset, performing a cost-benefit analysis can help parents weigh the costs against the short- and long-term benefits of improved brain health.
- Reliance on electronics as a "babysitter" in general is common, but overreliance suggests that parental support may need to be strengthened *prior* to initiating the Reset.
- Building support for the Reset takes time and effort, but it prevents burnout, improves ease and feasibility, and maximizes Reset effectiveness.
- Reset support can be built by educating others and creating win-win situations.
- Communicating your needs to others facilitates compliance with the fast and may lead to unexpected sources of support.
- A determined parent is a force to be reckoned with, and it's not always the parents with the most resources or perceived support that succeed — it's the ones with the most conviction, determination, and commitment.
- Review how much school-related screen-time your child is experiencing, and consider whether to ask for help from teachers or the school to limit this.

CHAPTER 9

ELIMINATION VS. MODERATION

A Game Plan Going Forward

When the sword is once drawn,
the passions of men observe no bounds of moderation.

— Alexander Hamilton

Let's say you've completed the Reset. *Now what?*

Before and even during the Reset, I always ask parents to focus on what needs to be done *now* — not on the future and what will happen afterward. I say this for several reasons: 1) the possibility that parents may need to eliminate or strictly reduce screen-time indefinitely may be overwhelming to consider; 2) parents need to *experience* the benefits — not just hear about or imagine them — before evaluating what they'll do next; and 3) parents are typically stressed prior to the Reset, and stressed people tend to be shortsighted in general. I want parents to be in a state of calmness and clarity — a state they'll be in *after* the Reset — so they consider the big picture in a careful way.

This chapter guides you in the decision-making process that follows a Reset, and it guides you in how to monitor and manage screen-time into the future. The truth is, parents will need to evaluate and adjust screen-time continually from here on; they will need to be both mindful of risks and flexible as circumstances change. As children grow older, as their brains develop, as life happens, and as unforeseen events occur, their needs and vulnerabilities will change, and so will their relationship with screens. You may need to repeat the Reset multiple times over the years, and each fast may result in new rules or realizations for how screen-time can be best managed going forward.

Immediately following a Reset, you have three choices: you can either extend the fast, decide to eliminate interactive screen-time indefinitely, or try reintroducing limited amounts. In the short term, you want to be cautious and conservative and proceed gradually. Over the long term, moderation needs may ebb and flow, and you'll need to continually assess whether to continue the status quo, relax or tighten restrictions, or regroup by embarking on another fast.

To Err Is Human: The Learning Curve of Healthy Screen Management

Even with the best of intentions, even in the most disciplined of families, human nature dictates that mistakes will be made — often repeatedly. Both immediately after the initial fast and over time, parents tend to allow too much too soon, and symptoms return. Your best defense against this is simply to be aware of this tendency, and to document what's happening, so you can look back and remember what life was like before and after a screen fast and to make appropriate adjustments from there.

What typically happens is that the Reset results in noticeable improvements, and parents experience relief and derive pleasure from seeing their child happy and blossoming. As they are lulled into a sense of complacency, however, wishful thinking begins: *Maybe my son can tolerate a little bit of gaming now. It breaks my heart when he asks to play, and he's the only one of his friends who doesn't.* Alternatively, doubt starts to creep in, as parents question whether "no screens" was really the reason for the improvements: *Maybe it wasn't the computer after all; maybe she's just maturing.* Whatever the reason, the tendency at this point is to relax the rules and allow some screen-time again. This often results in a sudden or more gradual return of the problematic behaviors and a realization that, from now on, screen-time needs to be restricted a lot more than anticipated. This is normal. Indeed, most families wind up experiencing a "learning curve" as they figure out how much screen-time their child can tolerate. Expect to hit a few speed bumps on the road to creating a "new normal" for screen-time in your family.

Jason: Good Intentions and Unintended Consequences

Jason's story provides an example of how things typically go in the months and years following an initial Reset, and it illustrates the need for ongoing vigilance. Jason was fourteen the first time his family agreed to do the Reset. Jason had ADD and tics, and he played video games for an hour or so a day. Jason was getting Bs and Cs in school, but he was quite bright, and really should have been an A/B student. With the first Reset, as expected, Jason's grades went up and his tics went down. Because he felt so much relief from his tics subsiding, Jason was on board with giving up video games altogether on a more permanent basis.

However, throughout the rest of Jason's adolescence, video games tended to sneak their way back into his life, and his tics would worsen or his grades would fall. More than once, I'd think he needed a medication adjustment, only to find out he was gaming again. In the midst of these exacerbations, his mother would sometimes admit that she had let Jason start playing again because he'd been so well-behaved and had been working so hard; understandably, she'd want to give him a treat and "let him be like the other boys." Ultimately, the family did three or four strict fasts by the time Jason graduated high school, with great results each time. By his senior year, Jason had become increasingly proactive about not gaming; he'd rally his friends to go outside and do something active instead, and he would even come home if they insisted on gaming anyway. Eventually his friends respected his choices more consistently, and Jason received nearly straight As that year.

After graduating high school, Jason began attending a four-year college as a biology major while continuing to live at home to save money. Jason did well his first semester, but that Christmas, he was given an iPad by his aunt. Jason's mom knew the iPad might pose a risk, but she felt it would be rude to return it, since it was a gift. "Besides," she thought to herself, "he's been doing so well, and he can use it for school."

Needless to say, things quickly went south. Jason started gaming again, just a little at first, then nightly online with his friends. He also was on

Facebook a lot more, so his total screen-time went up by several hours each day. By March, he was getting two Ds and an F in his classes, and his tics were so severe he could barely sleep. When his mom suggested they get rid of the iPad, Jason insisted he could handle owning it and promised to stop gaming. But a month later, exhausted and admitting he was out of control, Jason asked his dad to take the iPad to work with him. Jason began using a desktop in the family room for his schoolwork, and he was able to pull his grades up by semester's end. Meanwhile, he started working part-time in a job that required him to get up early, forcing him to go to bed early as well. By summer, his tics had lessened considerably, and he was sleeping much more restfully.

It's easy to see how this sequence of events happens. Despite seeing dramatic results from fasts over the years and being relatively mindful about screen-time, Jason and his parents could still become complacent and allow gaming and light-at-night to creep back in. Parents tend to forget how bad things were and how big a difference restricting screens can make. This is why tracking and journaling are so useful during the Reset. Parents always hope that children will outgrow or overcome their reactions to screen-time, or that they will learn to control compulsive use. Certainly, to one degree or another, both use patterns and sensitivity to screens can improve with age, but parents can't assume it will happen, nor rush how long it will take. In fact, the best way to maximize the odds of this happening as the child grows older is to protect the frontal lobe by limiting screens as much as you can for as long as you can. And remember, no one is ever inoculated against dysregulation — not even adults.

Elimination vs. Moderation: Decisions, Decisions

As I said, this chapter is devoted to helping you decide what to do after a Reset and to helping you manage screen-time over the long haul. First, I will describe the decision-making process itself, then some general rules of thumb, and then list specific risk factors to consider should you choose to reintroduce screens. Finally, I offer a guide for reintroducing screen-time, and I give an overview of the bigger issues that arise in regard to screen management as your child lives life and grows up.

The Post-Reset Decision Tree

To begin, ask yourself, how effective or helpful was the Reset? If you feel the Reset wasn't successful and your child is still dysregulated, then turn to chapter 7 and try to troubleshoot what might have gone wrong with the electronic fast. If you find that something undermined the fast, then fix the issue and continue fasting or try the fast again.

As a result of this process, if you've effectively eliminated electronics as the prime suspect in your child's dysregulation, the identity of other issues may now be clearer. However, if you do identify a new or stronger source — whether it be biological, psychological, or social — that better explains your child's dysregulation, I still recommend continuing to eliminate or strictly limit interactive screen-time while you get a handle on those issues, as this will render whatever else is going on more amenable to treatment.

Regardless, if you've seen some benefits from the fast, the next decision is whether to keep the restrictions in place, thereby maintaining and even building the benefits, or to allow modest amounts of screen-time to see if your child can maintain the benefits. If you decide to reintroduce screen-time, proceed very cautiously, using the guidelines in "Start Low and Go Slow" (page 231). If problems promptly return, you may need to fast again for a period of several months before attempting a reintroduction trial again. Conversely, if you reintroduce and problems don't return, then maintain the new screen allowances for *three months* while monitoring problem areas before adjusting screen-time any further.

Remember, even if your child can tolerate a moderate amount of screen-time after the Reset, that may change over time; new devices can upset the balance, and it's always possible for the effects to "build up" and become intolerable — which means another fast is in order. No matter what course you follow, keep documenting your child's behavior and progress in your Reset journal, noting what you're doing with screen-time and what effects this is having.

For an example of what the post-Reset decision-making tree looks like, see figure 8 (in the figure, IST stands for "interactive screen-time").

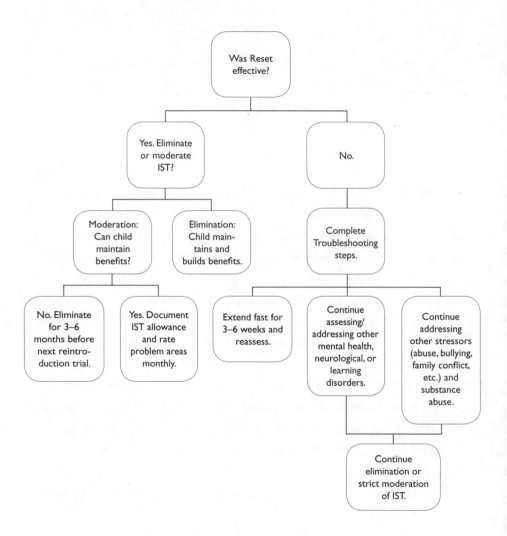

Figure 8. After the Reset: Eliminate or moderate?

Rules of Thumb for Healthy Screen-Time Management

Whatever you decide to do — and whether you and your child are fresh off the fast or it's months or even years later — here are a few rules of thumb to keep in mind as you evaluate your situation. There are many things to consider to determine what's best for your child; every situation and person is different. Use these guidelines in conjunction with the "house rules" outlined in chapter 10, which specify the everyday screen-time management rules I recommend, whether you're continuing the fast, eliminating screens long term, or allowing moderate use. These rules of thumb also function as guidelines for recognizing whenever your child or your family has "fallen off the wagon" when it comes to regulating screen-time. This happens to everyone occasionally — and when it does, all you do is dust yourself off, adjust, and move forward.

- The more symptoms your child has, the stricter you need to be.
- The more severe any given symptom is, the stricter you need to be.
- The more risk factors your child has, the stricter you need to be (see below).
- The younger your child is, the stricter you need to be.
- When "things aren't working" (your child struggles with learning, relationships, meltdowns, and so on), screen-time should be reduced or eliminated.
- You'll never go wrong with "too little" screen-time; when in doubt, pull back.
- A resurgence of symptoms or a regression in functioning often suggests that screens have "sneaked back in." Whenever you see signs of Electronic Screen Syndrome (dysregulation and hyperarousal), reduce or eliminate screen-time or do another fast.
- If dysregulation returns, before making other treatment decisions — especially medication-related or expensive ones — try another fast first.
- If your child suffers a return of insomnia or non-restorative sleep, repeat the fast and consider elimination.
- Don't compare your child's screen-time allowance to that of other children — most children use screens much more than is recommended.
- Media multitasking worsens attention, efficiency, and accuracy — even if total screen-time is low.
- Following the "house rules" described in chapter 10 will make following all the other rules easier.

Elimination vs. Moderation:
Factors and Consequences to Consider

When deciding whether or not to continue eliminating screen-time following the Reset, the most important consideration is appreciating possible serious long-term repercussions of continued exposure that are specific to certain preexisting conditions. It's also good to take into account how many underlying risk factors for developing Electronic Screen Syndrome your child has; the more risk factors there are, the more likely it is that your child may not be able to tolerate much interactive screen-time at all. In addition to these considerations, other factors to consider are how severe your child's symptoms are in general (both before and after fasting) and whether there are any safety concerns. Not surprisingly, the more difficulties a child experiences (in terms of feeling and functioning), then the more time it may take for that child's brain to heal by living screen-free. At the same time, safety risks should be taken into consideration, too; for example, if there are younger siblings who are at risk of harm if your child becomes explosive, then you may need to be extra conservative in how you proceed.

What follows, then, are two lists I've created to help you consider 1) possible future consequences of screen-time based on particular conditions and 2) how likely it is for ESS to recur — in other words, for your child to become dysregulated again — once screens are reintroduced. The first list describes "risks" you might be creating now or in the future by reintroducing screen-time, and the second list outlines "risk factors" that may already exist.

Conditions with Potentially Life-Altering Consequences from Ongoing Screen-Time

Some conditions have more severe, life-altering, and broad-reaching consequences from ongoing screen-time exposure than others. If your child has any of the conditions listed below, I *strongly recommend* permanently eliminating interactive screen-time altogether. The impact of screen-time on these conditions has already been discussed in chapter 3, but here I've highlighted the most serious long-term risks.

Although it may be overwhelming to consider a long-term ban on electronics, the way to view this news is to realize that by controlling your child's environment, you have control over your child's prognosis. Review chapter 4 to remind yourself how the brain benefits from being screen-free, and keep focusing on what you need to do to be as screen-free as possible *right now*. Living screen-free only gets easier the longer you do it. (Note: in this list, "screentime" primarily refers to *interactive* screen-time unless otherwise specified.)

Psychosis: Screen-time can trigger an existing genetic predisposition for a psychotic disorder (schizophrenia, schizoaffective disorder, or bipolar disorder with psychosis); it makes treatment more difficult; and it worsens long-term prognosis.

Autism spectrum disorders: Screen-time reinforces brain pathways and tendencies specific to autism; it increases risk of regression; it limits or hinders development of language and social skills; it suppresses right brain and frontal lobe development; and it may therefore limit job, relationship, and independence potential as an adult.

Intellectual disability: Screen-time may limit the potential for reading, writing, and math skills; it may stunt social-emotional maturity; and it may severely worsen the impact and prognosis of mental illness in a population that is more vulnerable to mental illness in general.

Internet or technology addiction: Continued screen-time exposure makes the addiction increasingly harder to treat or reverse; it increases risk of brain damage in white and gray matter that may be irreversible; it increases risk for other addictions; and it increases the risk for violence, delinquency, and other mental illness.

Reactive attachment disorder: Screen-time compounds hyperarousal; it slows down treatment or renders it ineffective; it creates a "hair trigger" response to stress; it limits the capacity for intimacy, empathy, trust, and compassion; and it effectively magnifies stress load on the adoptive family.

Alcohol or substance abuse: Screen-time further dysregulates the brain and worsens mental illness in those with other addictions; it synergizes addiction pathways; and it can compound brain damage.

Serious academic failure: Screen-time undermines academic progress, and academic failure can create a "downward spiral" that precipitates other social and emotional risks.

Antisocial behavior and conduct: Violent gaming further desensitizes the brain to violence; gaming and Internet use hinders development of empathy and compassion; and screen-time worsens impulse control.

Social incompetence: Screen-time worsens social anxiety and feelings of isolation, which leads to social avoidance and "escape" into cyber activities, creating a vicious cycle that self-perpetuates.

Explosive aggression: Screen-time aggravates aggressive tendencies, leading to risk of serious harm to self or others, and it adds to the dynamic of parents being paralyzed by fear.

Severe ADHD: Screen-time hinders both impulse control and attention, leading to dangerous behaviors (such as running into traffic or being a "daredevil"); it can render medications and other interventions useless; and it contributes to poor self-esteem due to academic and social failure.

Severe sensory dysfunction: Screen-time further hinders nervous system integration, which can lead to long-term emotional, cognitive, and physical deficits; it makes sensory integration therapy much more difficult.

Depression with suicidality: Screen-time worsens depression; screen-time and light-at-night heighten risk for suicidal thinking and behavior; and it increases risk for completed suicide.

Serious medical conditions: Both passive and interactive screen-time affect metabolism and may worsen diabetes, obesity, heart disease, and metabolic syndrome; interactive screen-time may worsen autoimmune illness via stress reactions; and radiation from EMFs may potentiate risk for certain cancers and other illnesses.

Risk Factors for Developing ESS

The following risk factors for developing ESS have already been discussed in part 1. These are factors that may have contributed to the development of ESS in the first place, and as such they also play a role in to how likely it is that your child will become dysregulated again should you choose to reintroduce. I've listed them so you can literally count the number of risk factors your child has; the more risk factors a child carries, the more prone the brain is to dysregulation. Consideration of risk factors is not an exact science, but in general, if your child has three or more of these, be extra conservative in your approach, and realize there is a chance your child might not be able to tolerate interactive screen-time without becoming dysregulated — at least for the time being.

Male gender: Boys' brains are more vulnerable in general* for many pediatric disorders — like ADHD, autism, tics, dyslexia and other learning disorders, and sensori-motor difficulties; boys are more likely to become addicted to screen-time; and boys are more likely to become dysregulated from smaller amounts of screen-time.

Younger age: Younger brains are still actively growing and developing, so they are more prone to dysregulation; infants and toddlers are most vulnerable of all, but consider age to be a separate risk factor if your child is twelve or younger.

Any psychiatric disorder: This includes mood, attention, behavior, anxiety, and addiction disorders.

Any neurological disorder: This includes tics, seizures, migraines, and genetic syndromes.

Any developmental disorder: This includes autism and intellectual disabilities.

Chronic medical conditions: This includes obesity, abnormal cholesterol levels, metabolic syndrome, diabetes, high blood pressure, musculoskeletal problems, pain conditions, allergies, and food sensitivities.

Any learning disorder: This includes reading, math, and writing disabilities.

Any sensori-motor disorder: This includes sensory processing disorder and fine or gross motor issues ("clumsiness").

Attention deficit issues: This includes attention difficulties for any reason, even if the child doesn't meet the full criteria for ADD/ADHD.

Performing academically below potential: This includes academic underperformance compared to peers and/or below the potential for that individual child.

Poor social skills: This includes social difficulties related to any condition, whether related to autism, shyness, a difficult disposition, sensory issues, and so on.

Family history of addiction or major psychiatric illness: A family history of schizophrenia, bipolar disorder, suicide or severe depression, alcoholism, or drug abuse indicates your child may have a more vulnerable brain in general.

---

* Having the extra X chromosome is thought to be protective for girls.

Pregnancy or birth trauma: This includes prenatal, perinatal, or postnatal injuries or "insults," including infections or other complications in utero, difficult labor or delivery, febrile seizures, and so on; these events predispose the nervous system to being more fragile, even if the child is considered to have fully recovered.

"But It's Their Culture..."

When discussing the possibility of eliminating screen-time, or even just video games, parents often protest that "*all* my child's friends do it. It's their culture." Parents fear that if their child stops playing or participating, they will be left out, won't have anything to talk about or do with friends, or worse, will be ostracized and left with no friends at all. However, I've worked with a wide range of children — some who were former gamers and some who never played much at all — and I've never seen a child's social life suffer from restricting screen-time. If anything, the opposite happens.

When children stop playing video games, they become more comfortable in their own skin and more comfortable relating to others. They have better access to emotions, become better at expressing those emotions appropriately, and develop a wider variety of interests. These skills help them develop richer and closer relationships with friends and later with romantic interests. If you worry your child won't have anything to talk about with his or her friends, don't fret — they'll be able to have longer and deeper conversations about other things instead. Your child will also naturally gravitate toward other children who don't game a lot — which is what you want! Teens who've given up gaming often end up prompting their friends to go outside instead — and eventually stop hanging out with the ones who won't.

I'm sure every parent reading this book has a child with a friend (or two) who plays video games nonstop, is pale and overweight, or skinny but out of shape, and who always seems distracted and disconnected — and would prefer their child didn't hang out with that friend. Ultimately, in the same way that removing video games allows space for creativity to blossom, weeding out friends who game all the time creates space for healthier children. Trust me. I've never seen a child who stops playing video games suddenly become friendless. Rather, they start to prefer the kids who make the best sorts of friends to begin with.

Reintroduction Trials: Guidelines for Mindful Moderation

If it were up to me, I'd love it if no interactive screen devices were introduced at all to children until age twelve, and after that only sparingly for computer skills. Further, I'd recommend that children who were having any problems in school or at home related to mood, cognition, or behavior issues have zero interactive screen-time, along with very limited television. That would optimize treatment — and make my job a lot easier!

But short of that pipe dream, my hope is to help parents who decide to reintroduce screens to do it in a careful and thoughtful way with built-in damage control. I'm aware that many parents — if not most — will hope that once the Reset is done, they'll be able to restore some level of interactive screen-time in their home. If you decide to reintroduce screens, keep the rules of thumb detailed above in mind and review the guidelines below for the best way to go about it. Be sure to implement all the house rules outlined in chapter 10 as well. Above all, consider any reintroduction as a test or trial: pay just as close attention to your child as during the Reset, and be ready to pull back if problematic behaviors or symptoms return.

Start Low and Go Slow

During my child psychiatry training, "start slow and go slow" was an oft-used expression that reminded us that children are more sensitive to medication than adults, and not just because of their smaller size; their brains are different in structure, function, and organization, and are continually being remodeled. The same strategy goes for screen-time management: once you quiet things down with the Reset, the last thing you want to do is create another storm by moving too quickly. Start low, and go slow.

To begin reintroducing screens, I recommend starting on weekends only after all homework and chores are done. Start with just *fifteen minutes once a week*, either on Saturday or Sunday (but not both). Set this period during the day, not at night, to minimize the melatonin suppression effect. Further, I recommend maintaining this limit for *at least three months* before considering further increases. Then, if you want to try allowing a little more, an appropriate increase might be thirty minutes total over the weekend, either all on one day or split into two fifteen-minute periods on both Saturday and Sunday. Take baby steps; it's easier to reverse a little bit of dysregulation than a lot.

In general, reintroduction trials are much more likely to be successful if they're contained to weekends only. Once you start adding back interactive screen-time on weekdays, you're asking for trouble. In contrast, by removing any possibility of interactive screen-time as entertainment during the school week, you'll effectively eliminate the lion's share of arguments and endless negotiations, plus you'll avoid setting your child up to rush sloppily through homework in order to get device time. As much as that, though, after a long day at school, *children need to move* and interact physically with their environment. Children sit so much now in school and have so much homework these days that it makes it even more critical for them to discharge pent-up energy and stretch the brain by interacting in the real, three-dimensional world as much as possible during the week.

Understand Dose and "Tipping Point"

Stress is a funny thing. Small amounts of stress can be stimulating and help performance due to increased arousal, which is why some children are okay with a little gaming. However, when the brain's capacity for dealing with stress is reached, it creates a cascade of negative effects, many of which I've described in this book. So I find that a useful analogy is to think of screen-time in terms of "doses," which isn't unreasonable considering all the physiological changes that occur with it. Your goal is to determine the "dose" your child can tolerate, both in a single sitting and over a given time period. If the dose is too high, stress builds, and sooner or later a "tipping point" will be reached, resulting in dysregulation. The tipping point where this shift happens will be different for every child, but by nature it will occur sooner for children whose nervous systems are already stressed for other reasons. This also explains why your child may be able to tolerate some screen-time better following a fast, but as the dose builds up over the next weeks or months, he or she may start to show signs of ESS again. Thus, even though how much screen-time you're allowing may not have changed, the dosage or exposure accumulates nonetheless, and another fast may be required for the system to reregulate.

A clear example of how dose and tipping point work is illustrated by Jack, a boy who developed OCD from playing the Wii (for his story, see chapter 3, "Obsessive-Compulsive Disorder (OCD)," page 91). Jack's mother initially did a one-month fast, then reintroduced games by letting her son play once a week (dose). When Jack's symptoms returned (tipping point), his mother ceased all gaming for an additional three months, then allowed him to play once a month for thirty minutes (adjusted dose, based on tolerability). That's it. Any more than that, and Jack would reach his tipping point and develop symptoms again.

However, compare Jack to Jason, whose story I tell at the start of this chapter. Jason had four risk factors — he was male, had ADD, had tics, and was underperforming academically — and he couldn't tolerate any gaming at all. Jack, on the other hand, only had one risk factor, being male (since his OCD developed only as a result of his gaming and quickly resolved, I won't count it), and he was performing well academically. Jack could tolerate small doses of gaming once a week because his brain was relatively less vulnerable. Jason, even though he was quite a bit older, would reach that tipping point much more quickly.

Treat Screens as a Privilege — Not a Right

Enacting a policy that screen-time can only be earned when homework and chores are completed *first* will yield two important benefits. One, the policy helps prevent children from becoming entitled; unhealthy entitlement is a recognized phenomenon with the current generation and it makes parenting that much harder. And two, the policy provides built-in protection for dosing screen-time appropriately, since a dysregulated child will have a difficult time getting homework or chores done in the first place — and thus he or she will be hard pressed to earn any screen-time. As such, the rule creates a "self-adjusting" environment. If up to now you haven't been assigning chores or monitoring whether homework is completed *and* turned in, this makes a good opportunity to do so. In terms of logistics, if you're not able to track homework assignment completion in real time, ask the teacher or a counselor to email you if assignments are missing, or have your child ask the teacher to sign them off. (If your child forgets to have them signed off, then screen-time wasn't earned — also self-adjusting.) Parents often complain that they don't know about missed assignments until a couple of weeks later; if you let the teacher know what you're doing and why, they may be more likely to help you stay abreast of homework status. If your child is consistently behind in homework, this is an indication that overall screen-time needs to be reduced further and kept that way.

Regarding chores, sometimes parents won't assign chores because they're concerned the child has so much homework that they don't have any time for chores, or because they want the child to focus all their energy on schoolwork. I recommend children have *some* chores, even if they're easy and don't take up much time, like making their bed daily and setting the table on the weekends. Aside from contributing to the family, chores force children to interact with the physical environment and teach attention to detail — things that kids these days need more of. Studies show that children who have chores do better in school and engage in less screen-time.[1]

Institute a Screen "Allowance"

A great strategy for restricting screen-time — while minimizing conflict at the same time — is to treat screen-time as an earned "allowance." Screen-time intervention studies show some objective support for this approach, and it's popular among parents. For instance, say you've agreed to allow a maximum of two hours per week of video games. By completing homework and chores, your child could earn thirty-minute "tokens," which can be "cashed in" for screen-time. Have the child "check out" the screen device, then set a timer for the appropriate amount of time. Many parents include television as part of earned screen-time, which works well and makes for fewer arguments and negotiations.

Parents' opinions vary widely on which methods work best. In fact, the best approach is to treat any given screen allowance as a test to see if it works and to determine how best to structure it. Let your kids know that the system might change depending on how things go — and that you and your spouse will be the judge of what's working, not them!

Types of Screen Allowance

1. Weeknights: No interactive screen-time, thirty minutes of TV per day after homework. Weekends: thirty minutes per day of passive or interactive screen-time after homework and chores completed.
2. If homework and chores are done, five hours per week of passive screen-time; no interactive screen-time except on special occasions (such as attending a birthday party).
3. No screen-time on weeknights; one hour of passive or interactive screen-time per weekend day.
4. If all homework and chores are completed, extra chores earn thirty-minute "tickets" for screen-time on weekends (passive or interactive), but only two hours total allowed per week.

The Reset aside, research shows that actively monitoring and restricting screen-time is associated with less total screen-time, more reading, more socially cooperative behavior, reduced aggression, improved sleep, and better grades.[2]

Track, Track, Track

To better support mindful monitoring, it's helpful to track whatever screen-time parameters you plan to work with. Get out your trusty Reset journal, and before you reintroduce any electronics, write down the date you plan to start your new trial. I recommend tracking the same three problem areas that you tracked during the fast, since post-Reset scores can serve as a benchmark. Rate them again once a month thereafter, and journal about your subjective impressions as well. Keep in mind problem severity might slowly increase as screen dosage builds and cumulative effects become more visible. If and when you reach a tipping point, pull back the amount you're allowing and double check there are no additional devices or opportunities sneaking in that could affect how you'll adjust going forward. Put a monthly reminder in your phone or on a wall calendar. Also, consider making tracking part of your ongoing Accountability Act with your child — that is, tell your child you'll owe "x" if you forget to document. That way, *your child* will help you remember to track.

On a monthly or periodic basis, review the tracking results with your spouse and with your child and consider together whether any adjustments will be made based on behavior, grades, chore completion, respecting adults, and so on. Be aware, though, that children may see these discussions as an opportunity to try to wear you down, so be sure to set limits regarding arguing or yelling at the outset. Including children in the discussion helps them understand the reasons for the rules, which makes it less likely they'll rebel against them. The meeting can also provide a safe place for your child to voice whatever may bother them about your electronics use, too.

To summarize, you'll want to track or document 1) how much screen-time is occurring per week and how it's doled out (passive, interactive, weekday, weekend); 2) the date a change started; 3) problem areas with monthly ratings; and 4) each time you change the parameters and why you did so.

Take Action Quickly If Behavior Slips

The moment you see that things are starting to slip, either pull back on screen-time or jump right into another three-week fast. Don't wait for things to become worse. If you act quickly, moderating alone may be enough to stop a backward slide. However, if things are snowballing or have returned to pre-Reset levels, don't bother trying to moderate. Be aggressive and go straight to another fast, since delays from attempting to moderate can compound damage to grades, friendships, and so on.

Don't Tolerate Lying or Defying

Since lying about and sneaking device use and being defiant with screen rules are signs of screen addiction, treat this behavior seriously. If the incident seems to be a one-time offense, you might try holding all screen-time for a week or two. But if the violations are flagrant and ongoing, this is a sign that you need to eliminate interactive screen-time altogether for a period of three to six months to interrupt and quiet those addiction reward pathways. After that, reassess or simply continue with elimination indefinitely.

EXERCISE *Cost-Benefit Analysis: Elimination vs. Moderation*

Before you decide for certain whether you want to extend the electronic fast, eliminate screens altogether indefinitely, or try reintroducing them cautiously, do another cost-benefit analysis like the one in chapter 8 (page 201). Include both immediate and long-term consequences of whichever course of action you're considering, especially if your child has one of the preexisting conditions or multiple risk factors listed above. Whenever you're considering a new course of action, you can refer back to this analysis to assist the decision-making process. If you want to reintroduce screen-time after a fast, take time to consider what you will gain and what you will risk by doing this. What seems convenient on a day-to-day basis might not seem so convenient if all hell breaks loose. Ask yourself: Is it worth it? In this case, you actually want to create two cost-benefit analyses: one looks at the costs and benefits of continuing complete screen-time restrictions, and the other examines the costs and benefits of reintroducing limited screen-time.

Even if you're certain you want to try reintroducing screens, one advantage of doing this exercise is that it forces you to consider exactly what's important to you. As you do, it may be that you realize there are alternatives that satisfy those needs that don't involve screen-time, and thus don't risk retriggering problematic behaviors. In other words, a cost-benefit analysis helps you define just how much risk you are willing to take and why.

Looking Ahead: Mindful Moderation Over Time

If all goes well, within three to six months after a Reset, you will have established a "new normal" regarding screen-time in your household. Congratulations! This is a major accomplishment, and both you and your child may be amazed at how different and better life is now that screen-time has been brought under control.

But alas, whatever that new normal is, it may need to reinvent itself. Life is dynamic and ever-changing, and so parents must be both vigilant and adaptable. Old problems may recur, and new problems may arise, particularly in relation to the following issues.

Your Child's Evolving Development

As your child's brain matures, he or she may be able to tolerate increasing (if still modest) amounts of screen-time without suffering side effects or full-blown ESS. In the case of Jack, after the Reset he at first could tolerate game play only about once a month without his OCD returning. About three years later, however, his "tolerated dose" became one day a week. Generally speaking, the younger the brain, the more sensitive it is, and the more vulnerable it will be to permanent change in potential or even damage.

That said, brain development in puberty deserves its own consideration. During puberty the frontal lobe begins to undergo rapid development, and brain cells and networks are "pruned" or weeded out depending on the experiences, lifestyle, and habits of the child. Hence, puberty may be an especially important time to keep screen stimulation at a minimum, since "what gets fired in the brain gets wired in the brain." This doesn't mean, however, that once your child reaches adolescence, you'll be able to suddenly allow unlimited screen-time; although a major portion of frontal lobe development occurs during puberty, active development of this area continues until the mid-twenties and beyond. Nevertheless, particularly if screen-time is kept limited, the further into adolescence or young adulthood your child grows, and the more integrated his or her frontal lobe becomes, the more tolerant your child will become. Just keep in mind that it's frontal lobe function — the very function that screen-time suppresses — that determines both sensitivity to screens and how disciplined one is when using them.

Lastly, it's worth mentioning that the American Academy of Pediatrics recommends limiting screen-time to one to two hours daily.[3] However, these guidelines don't distinguish between passive and interactive screen-time, and they apply to an ideal, "symptom-free" child, one who is well-rested, performing up to his or her academic potential, physically and creatively active, and enjoying healthy relationships with peers. Otherwise, be much more conservative, since this guideline is *way* too high for a dysregulated child.

Major Changes and Stressful Situations

Major life transitions or events — even positive ones like vacations or performing in a play — as well as typically stressful situations like studying for finals, working on a big project, or starting junior high can sometimes create enough stress that even small amounts of screen exposure become intolerable. In other words, the tipping point into dysregulation is reached not because of the amount of screen-time but because the nervous system is temporarily more vulnerable. Be aware of how the events in your child's life may be causing stressors that make current screen-time allowances unhealthy.

Consider pulling back during these periods (perhaps allowing only a little passive TV), until the event is over. In the meantime, emphasize other strategies to relieve stress: healthy snack breaks, green-time, shooting some hoops, leisure reading, playing cards, calling friends, and so on. For stressful homework assignments, remember that allowing even small amounts of interactive screen-time as a respite prior to tackling it will immediately worsen attention and organizational skills, so provide downtime with something more natural instead.

Naturally, negative or traumatic events produce stress and thus dysregulation, but they can also spark problematic screen-time use. This is in part because parents and caregivers tend to ease up on all rules during difficult periods — such as during a move, when parents divorce, when a loved one dies, and so on — and in part because the child may want to use screens more often as a means to escape. Out of sympathy, you may find yourself wanting to indulge your child during tough times, but remember that the stress response induced by screen-time will likely only add fuel to the fire. Instead, consider further reducing screen-time and spending more one-on-one time with your child, since bonding calms the nervous system — for both your child *and* you — and lets your child know you're there for him or her.

As an example, Carlie was a nine-year-old girl with ADHD who had been dysregulated until she completed a fast; she subsequently remained stable with twenty minutes of computer time a day. This screen-time dose was non-problematic for many months, as long as she didn't go longer than that. But after her favorite grandmother passed away, Carlie's emotional state was understandably more fragile, and any computer time at all would precipitate hours-long crying spells. Carlie's mom cut out all computer time for several months to allow the grieving process to proceed without screen-time complicating matters. Eventually, Carlie was able to tolerate her previous allotted screen allowance again without it affecting her mood.

Environmental Variables

If all stress boils down to oxidative stress at the cellular level, then combating stress with other healthy lifestyle choices may afford some protection in regard to screen-time tolerability for some children. However, among my patients, even when they start eating right, exercising regularly, and living in a relatively toxin-free environment,* they often still suffer from ESS from small amounts of screen exposure, especially if they suffer from an underlying psychiatric disorder.

On the other hand, if a child goes through a spell of not sleeping well, or isn't eating as well because of a change in environment, the sensitivity to screen-time can become much more pronounced. If you see that your child has become dysregulated again with a previously tolerated screen-time dose, try to ascertain if any environmental variables have changed, and adjust screen-time accordingly.

School-Related Screen Exposure

Generally speaking, children receive more screen exposure as they advance through school as homework and such becomes more Internet-dependent. In addition, schools vary markedly in terms of how much tech-based learning they implement. If your school district introduces a new computer-based learning program — such as one-to-one laptop or iPad programs in which each student is given his or her own computer — or adds WiFi to school buildings, which may complicate screen-time sensitivity (see appendix B on EMFs), be alert for a resurgence of screen-time issues for which you may have to compensate by reducing screen-time at home. See also chapter 11 for more on school-related screen issues.

New Technology

When I began developing this book, tablet computers didn't even exist. Now, iPads, iPods, e-readers, and tablets are commonplace. I recall when the iPod Touch first came along, and after the winter holidays, I had a slew of patients come into my office with symptom exacerbations, which invariably led back to them receiving the device as a present. The same thing has happened again with iPads and tablets, but the resulting problems have become much bigger, particularly since companies are marketing now to very young children. What will happen next — perhaps even before this book hits the shelves?

---

* Typical means of minimizing toxins include drinking filtered water, eating organic foods, using air filters or purifiers, reducing use of plastics, and reducing exposure to chemicals from self-care and cleaning products.

Who knows, but considering the current trend is wearable computing, the next wave of devices might make today's screen-time problems seem laughable. When parents are reluctant to put tablets away for a fast, or when I discover that a new iPad is the source of a relapse after months of hard-won gains, my response is often: "The iPad is the devil." *Of course* the iPad is convenient. That is perhaps its sole reason for existence. But don't be fooled. A penny's worth of convenience will cost you a pound of problems. What's true for fast food, convenience stores, remote controls, and so on also applies to new screen devices. So be wary when the next new technology comes out and steer clear of adding new devices to the home. It's harder to have and give up than never to have at all.

Chapter 9 Take-Home Points

- Parents will need to determine whether to eliminate or moderate screen-time immediately following the Reset, and they will need to decide on a continual basis thereafter whether to eliminate, moderate, or do another fast.
- If parents decide to reintroduce screen-time, it should be earned as a privilege, and decisions must also be made regarding amount, frequency, and consequences of rule violations.
- Rules of thumb and the Reset decision tree can be used when contemplating specific screen-management questions.
- In regard to screen-time decision making, err on the conservative side; pulling back will never be wrong.
- Certain factors should be considered high risk in terms of long-term consequences, and therefore they may justify elimination in lieu of moderation of screen-time.
- Reintroducing screen-time with the hopes of moderating use should be thought of as a trial run and presented as such to the child.
- Moderating screen-time allowances may change over time, based on developmental stages, current or ongoing stressors, and general health status.

PART THREE

BEYOND THE RESET

Action Plans for
Home, School, and Community

CHAPTER 10

EVERYDAY HOUSE RULES
AND PROTECTIVE PRACTICES

All medicine comes down to this:
Find out what's bugging you; get rid of it.
Find out what you need; get it. The body does the rest.

— Mark Hyman, MD

Part 3, as the title says, goes "beyond the Reset" to describe what we can do to protect our children from screen-related stress by promoting mindful screen management at home, in schools, and within our community. Screen-time negatively affects all of us, not just those children who struggle with Electronic Screen Syndrome. If we all were more aware that screen-time stresses the brain, and we developed healthier practices with our increasing array of technological devices, then all of us would enjoy healthier lifestyles, and we would maximize the potential of all children while protecting those most vulnerable.

A healthier relationship with screens begins at home. In this chapter, I present what I recommend as the best approach to living with technology and managing screen-time on an everyday basis, whether you are doing the Reset or not. These practices will reinforce the results of the Reset and help prevent ESS from returning, and they provide health and brain benefits to everyone in the family who practices them. Whatever the rule or practice, the overarching theme is to keep play, stimulation levels, and the sleep environment simple and natural — to soothe rather than irritate the nervous system.

I have divided this advice into three sections: one on making adjustments to the environment, one on recommended everyday "house rules" for screen-time, and one on activities that promote brain health integration. Whenever these topics reflect issues that are addressed during the Reset Program itself, I have kept explanations short and cross-referenced earlier discussions for more detail.

Toward Nature: Adjusting Your Child's Environment

Whatever screens you have in your home, and whatever rules you institute for their use, you can still create an environment that resonates more closely with nature by making certain adjustments. Most of all, these adjustments help mitigate the impact of the intense, blue-toned light that all screens emit. In other words, implementing these practices will minimize overstimulation and hyperarousal, and they will help prevent your body clock from going "out of whack."

Go Wired

Using wired-only connections — especially Internet connections — will kill several birds with one stone. First, use of wired Internet and wired power effectively makes it so kids can't plop down a laptop or tablet anywhere, any-time they please. Reducing ease of access reduces overall use. Second, while it may not seem like you want this inconvenience, you do: it's a whole lot easier to maintain and enforce screen-time "house rules" (per below) if all devices are "wired only" and restricted in location. This practice reduces arguing and limit-pushing, and it helps adults keep their use in check, too. Third, elim-inating wireless communication greatly reduces manmade EMFs. Desktop monitors and detached keyboards emit far less radiation than their mobile counterparts, and EMFs from a wired (cabled) Internet connection are neg-ligible compared to those emitted by WiFi. The "wired" rule can apply to phones, too; go old-school and make it a habit to use a corded landline when-ever possible. (For more on EMFs and potential health risks, see appendix B.)

Reduce Artificial Brightness

Televisions, computer monitors, mobile devices, and smartphones typically have brightness controls that are adjustable. For phones and other devices, the "automatic" brightness setting may or may not be natural enough depending on the device model and version; in some devices, this setting is still way too bright. Lower the screen brightness to more closely match the surrounding environment to reduce overstimulation, eye irritation, and melatonin suppression. If you or your children work on a computer in the evening (or after dark), minimize sleep issues by turning down the brightness control *below* whatever the automatic setting is. For most monitors, the lowest end of the brightness scale is plenty bright.

Aside from light's effect on arousal, our eyes aren't meant to look directly *at* light; they're meant to look at things that reflect light. Studies show eye strain from electronics may eventually result in retinal damage. If you notice you're turning up the screen brightness or contrast so you can see better, this is a sign your eyes need a break.

Download f.lux

Download and use f.lux, a handy and free software application (available at https://justgetflux.com) that gradually changes the screen's appearance by adding warmth (red tones) and reducing brightness as night falls. This idea is based on research that blue-toned light suppresses melatonin more potently (about twice as much) than red-toned light does.[1] As discussed in chapter 2 (in "The Eyes," page 36, and "Disruption of the Body Clock," page 40), because electronic screens emit bright light rich in blue and white tones, it mimics outdoor lighting (think blue skies), which tricks the brain into thinking it's daytime. As noted throughout, the brain responds to these signals by remaining or becoming alert; melatonin is suppressed, and disrupted sleep results. While I recommend making a habit of not using or allowing interactive screens after dark altogether, when this can't be avoided, f.lux may partially mitigate the impact on sleep. I began using f.lux while writing this book and found it soothing.

Although some users complain that the red tones affect the appearance of graphics, it should not affect what your child needs to do for school. (In other words, if you get complaints, "too bad!")

Use Smaller Screens and View from Farther Away

When it comes to screens, bigger isn't better. You may recall that larger screen size is one of the factors implicated in higher arousal levels. With screen sizes becoming larger and larger in everything from televisions to computers to smartphones, this is a factor you'll continually need to watch out for. Fight pressure from others in your family and from advertising to keep sizing up. This is one of those areas that's relatively easy to control but can make a big difference in stimulation levels, especially over time. Whether it's a touch-screen device or a television set, the issue boils down to how much of the visual field is taken up by screen content, as well as how close the screen is to the eyes.

For passive TV and movie viewing (for more, see chapter 5, "Reset Rules for Television," page 156), the rule of thumb is to view from a distance that is 2.5 to 3.5 times the size of the screen (measured diagonally). When purchasing or moving TV monitors around, keep in mind the dimensions of the room a screen will be viewed in. For computers, this is another reason to use only desktops, since you naturally sit farther away from the monitor. Desktops also allow for better ergonomics. If you only have laptops in the home, I recommend obtaining a separate, wired keyboard and putting the laptop on a stand atop a table or desk, thus treating it like a desktop. This gets the device off of the lap and away from the body, gets the monitor away from the eyes, and removes the hard drive and battery out from under the hands. (See also appendix B; heat and EMFs from laptops have been shown to impair reproductive function in boys, and it may damage other developing organs as well.) In general, *never* let a child use a laptop or tablet on his or her lap.

Maintain a "Sleep Sanctuary" and Optimize Bedroom Lighting

Ideally, a child's bedroom should be for sleeping or relaxing only. In reality, however, children use their room to play, read or do other leisure activities, do homework, and socialize. Nevertheless, the bedroom should remain free of electronics, meaning no television, computers, gaming consoles, or mobile devices, including e-readers. This is both a "house rule" and an environmental adjustment. The bed itself should be cozy and comfortable and made each day. The bed, bedside table, and area surrounding the bed should be clear of clutter. These environmental adjustments send conscious and unconscious cues to the brain that it's time to rest and that it's "safe" to do so, while an electronics-cluttered environment tells the brain to stay on the lookout.

Use of low lighting beginning for an hour or so before bedtime helps the brain and body wind down before drifting off to sleep. Candlelight or other dim lighting can help achieve this effect, and it provides a warm, relaxing atmosphere. Recent research out of Harvard suggests using a red lightbulb for bedroom lighting in the evening helps quiet the brain by removing blue light tones.[2] Per chapter 7, "Unhealthy Lighting" (page 197), avoid exposure to CFL and LED bulbs in the evenings and never use them in bedrooms, as they emit more blue- and white-toned light. Use incandescent or halogen bulbs instead. CFLs irritate the nervous system in other ways, too, and may contribute to insomnia even when used in other areas of the house.

For optimal melatonin release, your child's room should be pitch-black during sleep time. Sleep masks work well in achieving this total darkness state and studies show them to be a simple but effective remedy. In my experience even younger children don't mind wearing them; they will even seek them out at bedtime if they find the mask comfortable. Silk masks are best and can be found at any drugstore; Target carries child-size masks as well. When it comes to counteracting tech-related overstimulation, for less than $5 sleep masks are a no-brainer intervention.

Minimize Screen-Time after Sundown

To best imitate the natural day/night cycle, minimize screen-time after sundown and avoid interactive screen-time altogether. Particularly for children, make a concerted effort to avoid highly stimulating screen-time, including violent or excessively exciting content, fast-paced cartoons, all video games, and Internet surfing. Have children do any computer-related homework as early in the afternoon or evening as possible. For computer use at night that can't be avoided, in addition to downloading the f.lux software (see above), you can try blue-filtered glasses ("blue-blockers"), which have been shown to reduce screen-induced melatonin suppression as well as hyperarousal before bedtime.[3]

House Rules:
Everyday Screen-Time Guidelines and Boundaries

These house rules essentially expand the Reset Program rules and work as ongoing, everyday screen-time rules for the whole family. You may not follow each and every "rule" perfectly all the time, but they make an ideal to aim for, and you should always return to these guidelines whenever any mood, behavior, cognitive, or sleep issues emerge or worsen.

Keep Bedrooms Screen-Free

As with using only wired devices (see above), the simple rule that bedrooms are screen-free zones provides a lot of mileage — it reduces evening and overall screen use and is associated with improved sleep, better grades, less depression, and healthier weight. Despite it being one of the most universally recommended rules with an extensive research base to back it up, most households in America don't abide by it, and in my experience it's a hard step for many parents to take. If you have never used or allowed electronics in the bedroom, don't ever start. If you have till now, break the habit and *remove the devices themselves* from all bedrooms. It's nearly impossible to manage screen-time without doing so. It'll mean a lot to your child if you follow the same rules for your own bedroom, too.

If there is only one rule you take away from this book, make it this one.

Create a Family Workstation

The benefits of having children use a communal workstation in a public space are numerous: It automatically reduces screen-time and homework completion time as well as media multitasking. It also reduces EMF exposure, particularly if all connections and Internet access are wired. And it effectively discourages children from viewing inappropriate websites (with content that is pornographic, violent, and so on) or from engaging in inappropriate social media interactions (such as sexualized texting, bullying or being bullied, oversharing highly personal matters, talking to strangers, and so on). Keep in mind that children and teens don't yet have the frontal lobe capacity to control impulses or to consider consequences before acting on them, so we can't expect them to. Moreover, the anonymous nature of the Internet permits children to push boundaries that they normally wouldn't push — getting them into all sorts of trouble. Although it's difficult to prevent children from engaging in these activities completely, requiring them to use the Internet and social media where they can be seen is more effective than other interventions, including blocking devices and software. It also provides an opportunity to talk with your children about appropriate and inappropriate Internet use.

Lastly, using a wired family workstation encourages family members to complete computer tasks in discrete chunks of time rather than spreading them out throughout the day or evening. This teaches time management and provides everyone with longer breaks of being screen-free.

Match Screen-Time with Exercise Time

Another good way to ensure a healthier balance is to require that all children engage in an hour of physical activity at home before they earn or become "eligible" for any screen-time that day. This does not imply, of course, that a day-long soccer tournament means a child could later play video games for five hours straight. Daily and weekly limits should still apply, and interactive screen-time should only be allowed when children are symptom-free, performing well academically, and completing homework and chores. However, it's a good idea to make daily exercise an everyday "given" for earning screen-time in general, regardless of the amount you're allowing.

Screen-Time Is a Privilege, Not a Right

As discussed in chapter 9, screen management will be easier and more effective if you treat screen-time as a privilege to be earned, not an automatic "right." Set standards that must be met before any screen-time is allowed, including completion of homework and designated chores. I also recommend adding a behavior standard, such as "being respectful," especially if entitlement and lack of respect for rules in general are ongoing issues. Thus, even if a child has done everything else he or she is supposed to but then disrespects the parents in some way (for example, by name-calling or belittling), the child would still lose screen privileges for a particular period, which can then be extended if the child does it again before the time is up. The trick is following through, since parents who deal with this issue have typically been letting this behavior slide for many years, and they often feel guilty about suddenly setting limits in this regard. However, this is a highly effective way to get rid of disrespectful behavior when applied consistently, even if you make errors along the way. Incidentally, it's not just children who are bullies or who are troublemakers who engage in these behaviors. Plenty of otherwise pleasant children act this way, and sometimes children literally tell their parents to not let them get away with it because they don't like how it makes them feel.

Regardless, whatever criteria or rules you establish for earning screen-time, review them with the whole family, and even write them down and post them where all can see. Check in with your spouse regularly about how it's going; discussing it will help you learn from instances that could have been handled differently. Studies show children respond best to a parenting style that combines consistent rules with nurturing. Children need to be "safe and seen" to grow into secure adults, and practicing good boundaries helps them get there.[4]

Ban Media Multitasking

Ban the practice of using multiple types of media simultaneously. This is another factor that magnifies screen-time stress. Media multitasking fractures attention and magnifies hyperarousal, and it's been shown to adversely affect the efficiency and accuracy of task performance and completion.[5] Naturally, this rule is important for homework, when many children engage in the activity, but also the practice in general contributes to brain fatigue and poor focus because of the demand it puts on the brain. If your child insists on using another form of media while doing homework, you can allow classical music. All other forms of media, including other music styles, have been found to impede attention.

Designate Screen-Free Times and Zones

In addition to establishing screen-free zones and times, designate a "device basket" to place electronics in as soon as family members walk in the front door. This area should be away from other communal areas, if possible, to reduce the accessibility of devices, and it can also be used to make sure devices are checked in before bedtime.

Then establish certain times that are always screen-free. Recommended ones are meal preparation, mealtimes, car rides, mornings before school, family and one-on-one outings, holidays, birthdays, and other special events. Also, designate windows of time that screens can be used (whether earned or for homework for the kids, and work and leisure times for parents), as well as a time in the evening when everything is turned in and shut off. Try designating at least one screen-free day every week and see how nice it is to just talk, hang out, and go to bed early. You'll be more compliant with this rule if you make this the same day each week.

In addition, establish specific device-free zones, or places where devices should never be used. Recommended ones include the dinner table, the car, restaurants, and bedrooms. With today's hectic schedules, car rides also represent an opportunity to talk and connect with one another. Parents often report that their children tend to share more when riding in the car, so allowing device use during these times could be robbing you of precious moments.

Walk the Talk

At the risk of beating a dead horse, allow me to remind you that it's nearly impossible to govern a child's screen-time if parents' own screen-time is not adequately managed. Aside from being less aware of your surroundings when engrossed in a device, the impact on the frontal lobe makes it more difficult to follow rules and keep track of things. (For more, see "Six Reasons to Reduce Your Own Screen-Time During the Reset," page 149.) Use the Reset as an opportunity to be super strict with your use — or do a complete fast yourself — then commit to rules you all can live with that don't affect your sleep or health. As with children, sometimes making drastic cuts works better than simply trying to reduce.

If you absolutely have to do work-related screen activities when your children are home, pick a designated time slot and stick to it. Try to really limit or eliminate leisure screen activities like Facebook when you're with your kids, and as mentioned earlier, I recommend checking in with your children about how they perceive your use. Many of the kids I see become tearful when this subject comes up because they feel like they have to compete for their parents' attention. All of us can benefit from cutting back and being more present with loved ones, so establish rules for parents, too.

Utilize the Accountability Act

During the Reset, I suggest creating an "Accountability Act" (see chapter 5, page 148), which gives children the ability to hold parents accountable for living up to promises and following rules. Violating rules or breaking a commitment requires parents to pay a "tax" of some kind, typically one that rewards the child or the family as a whole. After the Reset, you can continue to use this for general "house rules" and anything else that requires follow through and accountability. Children get a thrill out of holding a parent accountable, so the policy keeps everyone in line quite efficiently. Naturally, you can have your children pay a tax for violating rules, too, and the act can also be used to hold spouses mutually accountable for responsibilities.

Use Timers and Checkouts

If you have designated screen-free times, and are using screen-time allowances with your children (see chapter 9, "Institute a Screen 'Allowance,'" page 234), then get in the habit of using timers and checkout sheets to keep everyone honest and in line. Checkout sheets work particularly well in conjunction with a communal workstation ("Create a Family Workstation," page 250) and/or a communal basket for handheld devices ("Designate Screen-Free Times and Zones," page 252). This way mobile devices are not allowed to float freely around the house, which will greatly reduce miscellaneous screen-time.

In the spirit of keeping screen management low-tech, I prefer using simple kitchen timers rather than parental controls on the computer. A timer also guards against "slippage" and helps keep children from going over their allotted amount; parents don't need to watch the clock themselves, just listen for the beep.

Toward Resilience:
Promoting Brain Health While Preventing ESS

The following activities protect the nervous system from stress, promote brain integration, and reduce risk for ESS. In essence, these measures are all about getting back to our natural roots.

Greenery, Nature, and Sunlight

Numerous studies have found that green surroundings enhance mental health and learning capacity by lowering stress levels, both immediately and over time.[6] *Attention restoration theory* posits that green scenery produces "easy attention" by drawing the eye while calming the nervous system, creating a state of "calm alertness." This state is considered ideal for learning and is in contrast to stress-based alertness, which depletes attention.[7] A growing body of research tells us that greenery improves learning, raises grades, and reduces aggression, all due to its restorative effect on attention and arousal regulation.[8] Indeed, this dynamic regarding arousal, attention, and aggression is the exact reversal of the ESS process.

Take advantage of this fact by placing greenery around and throughout the home, including in bedrooms. As an added bonus, plants in the home reduce toxic emissions in the air, including those emitted from electronics. For restorative window views, arrange bushes, flowers, and trees outside in such a way that lushness is viewable from wherever your child does homework and from frequently used areas in the home.

Of course, regular physical activity *in* green spaces, such as parks, fields, and nature areas, is even more powerful. Closeness to nature and having the freedom to run and play outside may be the reason that children who live in rural environments have lower rates of attention deficit disorder and autism than do their urban counterparts. Help your child engage with nature by planting a vegetable or flower garden, visiting city parks and zoos, going on nature walks, and interacting with animals. For urban dwellers, drive out to the countryside as often as you can.

The subject of artificial light's negative effects on health is discussed throughout this book, but what about natural light's positive effects? *Chronobiology*, the study of how the body clock affects health, is a rapidly growing area of research. Exposure to sunlight may help reduce attention deficit symptoms,[9] and abundant bright light first thing in the morning can help restore disrupted circadian rhythms, improve mood, and enhance restorative sleep.[10] Many children go right to school in the morning without seeing much natural daylight, and at the end of the day they have too much light-at-night — exactly the opposite of nature. Resynchronize rhythms by having your child spend fifteen minutes or more outside each morning (or at least sit next to a window that lets in direct light) and by reducing light-at-night.

Movement, Exercise, and Free Play

In his fascinating book *Spark*, Harvard psychiatrist Dr. John Ratey describes how stress and exercise affect the brain: "Toxic levels of stress erode the connections between billions of nerve cells in the brain...[while] exercise unleashes a cascade of neurochemicals and growth factors that can reverse this process, physically bolstering the brain's infrastructure."[11] Exercise literally changes and grows the brain; it fights depression, poor focus, insomnia, addiction, and anxiety by raising and balancing the very brain chemicals and hormones that become imbalanced from using electronics. Exercise even affects what genes get expressed. For team sports that keep kids moving nearly constantly, try soccer, basketball, tennis, and volleyball. Running has also been found to have dramatic effects on brain function.

Aside from aerobic exercise, *movement* and *free play* are also essential to learning and are in fact requirements for healthy brain development.[12] Unstructured play is not just for fun — it is an integral aspect of development and encourages brain integration, mastering of new skills and roles, grasping others' mental states, cause-and-effect thinking, problem-solving, and managing conflict. Active play also develops core muscle strength, stimulates the vestibular system (affecting balance and body awareness), and discharges pent-up energy — all things that are required for learning. Children with sensory issues, ADHD, and autism often have an even greater need to expend energy, and they may need several hours a day to do so.

I've said it before and I'll say it again: *movement and play are more important than homework*. If you feel homework time is cutting into time your child needs to unwind and discharge physical or creative energy, see if you can get homework reduced or even eliminated, at least temporarily. Encourage and allow both structured play (such as team sports) and unstructured play, and you'll reduce risk for ESS as well as obesity and other chronic stress health issues while strengthening your child's brain.

Deep Sleep and Clean Diet

Virtually all mental health issues impact sleep, and non-restorative sleep can precipitate numerous cognitive, mood, and behavioral issues no matter what the source. Conversely, restorative sleep is reparative; it's a powerful healer across the board. Help promote deep sleep by following this chapter's guidelines and by establishing a regular sleep-wake schedule. Research shows that parent-set bedtimes are associated with better sleep and improved daytime functioning in children.[13]

In theory, a clean natural diet will provide the antioxidants the brain needs to fight screen-related stress inflammation. However, I've worked with many families who maintain a very healthy diet but who nevertheless have a child with ESS. Thus, like exercise, a good diet may be "necessary but not sufficient" to protect against ESS.

Creativity

Creative activity helps stimulate the right brain, which is often underactive in our information overloaded world. But the creative process also activates numerous areas throughout the entire brain, facilitating whole-brain integration and brain-body integration as well. Moreover, flexing our creative muscle helps build problem-solving skills. Obviously, however, "creative" video games (such as games in which you build things) do not count toward protective measures.

In fact, studies show that screen-time diminishes imaginary play. When the brain is fed a constant stream of stimulating entertainment that saturates the senses, it deadens the creative drive, as does viewing a two-dimensional screen with flat, unnatural light. In contrast, reduced levels of stimulation enhance creativity,[14] and varying depth of field and the interplay of natural light and shadow in a three-dimensional world stimulate the seer's mind to wonder, "What's there?"[15]

Mindfulness and Meditation

It's tricky getting children to engage in mindfulness techniques, but without exception, when a child *does* start practicing a mindfulness activity — such as kids' yoga — they are calmer, less easily frustrated, and better rested. Like reducing or eliminating screen-time, practicing mindfulness will provide your child a lot of bang for your buck. Nor does it have to be expensive; practice with them at home.

How does mindfulness benefit thee? Let me count the ways....Meditation and yoga quiet the brain and reduce stimulation. As this book makes clear, electronic stimulation plus our stress-driven society invariably means that our brains get *too much* intense stimulation. As for cognitive benefits, research suggests that meditation is associated with increased thickness in areas of the frontal lobe cortex associated with attention and emotional regulation.[16] Not surprisingly, a study on second- and third-graders who were taught mindfulness techniques showed an improvement in executive function, particularly in children with attention problems.[17]

Bonding: Human Touch, Empathy, and Love

It is well-documented that children who receive healthy nurturing early on — such as being held, rocked, soothed, and attended to by an "in tune" empathic parent — have larger brains than children who do not receive adequate nurturing or who are outright neglected. As children develop, eye contact, face-to-face interaction, touch, and learning body language are all critical for development, including learning how to regulate emotion and arousal, developing a sense of self, and capacity for intimacy.[18] Spend time with your children in ways that promote physical and emotional closeness. Healthy attachments and a strong support network will also protect your child against delinquency and addiction, including screen addiction.[19]

Aside from receiving nurturing, expressing feelings of love and compassion for others has benefits as well; research shows that practicing these feelings can stimulate the frontal lobe, fostering emotional regulation and executive function development.[20] In fact, integrative medicine physicians cite *love* as one of the pillars of evidence-based natural healing. Additionally, altruistic activities can improve a child's self-esteem and can facilitate empathy skills; I've found that arranging for a child to mentor or tutor children one or two years younger has enormous benefits. Schools are often willing to work out something like this, and it creates a win-win for everyone.

Finally, human contact promotes brain integration and academic learning. One of the most consistent determinants in how well children learn to speak, read, and write is access to face-to-face conversations with an adult.[21] Likewise, older children with at-risk behaviors and low grades benefit from healthy supportive adult relationships, including with teachers.[22]

Chapter 10 Take-Home Points

- Healthy screen management boils down to following Reset rules and guidelines, making environmental adjustments, and implementing counteractive (protective) measures.
- Following these practices will help normalize stimulation levels, mitigate the stress response, and promote brain integration.
- Adjustments can be made to lessen nervous system irritation and lower arousal levels by adjusting screen brightness levels, using smaller screens, and avoiding media multitasking, especially before bedtime.
- Screen-time rules and guidelines include maintaining an electronics-free bedroom, setting up a desktop in a common area, balancing screen activities with physical and outdoor play, and completing homework and chores in order to earn electronic play.
- Reset guidelines should always be followed, including reducing screen-time and/or implementing fasts when your child becomes dysregulated or is falling behind in school.
- Everyday screen-time management should be a holistic approach to overall health, promoting healthy frontal lobe growth, integrating brain and brain-body connections, restoring attention, and developing healthy attachments.
- Three "rules" are most important: keeping the bedroom free of screen devices, using a wired desktop workstation, and modeling the screen rules yourself.

CHAPTER 11

SCHOOL DAZE

Concerns in the Classroom

*There seems to be a direct conflict between the advocates of [technology]
in early years education, on the one hand, and the warnings arising
from studies in paediatric medicine and biology, on the other.*[1]

— Aric Sigman, health advisor to the European Parliament's Quality
of Childhood Group on the Impact of Screen Media on Children

Presently in our society, there is a growing mismatch between what children's
brains and bodies *need* to learn and to develop optimally and what is actually
being *provided* by the public school system. In fact, the modern-day classroom
is far from ideal; it contains a variety of potential hazards that put stress and
pressure on children's nervous systems, which can impede or undermine cognitive, emotional, and social development. Some of these negative influences are
related to too much screen-time and an increasing reliance on computer-based
learning, and some are part of what our society has come to accept as a "normal" classroom-based education, in which students spend too much time sitting indoors and not enough time playing, interacting with nature, and being
creative.

Fortunately, by doing the Reset and creating a brain-healthy environment at home, you will be affording your child powerful protection against
many of the school-related hazards he or she will face. This chapter surveys
some of these hazards to illustrate how off-track our education system has
become as well as to underscore the importance of minimizing technology

elsewhere in your child's life. It will also provide guidance about effective approaches for communicating with your child's school, including how to go about obtaining screen-time accommodations for the Reset and in general.

As I write this, most of the time the Reset will be effective without addressing school-related screen-time, but as discussed in chapter 5 ("Reset Planning and School," page 158), some parents will need to tackle school-related screen issues to obtain a "cleaner" fast or because school *is* the main source of screen-time. In other cases, parents may want to address what's happening at school as a troubleshooting issue. In fact, beyond the Reset, the school environment will likely present you with various ESS risks that you may have to contend with periodically as your child grows up. Whether and how you address school-related electronic stress depends on several factors: how dysregulated and how sensitive your child is, how your child responds to the Reset at home, how much exposure your child receives at school, and your child's unique balance of risk factors.

What If My Child Gets Left Behind?

When parents contemplate extending screen-time restrictions to the classroom for their child, some worry: "What if my child gets left behind as other children learn and know more about computers?" I understand where this fear is coming from, since no parent wants to potentially handicap their child's future. But the concern is unfounded, since it is frontal lobe functioning that determines academic and social success. Supporting brain integration by being screen-free means you'll be optimizing your child's learning ability, no matter what the subject matter. In contrast, a child who has great computer skills but poor frontal lobe functioning will have trouble advancing in anything, since good frontal lobe function is needed to "get things done," tolerate frustration, and develop a strong social network.

Further, compared to trying to learn to read, write, and do math, research shows that learning computer skills is relatively easy. Studies on rhesus monkeys have shown they can easily learn how to use a touchscreen or joystick to problem solve on a computer, and dolphins and apes have been taught to use iPads.[2] And how much technology do kids really need to know that they don't know already in order to succeed — or that won't be obsolete by the time they graduate? Studies show computer skills don't translate into better wages,[3] and most kids are plenty tech-savvy already. Worst-case scenario, your child will be able to catch up later.

Moreover, based on the fact that early screen-time exposure is associated with language and reading delays,[4] there appear to be critical and potentially long-term benefits to *delaying* screen technology until the brain is better able to tolerate it. Nor am I the only one who suggests it's wise to delay technology's introduction; top-notch private schools like Waldorf schools, renowned for their natural teaching methods, don't introduce any computer training until sixth grade.[5] Tellingly, many CEOs and executives of Silicon Valley tech companies prefer low-tech "nature-based" education, including Waldorf, for their own children.[6] Steve Jobs, of all people, reportedly strictly limited his kids' access to electronic gadgets, and apparently so do numerous other execs and wealthy venture capitalists around the country.[7] If the people at the top of their game in the tech and finance world — who have access to the very best resources — want to delay introducing technology to their own children, what does that tell you?

If you find yourself struggling with the concern that your child may get "left behind," always remember: *First, do no harm.* Weigh carefully the risks of electronics exposure on a growing brain against reassurance that your child is keeping up with technological advancements. The latter is akin to "keeping up with the Joneses."

Who will be left behind? The child who can't concentrate.

The Encroachment of Screen-Time and the Disappearance of Developmental Support

In the United States, children are in school — mostly sitting — for seven-plus hours a day, and they are typically given anywhere from a half hour to three hours of homework each night. Meanwhile, physical exercise, recess, exposure to nature and greenery, and free play are all disappearing, even though each of these is proven to improve cognitive skills.[8] Furthermore, the American Academy of Pediatrics has recommended school-age children receive no more than one to two hours of screen-time per day,[9] yet school-related screen-time can easily add up to several hours daily on its own. As I've shown, there is no functional distinction between screen-time that's "educational" and for "entertainment" when it comes to impacts and health risks, and schools themselves are driving an increase in screen-time for all children on average. Children of all ages are increasingly being taught computer skills, assigned homework that requires online research or electronic methods of completion or delivery, viewing lectures via electronic whiteboards or other types of interactive media, and being told "educational" screen-time is okay, or even helpful, despite evidence to the contrary.[10] Then, at home, as children do their homework electronically, they often engage in media multitasking, communicating with friends and entertaining themselves as they work: texting, instant messaging, Skyping, checking Facebook, listening to music, and watching videos and TV.

On top of all this, an increasing number of school districts are installing wireless Internet access, despite warnings regarding possibly harmful biological effects from leading medical experts and organizations. Did you know that other countries such as France, Italy, Sweden, Germany, and Australia are concerned about exposing children to EMFs, and that some countries have outlawed WiFi in schools, daycares, and preschools entirely?[11] Did you know the official recommendation from the American Academy of Environmental Medicine is that children use *wired only* Internet access?[12] Did you know that the American Academy of Pediatrics has written several letters to the FCC asking for updated acceptable radiation exposure levels for children because of the dramatic growth of wireless communication, stating, "Children are not little adults and are disproportionately affected by all environmental exposures"?[13]

Probably not, and probably no one at your school has either. Following are some of the major areas of concern. Consider them and keep them in mind when talking to teachers and school administrators about reducing your child's risks from exposure to electronics.

Computer Devices and Internet Use

In the not-so-distant past, computer use in school was limited to learning skills in a computer lab, using wired Internet access only. Now, laptops, iPads, tablets, and other mobile devices have become commonplace, including in early-years classrooms. School districts continue to introduce one-to-one iPad or laptop programs, despite no clear benefits, substantial and documented risks related to computer use, and enormous monetary cost. Laptop and iPad use also presents unnecessary additional screen-time and various distractions for students as well.

Recently, the struggling Los Angeles Unified School District handed out its first wave of iPads in a pilot program to give every student in the district a school-dedicated computer. What did many students do? They quickly disabled security filters to play video games and surf the Internet. The projected cost of the program for its estimated three-year lifespan is over a billion dollars — paid for by twenty-five-year bond funds — and yet the LA district schools go without badly needed repairs for things as basic as drinking water, functioning bathrooms, and safe and stable classroom infrastructure, not to mention "extras" like lights on soccer fields so the kids can have night games.[14] It's absurd.

Laptop and other mobile computers create substantial risk over desktop ones, particularly if placed on the lap. As I describe in appendix B on EMFs, these issues include heating and non-heating radiation effects that may damage reproductive organs in children and cause skin inflammation. Aside from increased radiation exposure, laptops and tablets are terrible for posture and can create neck and back problems. Desktop computer use causes posture problems, too, including "forward head posture" that is now endemic in young people, but with laptops it is virtually impossible to be in an ergonomic position due to the keyboard being attached to the monitor.[15] That schools are adding to these problems is a serious public health issue.

A variety of issues arise when schools require students to use the Internet for schoolwork. For starters, it promotes media multitasking, provides easy access to all sorts of entertainment, and creates opportunities to access inappropriate content. These temptations are distracting for many students, but they are especially so for children with poor impulse control. Further, studies show that reading hyperlinked text tends to produce fragmented understanding of material, due to a heavier cognitive load from increased decision making and visual processing.[16] Internet use also contributes to hyperarousal from frequent page changes and sensory overload. Lastly, studies suggest that use of Google and the Internet for researching assignments has led to a rise in plagiarism, the practice of which is next to impossible to monitor.[17]

To better grasp how school-related computer use impacts your child, talk to teachers and find out how much time is delegated to learning actual computer skills and how much time is spent using computers in class, for research and for homework. For Internet use, find out if the kids have unstructured or unmonitored access and what safeguards are in place. Since early and regular Internet use is a risk factor for problematic screen use as well as cognitive delays, ask teachers if assignments can be modified to minimize computer use at home and at school. Elementary school children should ideally have computer lessons no more than once a week, and even high school students seem to do better when school computer availability occurs just once or twice a week.[18] Also inquire about library time, study periods, and breaks, where your child may be logging in a lot more screen-time than you realize, as well as whether the students can earn computer or video game time as a reward.

School cell phone policies should also be examined. Each teacher's attitude is relevant, as some are quite lax about cell phone use even if the school's policy is strict, and vice versa. Many children text and use the Internet on their phones, during recess as well as during class, in spite of school policies. Needless to say, the explosion of smartphones in young hands has compounded this problem, and children should not be expected to control this behavior on their own. Then again, per the Reset guidelines, whether your child has a smartphone — or any phone, for that matter — is a parenting issue, so if unwanted phone usage is occurring at school, whatever the school's policy, parents can handle this by eliminating the phone.

"Interactive" Media: Electronic Whiteboards

Interactive electronic whiteboards represent yet another source of unnatural stimulation designed to keep children "engaged." But research doesn't support their use, and they're exorbitantly expensive. A 2007 study at London

University's Institute of Education found that whiteboards provided no impact on student performance in the first year of use, that any increase in motivation from the initial intrigue was short-lived, and that some children became distracted by the technology. The study also showed that the pace slowed in classrooms with lower ability students, where there was a tendency to overemphasize the "interactivity" by letting all the children take turns at the board.[19] Once again, the most vulnerable kids suffer the most, while precious dollars are spent needlessly.

Paradoxically, these so-called "interactive" methods lead to reduced human interaction, as children's eyes are glued to the screen instead of to the teacher. The teacher in turn becomes more and more reliant upon using high-tech presentations to stimulate and entertain the audience, creating a vicious cycle. They also contribute to media multitasking because children are forced to attend to various visual and auditory stimuli while answering questions or taking notes and attempting to absorb the lesson at the same time. As mentioned in the previous chapter, media multitasking fractures attention and impairs performance, both immediately and over time.

Less Movement, Outdoor Time, and Creative Expression

Accompanying the steady increase of technology in the classroom has been the steady decline of gym class, art and music lessons, recess, free play outdoors, and occupational therapy services. Because of tighter budgets and pressure to "teach to the test," schools have cut back on these areas. They have also cut back after-school sports and coaches' salaries, making it difficult for children to have regular and free access to organized sports. Further, there is altogether too much sitting, too much "busy work," and too much homework. All these factors contribute to declines in movement, creative expression, healthy socializing, and time spent outdoors — the very things known to support mind, body, and brain development.

As discussed in chapter 4, these are the "right brain" activities that help integrate the entire brain, including the frontal lobe, by providing all the proper ingredients: utilization of all five senses, human interaction that fosters a sense of competence and of feeling cared for, exposure to nature and sunlight, and actively experiencing a three-dimensional physical environment. By emphasizing and putting resources into more technology, schools undermine the cheapest and most effective ways to foster development in our children.

Exposure to EMFs from WiFi

While I have largely restricted the discussion of electromagnetic fields (EMFs) to appendix B, including what they are and how they may possibly cause harm, the growing use of WiFi (wireless Internet access) in schools bears mention here. Because of the explosion of electronics and wireless communication, we all now live in a sea of manmade EMFs. However, that doesn't mean we shouldn't try to minimize children's exposure. WiFi compounds EMF exposure many-fold — and its usage is *optional* in a school setting. Even if we were to suppose that there are no health risks, why is money being spent on its installation and use when wireless access leads to unmanaged screen-time for students and teachers alike, who could simply use wired Internet access instead? For that matter, why can't all computer-related assignments be completed during designated school hours, which would reduce cost, diminish back pain from carrying around laptops, and reduce light-at-night effects?

But, in fact, a case can be made to consider WiFi's impact on the developing brain because it is literally impossible to determine that exposure to WiFi is safe. Even minuscule changes in a developing nervous system can amount to large changes in function over time, and because WiFi is new, we *can't* know the impact of what's happening now until several decades into the future. That said, there are already thousands of existing studies demonstrating biological effects from EMFs, and current government safety exposure limits are outdated and based on adults — not children, whose growing brains are substantially more sensitive. [20] Further, exposure to EMFs from WiFi in a classroom is constant, occurring all day every day, because signals are emitted by the access hubs even when devices are not in use. The signals produced are also much stronger than those produced by your average home WiFi hub because of the amount of bandwidth required to accommodate a large number of users. Lastly, in a school setting, multiple devices tend to be in use at once, which causes EMFs to reverberate and magnify one another.

This makes WiFi use in schools a serious public health matter, one that the US government has been slow to recognize and address. Meanwhile, there is a burgeoning outcry from medical and science experts, such as pediatric neurologist Martha Herbert, PhD, from Harvard Medical School, and Martin Blank, PhD, of Columbia University, who are taking a public stance against WiFi installation in schools. [21] Medical organizations in the United States,

Europe, Canada, and Australia have all made objections.[22] The board of the American Academy of Environmental Medicine takes this position:

> Adverse health effects, such as learning disabilities, altered immune responses, headaches etc. from wireless radio frequency fields do exist and are well documented in the scientific literature. Safer technology, such as hard-wiring, must be seriously considered in schools for the safety of those susceptible individuals who may be affected by this phenomenon. [23]

Meanwhile, the Parliamentary Assembly Council of Europe (PACE) made the following statement regarding WiFi use in schools:

> As regards standards or threshold values for emissions of electromagnetic fields of all types and frequencies, the Assembly strongly recommends that the ALARA (As Low As Reasonably Achievable) principle is applied.... Moreover, the precautionary principle should be applied when scientific evaluation does not allow the risk to be determined with sufficient certainty.... For children in general, and particularly in schools and classrooms, give preference to wired Internet connections, and strictly regulate the use of mobile phones by school children on school premises.[24]

Why should we in the United States — to whom the rest of the world looks in regard to technology *and* health care — want to be on the wrong side of history? For more on the subject, including a discussion on vulnerabilities specific to autism, please turn to appendix B.

Other Unhealthy Factors in the Classroom Environment

In a word, today's classrooms represent an environment of *unnatural* influences. There are unnatural foods (sugary snacks and beverages and fast food in the lunchroom), unnatural lights (from screen devices and fluorescent overhead lights), unnatural sensory input (from electronic stimulation), and unnatural activity levels (prolonged sitting, interacting with screens, and reduced exercise). In some areas, there may also be air pollution and a lack of access to clean drinking water that further harm children.

Overhead fluorescent lights exist in virtually every classroom. I discuss some of the effects of fluorescent light on stress, sleep, and general health in chapter 7 ("Unhealthy Lighting," page 197), but there are a few smaller studies on classroom behavior and performance as well. One study showed increased stereotypic repetitive behaviors in autistic children under fluorescent light compared to incandescent,[25] consistent with clinical experience and parental reporting of some autistic children. Another demonstrated reduced blood pressure and aggression with full spectrum lighting compared to fluorescent light in a study with severely developmentally disabled children — including two who were blind,[26] suggesting the effects were occurring via non-visual pathways (as is the effect on melatonin suppression). Parents sometimes report that their child's behavior (for example, hyperactivity, irritability, or tics) is worse when the child is exposed to overhead fluorescent lights. Some clinicians minimize or discount this observation, and they suggest that these exacerbations are more likely to be due to a child having to sit in school all day. But the research as well as anecdotal reporting suggests that classroom lighting poses its own risk.

Although it's perhaps unrealistic to change lighting in a classroom, if the classroom has large windows letting in abundant natural light, ask the teacher if at least half the overhead lights in that half of the room can be turned off, then ask to have your child sit near the windows.

Technology to Teach: Pressures and Impacts

In addition to an overemphasis on teaching computer skills, there exist enormous social forces that pressure educators to use technology to engage students via "interactive methods," to provide laptops and Internet access to "level the playing field for all students," and to "take advantage" of technology to overcome writing, learning, or literacy issues. Yet these steps are taken without regard to effectiveness, without utilization or knowledge of outcome measures, and are given a higher priority than evidence-based teaching methods. Aside from the fact that whatever computer skills are taught and whatever devices are purchased are likely to become obsolete by the time students graduate, research shows most children *do* have access to computers and the Internet, including those in low-income families.[27] Thus, the so-called digital divide — the concern that poor or rural children will be left behind because they don't have broadband Internet access — is essentially a non-issue. In fact, the race to close the supposed gap by providing universal access has contributed to tech overuse, which has inadvertently *widened* the gap, since disadvantaged children are affected by this phenomenon disproportionately.

Innovation ≠ Superior Education

There is a certain seductive quality to innovation and to the "coolness" of technology — but this can lead to short-sightedness. As I reviewed the research for this chapter, when I read about the "promise" ed-tech companies were serving up and how impulsively taxpayer dollars were being spent, it made me extremely uneasy. I couldn't help thinking that educators and policy makers had somehow been spellbound, by either spectacular presentations or the prospect of how much money could be saved, because the promises fly in the face of everything we know about how children learn. Apparently, education professor emeritus Larry Cuban of Stanford University agrees; in one of a series of articles taking a critical look at technology in education published in the *Washington Post*, Professor Cuban remarked:

> Magical thinking about transforming teaching and learning — dumping teachers and traditional schools disappearing — is close to make-believe even when children have these powerful devices in their hands....Vendor-driven hype and wishful policy thinking...feed private and public fantasies about replacing teachers and schools.[28]

Cuban also contends that technology enthusiasts "[equate] access to information with becoming educated," and that "there is hardly any research that will show clearly that any of these machines will improve academic achievement. But the value of novelty, that's highly prized in American society, period. And one way schools can say they are 'innovative' is to pick up the latest device."[29]

"First to Worst": The California Literacy Disaster

In the 1950s, California schools were the pinnacle of effective public education. At the time, reading was taught using phonics, which is still the best proven method today. But because of a series of events in the sixties and seventies affecting how school districts were funded, the state's power over education grew, and local government control weakened. During the 1980s, state policy makers decided to implement a "Whole Language" reading program after being seduced by enchanting presentations involving the use of storytelling to teach reading, without regard to whether the program worked or not. Schools across the state were effectively forced to implement the state-funded program in order to receive funding, and literacy scores plummeted. When state officials finally realized what a debacle the program had caused, the damage was done. This and other factors led California schools to fall from first to last place, "equaled only by Mississippi and Guam."[30]

Historically, at the state and federal level, government mandates have been known to complicate rather than solve problems in education. Too often, unproven "new ideas" are expensive to implement and are often inferior to what's "tried and true." Furthermore, big business, technology companies, and powerful lobbyists for special interest groups can influence politicians to enact education policies that benefit industry first and students not at all. Since government-based research dollars are limited, most tech-education research is funded by media industry dollars, creating an inherent conflict of interest.[31] Lastly, schools are often cash-strapped, and so they typically welcome dollars offered by corporations in exchange for trying out or endorsing new programs.

Let history be our teacher. Changes in education should be made based on evidence-based peer-reviewed research, including outcome studies — not on ideas that "seem like a good idea at the time."

Computer Use Detracts from, Not Enhances, Learning

There is mounting evidence that computer use and electronic-based learning not only doesn't assist learning but seems to hinder it. In the introduction to chapter 4, I describe how several IQ studies have documented that children and young adults have been declining in performance over the last two decades. Why? Studies suggest these declines may be related to delays in individual cognitive development imposed by technology exposure.

For instance, a 2010 study out of Duke University following 150,000 middle school students found that acquiring a home computer negatively impacted reading and math scores, and that regular access to computers in general was associated with lower scores.[32] Another large 2004 study in over thirty countries found that fifteen-year-olds who used the computer several times a week performed worse in math and reading compared to those who used computers less frequently.[33] And a 2010 study out of Romania found students provided home computers by the government scored higher in computer skills assessments but lower in language, reading, and math.[34]

Still, acquiring computer skills must make a difference in the workforce, right? Actually, not so much. A careful analysis of labor force data in the United Kingdom suggested that computer skills make no difference in wages, while writing and math skills do, all other things being equal. The authors of one such review in 2004 state that "the ability to use a computer effectively is not of great importance for a worker's performance in a job, implying that there is no evidence that computer skills are becoming a new basic skill important to teach at school. Rather, it seems to be the case for most jobs, that once computers have to be used, the necessary skills to do so are acquired relatively easily requiring little investments, if any."[35] So much for "leveling the playing field" by providing computer and Internet access to low-income students — which seems to hurt children in areas that really count instead.

Regarding literacy, research suggests early and regular screen-time exposure reduces time spent reading, and that time spent gaming tends to worsen reading scores.[36] Fewer children read fiction than ever, particularly boys, and comprehension skills are diminishing.[37] Furthermore, boys have always lagged behind girls in reading ability, but they are now "falling off the curve," and experts speculate this is due to computer time and video games.[38]

Research on college students has shown that those who read books more and use electronic media less have higher grades and better focus.[39] In general, print reading for recreational purposes is correlated with achievement and other benefits across all age groups.[40]

What about learning how to read in the first place? Many educators jump right to software programs to "teach" children how to read, without realizing that the electronic screen itself inhibits the reading process. A 2002 study comparing e-learning versus book-based reading programs showed that although word count was the same with both methods, children who learned to read from books had better comprehension.[41] Early literacy is dependent on parent-child dialogue, and reading, speaking, and writing skills are largely dependent on face-to-face conversations with adults.[42]

Lastly, we know from studies on toddlers that learning a task from screen media does not translate easily into real-life learning.[43] Other research suggests that early screen exposure affects play length and focused attention during play and slows language acquisition.[44] Since toddlers and grade-school children learn through imaginary and social play, educational software programs may be dangerous, not only because of screen-related factors, but because using them is associated with reduced imaginary play and reduced interaction with parents and teachers.

The Importance of Writing by Hand for Learning

Increasingly, students who have trouble printing or writing are allowed to use computers instead, but research suggests that adopting this practice too early may cause additional setbacks. Sensory integration specialists and child development experts assert that children who can't hand print well don't learn to read easily because they don't have as strong a visual-motor "imprint" for letter recognition. In contrast, practicing and becoming proficient in printing makes both printing and reading more fluid and automatic, freeing up mental energy to work on other subjects like math and spelling.[45] More generally, printing and cursive writing stimulate the brain and mind in unique ways that typing does not, including hand-eye coordination, self-discipline, attention to detail, and global engagement of thinking, language, and working memory areas.[46] Yet increasingly, schools bypass this critical skill and rush to let a child use a keyboard at the first sign of struggle; teaching cursive is no longer a requirement of the national Common Core standards.

What's more, studies show that laptop note-taking produces a more shallow understanding of the material compared to taking notes by hand, and that laptops are distracting both for users and for their neighbors, even when they're being used in an appropriate manner.[47] Other research has shown that students using laptops to take notes don't perform as well on exams compared to longhand note-takers.[48]

In a compelling 2007 report advocating the banning of laptops in the classroom,[49] professor Kevin Yamamoto of the South Texas College of Law presents a litany of research supporting his case, including that the use of laptops in law classrooms is linked to a lower pass-rate of the bar exam. In a study on his own classroom, he found that laptop use reduced student-teacher eye contact, created an overreliance on looking up material instead of internalizing concepts, hindered critical thinking, and erected a mental and physical barrier between himself and the students. He also found that students were frequently not following along, making discussions maddeningly inefficient. In contrast, after banning laptops, Professor Yamamoto noted there were more questions from students and more in-depth discussions, as well as higher exam scores and overwhelmingly positive feedback from students (nearly 90 percent felt positive or neutral about the ban). Interestingly, Yamamoto noted that the ban made the administration very nervous, and he was discouraged from making such a bold move.

The Needs of "Visual Learners"

Because of the primitive survival instincts, visual input will always be attended to over auditory input when presented together. Yet children who have trouble following verbal directions are often labeled as "visual learners," with the result that auditory skills aren't developed as instead attempts are made to provide a workaround with stimulating visual cues. This leads to an overdependence on visual learning and understimulation of auditory processing, resulting in attention difficulties.[50] Considering that children with attention problems are more severely impacted by screen-time, more emphasis should be placed on developing listening skills and auditory attention along with less emphasis on electronic visual input. If a child does require visual cues as an aid, such as pictures or word prompts, they should be non-electronic and simple.

Measures to Promote Academic Success and Healthy Development

While we need to be aware of the shortcomings of the modern-day classroom, research tells us that certain factors are associated with improved attention, academic success, and social well-being. Luckily, you'll already be implementing them by doing the Reset Program. These factors include less screen-time, chores, rituals and routines, restful sleep, exercise, exposure to nature, family time, one-on-one time, and firm boundaries.[11] These are the same practices that are presented in chapter 10, so turn there for more detail.

Working with Your Child's School: Effective Attitudes and Approaches

Whether you're trying to address temporary school-related screen-time for the Reset or to create more permanent change in your child's school, begin by asking questions. Ask both your child and the teacher how much the teacher uses computers, the Internet, and electronic whiteboards as teaching tools on an everyday basis. Try to estimate what portion of your child's homework requires computer use. Find out if students have days in a row where they don't use computers or electronic tools at all, or if they're exposed daily. If you can, sit in on your child's classroom for a day. If you can't, ask the teacher about his or her teaching style and what kinds of teaching methods they use. For older children with multiple teachers and classes, meet as many of the teachers as you can. Keep in mind that you'll meet a mixed group — some of them will see any screen-time as the enemy, and others will sing technology's praises. You can also speak to the special education or resource teacher, psychologists or other therapists, academic counselors, the principal and vice principal, coaches, and so on.

If you approach school personnel with a request and someone tells you, "You can't do that," don't get too discouraged. If you think your request is feasible and would not detract from your child's (or others') education, keep trying. School systems embody a lot of bureaucracy, and initial denials can be knee-jerk responses. Many times I have made requests to change a child's school environment only to be told no at first. Yet once the parent and I have made sure that staff understand the reasoning behind certain requests, and if we make the changes easy enough for the school to implement, they eventually come around.

At the risk of stereotyping, you may find that female teachers resonate more with the screen-time message; in general, male brains are more intensely drawn to technology. But male teachers and male coaches who support screen-time reduction can be highly valuable and influential allies, with both children and the administration. Nurture these relationships, and don't waste too much energy on those who are defensive about the topic. However teachers react, know that seeds of awareness are being planted. Eventually those seeds will produce roots and germinate, strengthening your position. There is strength in numbers, whether support comes from other parents, teachers, or coaches.

Be firm but respectful in your approach. The squeaky wheel gets the oil, but nobody likes entitled parents who blame the school for all of a child's difficulties. Volunteering or contributing in other ways helps, too; being liked makes a difference in terms of teachers and other staff going out of their way to help your child.

Ben: A Reward with No Gains

Melissa was a stressed-out mother who decided to try the Reset with her teenage son, Ben, who spent the majority of his free time at home online. When the Reset didn't seem to work, we discovered that Ben had been texting at night. After establishing a new rule that he hand in his phone by 7 p.m. and disabling its Internet access, we waited to see what would happen. Ben began turning in more homework, but he was still extremely moody at home and refused to participate in anything the family was doing as a unit. For example, when Ben's dad took the kids to pick out a Christmas tree over the holidays — a ritual Ben normally enjoyed — he refused to go. Later, when Melissa turned on some music and she and Ben's siblings set about decorating the tree, Ben became irritated and rude, then withdrawn and apathetic, isolating himself in his room.

Since Ben was receiving a full range of mental health services and was under strict screen management at home, I suspected we had overlooked some screen exposure, but I could not figure out where or when. Finally, I asked Ben about computer use at school. When he answered, "We use it a little bit, but not really," I knew he was probably minimizing. I suggested to Melissa that she investigate the matter a little further, and she promptly asked for a meeting with Ben's teacher.

Ben attended a small private school, and he had the same teacher throughout the day. Melissa learned that the teacher — trying to be helpful — had made a deal with Ben that if he got to school on time and turned his work in, he'd earn computer time. He could also use it during his lunch break, so Ben was essentially getting a couple hours' worth of either Internet or computer game time every day. Melissa explained what we were trying to accomplish, and the teacher started awarding Ben with non-screen rewards instead. Ben's mood lifted, and he began engaging more with his family.

Be aware that school-related screen-time can add up quickly. On the one hand, this child "forgot" to mention his computer time at school, so it was overlooked. On the other hand, we thought his teacher might be resistant to changing Ben's reward system, but once Ben's mother explained what we were doing and why, the teacher proved to be an ally instead.

"We Need a Doctor's Note": Obtaining Reset Accommodations at School

Let's say you want to eliminate computer use at school before you start the Reset, or you wind up wanting to do so as a troubleshooting intervention. To accomplish this, sometimes a parent need only make the request in writing that his or her child be taken off computers for a few weeks, but sometimes the school will request a doctor's or therapist's note. Depending on the school's policies, they may require the note to be signed by an "M.D.," as this effectively makes the request an order to be implemented "out of medical necessity." Whether you ask a pediatrician, psychiatrist, or therapist, it is helpful to provide a template, though he or she may want to edit or rewrite it. See chapter 5, "Reset Planning and School" (page 158), for an example, and visit the book's website to obtain a downloadable form (use the password "resetdocs").

Even if your child's physician has little knowledge of screen-time effects, he or she would be hard pressed to deny this request, as the fast presents zero risk and potentially large benefits. Rather, it's more likely to be denied because of the hassle-factor or out of confusion, which is why the template is helpful. If you're requesting this from a physician, I suggest calling or emailing the doctor's office first to explain what you're requesting, then making an appointment to visit the doctor in person to explain the reasons why and to have it signed. You can attach references as needed (see the next section as well). For more help, visit www.ResetYourChildsBrain.com.

Making a "Disability" Argument for Electronic-Related Accommodations

Children with a disability (mental, physical, or learning) that is affecting educational performance are technically eligible for an "individualized education plan" (IEP) or a 504 Plan that is tailored to assist the child in school in a manner specific to his or her needs. An IEP or 504 Plan outlines any accommodations the school will provide to make learning or schoolwork easier for that child. If you want your child to benefit from long-term accommodations above and beyond a Reset time frame, and your child already has an IEP or 504 Plan, you can request that tech-related accommodations be formally included in the plan. Without such a plan, you can still request such accommodations, but even if the teacher agrees to them, they aren't legally enforceable.

Examples of tech- or electronic-related accommodations include being able to complete and turn in assignments without having to use the computer and/or the Internet, not being allowed video game play or computer time as a reward or during recess, restricting the number of hours of computer or screen-time per week, opting out of "pilot programs," such as those that incorporate iPads, and moving to a WiFi-free classroom. Other accommodations that can mitigate electronic-related stress include being seated near a window to increase exposure to natural sunlight, having more breaks outdoors, being allowed to move about the classroom more often, and reduced or eliminated homework.

How does one go about getting screen-time or WiFi-related recommendations incorporated into an IEP or 504? Since ESS and sensitivity to EMFs aren't formal diagnoses, you would need to make an argument that ties the request to a formal disorder or disability that your child already has or is suspected of having. Since 504s and IEPs are based on law, an effective argument would need to do the following:

1. Link the child's current recognized or suspected disability to sensitivity to electronics (such as to screen-time in general, computer use, EMF exposure, or light-at-night);
2. Show that the sensitivity leads to an exacerbation of your child's symptoms;
3. Show that the exacerbated symptoms in turn result in impaired academic performance; and
4. Show there are reasonable alternatives or accommodations that can be made.

To strengthen your argument, attach references from studies, reports, and books that cite screen-time effects relevant to your child's case; all the research referenced in this book can be found in the endnotes. Naturally, you may also need to provide documentation from your child's treatment providers, including a letter from a physician or therapist supporting the recommendation. In terms of complying with the request, in my experience some schools care more about research references, and others prioritize written recommendations from a treating clinician.

For example, let's say your child has ADHD and has an IEP, and one year your child gets enrolled in a classroom that utilizes iPads for numerous "educational" tasks, homework, presentations, and so on. To obtain accommodations to opt out of this practice, you could make the argument that, for children with ADHD, even modest amounts of screen-time can affect attention, memory, sleep quality, and impulse control. For each of these impacts, you might reference published research by providing a citation (the basic information such as title, authors, and date), an abstract (a formal summary of study findings), or an entire article; many studies are available for download these days to the general public. If you wanted to include eliminating exposure to WiFi, too, you could cite research linking EMF exposure to impaired behavior, learning, and memory in human and animal studies, and provide the official recommendation from the American Academy of Environmental Medicine that for safer technology use, hard-wiring is preferred.

If your child doesn't have a formalized plan already in place, he or she may be eligible for one. Indeed, children with mental health or behavior disorders often *are* eligible, but they are more likely to have fallen through the cracks because of stigma and other reasons. Any parent can request an eligibility assessment by making a request for an IEP in writing to the school principal or vice principal. Though it might seem like a hassle to get it set up, education plans give your child more options, which will become increasingly important if current trends in education and technology continue.

Chapter 11 Take-Home Points

- Don't neglect the school day and homework time as significant sources of screen-time, but the Reset is usually successful without eliminating school-related screen-time if fast guidelines and house rules are strictly followed.
- You may need to assess and address school-related screen-time if the Reset is unsuccessful or if your child's classroom or curriculum is tech-heavy.
- Don't be seduced by "cool" or "innovative" tech-related methods of teaching that claim superior results. Educational technology studies are largely negative or neutral at best.
- Don't be concerned about your child being left behind if he or she has less technology exposure compared to peers. Computer skills are relatively easy to learn, but poor attention and dysregulation from a poorly developed frontal lobe make it hard to learn or accomplish anything.
- Media multitasking leads to a slowing of work, reduced accuracy, and impaired attention.
- Movement, human connection, and exposure to nature improve learning and support nervous system development.
- If your child's school is tech-aggressive, it's extra important to balance this by creating an *au naturale* environment at home.
- If your child has or needs an IEP or 504 plan, you may be able to obtain electronic-related accommodations by arguing that electronics exacerbate your child's disorder or disability.
- Don't be passive with school-related technology issues; parents have a voice. Plant seeds, band together, and teach others.

CHAPTER 12

FROM GRASSROOTS
TO GLOBAL AWARENESS

Building Support for Overcoming ESS

*It's just human nature to take time to connect the dots. I know that.
But I also know there can be a day of reckoning,
when you wish you had connected the dots more quickly.*

— Al Gore, *An Inconvenient Truth*[1]

*Here's good advice for practice: go into partnership with nature;
she does more than half the work and asks none of the fee.*

— Martin H. Fischer, on the practice of medicine[2]

We create our children's futures. We don't know what the next wave of technology will bring, but surely being mindful of vulnerabilities specific to children, and to mental health in general, can help us to adapt to technology in a more graceful and balanced manner in the future. If we were all more aware of the magnitude, severity, and variety of electronic-related stress that most of us are exposed to on a daily basis, and we all took action accordingly, we would not only reduce suffering from mental and physical illnesses, but we'd dramatically reduce the costs associated with these illnesses. This, in turn, could free up resources to provide what children, families, and communities *really* need to thrive.

Lessons from Big Tobacco

If we keep in mind that technology is an *industry* — with associated corporations beholden to shareholders, not the general public — we can begin to build the framework needed to change how we view and use technology. We need to be conscious of the fact that, ultimately, corporations and even small businesses are driven by profits, not good will. This is not a bad thing in and of itself; the tech industry — with its related ed-tech, entertainment, communications, information, and medical components — creates an enormous number of jobs and helps drive the economy as a whole. But financial incentive does need to be considered. Indeed, it can *become* a bad thing if messages conceived to drive profits impact health and education. With the tobacco industry, this kind of realization — that the industry was motivated by profit, not scientific truth — is what helped shift attitudes toward smoking, since it allowed the dangers of smoking to be brought to light and helped the public and health agencies to appreciate that "evidence" denying these dangers was being manufactured. As such, let's look at a page from the tobacco story.

Early tobacco warnings regarding health risks were undermined by a powerful industry whose strategy was to create doubt and confusion. They accomplished this by repeatedly sending the message to the public (via the popular press) that there was a lack of consensus about whether or not smoking caused health risks, and by funding "research" at respected institutions with hand-picked unscrupulous researchers whose findings were communicated to Congress.[3] Other strategies included aggressive marketing to younger and younger consumers — thereby acquiring addicted lifelong customers — and manufacturing "healthy" (filtered) cigarettes, while simultaneously altering cigarette composition to make them more addictive. Tobacco marketers decried government regulation proposals as both a violation of personal freedom and a belittling of one's capacity to be responsible for one's own health. Since then, we've seen many of these same arguments and marketing tactics being used in various industries, including the chemical and food and beverage industries.[4]

The technology industry uses these tactics, too — masterfully. For starters, concerns about screen-time affecting attention and brain development are held at bay by industry-funded research claiming the opposite. The mountain of evidence of screen-time's harmful effects on cognition *appears* to be the same size as the evidence for "positive" studies, but only because the peddlers of the studies on positive findings have mountains of money to publicize them. In reality, there is probably a 20:1 ratio between negative and positive studies, and it's probably higher than that if you exclude nonbiased research. Other health concerns are equally discounted or are quieted by a new spin: just as "safe" cigarettes were made, "healthy" video games and "educational" software are made; worry that screen-time makes us lazy is met with arguments about the stimulating effects of "interactive" screen-time; and concerns about technology making us disconnected and lonely are fought with reassurances that the Internet and social media "connect us all." Meanwhile, video game designers purposely hook players into games that never end, and electronics advertisers market to younger and younger children, who then become dependent on devices for the rest of their lives. Perhaps most disturbing of all is that the infusion of technology into public education has created an ongoing "need" for more equipment and more products, making schools themselves dependent on the tech industry.[5]

Then there are the parallels regarding "personal choice" tactics. People — and especially Americans — don't like their freedom being restricted. But how free to choose is a child who has become addicted to technology before his or her brain has finished developing, making the addiction a much bigger beast to tame? We adults determine the environment our children grow up in — but children have no choice. When suggestions are made to limit children's screen-time, we are reminded that this threatens our personal freedom, that Americans do not want the government in their living rooms telling them what to do, and yet ironically, at the same time our children are being forced into using technology in public schools — largely because of government mandates such as the Common Core — whether they like or not, whether it brings inherent health risks or not, and whether it helps them or not. On top of that, their data is being mined in the name of education, but in reality it's used and sold to make more profit. Are Big Tech companies really benevolent, really free of conflict of interest, when they "donate" equipment and software in exchange for contracts to use their technology? With taxpayer dollars, no less?

When tech corporations play to our emotions by selling the promise of individualized education adapting to each child's specific needs, or of creating "readiness for succeeding in today's world," they create an atmosphere that makes us feel we can't possibly survive without them. This is despite evidence that the majority of kids — with and without special needs — are hurt and not helped by tech in the classroom. Since when are evidenced-based methods of learning no longer the gold standard?

While contemplating these issues might make us uncomfortable, it's important to be conscious of them and to remember how powerful and sophisticated marketing tactics are these days. Be clear about the fact that politicians, governing bodies, and corporations don't always (or perhaps even usually) have our best interests in mind; that's just the reality of it. Ultimately, no one cares about your children more than you do. But that doesn't mean you're powerless; it just means you have to make decisions about your child's future consciously, take advice regarding the "benefits" of technology with a grain of salt, and make healthy choices where you can.

In fact, by doing so, you help others to do the same — which takes power away from deceptive practices, and brings truth to light. The benefits of technology can still be realized, but the impact of technology needs to be taken much more seriously and viewed more realistically.

The Butterfly Effect: Practical Ways to Raise Awareness and Enact Change

One of the more interesting laws of nature is that small changes in energy can create large forces over space and time. Scientists have found this phenomenon exemplified in weather systems, where small breezes collectively alter currents that span the globe. In theory, an insect flapping its wings could contribute to weather patterns that eventually become strong enough to cause a hurricane or tornado thousands of miles away: hence, the "butterfly effect."

My hope is that everyone who practices the Reset principles and mindful screen management will together effect a change that can grow until it changes our culture's practices regarding technology. Each time you consciously act to reduce screen influences, you send a message to others — even if you don't share information verbally. Each time you approach another parent about doing an electronic fast together, he or she may mention the idea to someone else. Each teacher you speak to has influence over numerous students, year after year, while each doctor or therapist has influence over dozens, hundreds, or even thousands of children over time. Just as changing your child's screen habits now will affect his or her life trajectory, so do small efforts to raise awareness extend beyond your initial action. It's a law of nature!

Here are some ways to initiate your own butterfly effect. You may wish to revisit this section after you've already done the Reset with your own child. When ready to share, you can access fact sheets and other resources at www.ResetYourChildsBrain.com.

Mentor a Fellow Parent

Sharing your Reset experience with another mother or father can be a powerful method of raising awareness. Word-of-mouth from mother to mother conveys particularly strong testimony — stronger than I could ever give by telling you my experiences with patients. If you know another parent who might benefit, share your experience, loan him or her the book, and offer to help. This help might be offering screen-free activities for their child and yours, babysitting, or taking the parent out for a break. You can also offer phone support during the fast as questions or problems arise.

Form a Reset Club

I first mention utilizing preexisting communities to do the Reset with a group of parents in chapter 8 ("Parenting Communities," page 213); here is an expanded description of what to do. A community Reset is a highly effective approach, but it requires some organization. It can be done the first time you do the fast, during subsequent Resets, or simply as a way to maintain ongoing screen-time limits within a like-minded group of friends and neighbors. Forming a Reset "club" within your own community creates a win-win for everyone involved, as each child's improved functioning creates virtuous cycles within and between children, and more and more parents conduct screen-free child care.

As with any productive group endeavor, each meeting should embody three elements: a mission or vision statement, goals, and an action plan. Begin recruiting by putting out feelers for interested parents among friends, neighbors, and your child's playmates' parents. Tell them you want to start a club to support healthy play and reduce screen-time, and if appropriate, add that it'll be particularly helpful for kids with behavior, mood, or attention problems. PTA meetings and neighborhood get-togethers are good places to find prospective members. For parents interested in participating, provide information about the book or the book's website and ask them to read part 1 prior to the first meeting. You can also offer to loan or share copies.

For interested parties who don't want to read an entire book, ask that they read the email course available at www.ResetYourChildsBrain.com and a few of the key articles on my *Psychology Today* blog, such as "Electronic Screen Syndrome," "Gray Matters," and "Wired and Tired."[6] One reason to suggest this "homework" is that it will help you screen for parents who are highly motivated and who won't balk at the idea of a strict fast. I recommend keeping the group small, say two to six parents, and not more than ten or so. Once you've recruited some like-minded parents, here are some tips that'll give your fledgling Reset club some legs:

1. *Recruit a cohost.* Prior to the first official meeting, see if you can get at least one other mother or father to cohost with you. Hearing ideas from two parents can be more convincing than just one, and the extra support will help you, too.

2. *Establish a clear agenda.* Keep a Reset club notebook and ask someone to volunteer to take notes during each meeting. Begin each meeting with the purpose of the club and your goals, followed by meaningful discussion (educational, brainstorming, planning activities, and so on), and ending with action items.

3. *Identify individual and group goals.* For the first meeting especially, have each parent verbalize and write down what problems they're experiencing and what they'd like to see instead. For each meeting, talk about individual goals ("Joey will display fewer tantrums") as well as group or community goals ("Incorporate more outdoor play each weekend").

4. *Educate and support one another.* During the first meeting, the host(s) can lead a discussion about the mechanisms and effects leading to ESS and ask each member how this has impacted home and school life. During the first or second meeting, brainstorm activities and how you can help one another with child care as well as breaks.

5. *Have specific action items, delegate, and take turns.* Each meeting should end with a clear plan. Delegate tasks as appropriate, with the shared understanding that some weeks may require more time and energy than others. Plan activities the children can do by themselves, with the family, and as a group, and get down hard dates as much as possible.

6. *Chart results.* Following the fast, schedule an in-person meeting where you document each child's results (see chapters 5 and 7). Tracking, appreciating benefits, and obtaining validation and praise from others are highly reinforcing for long-term screen management, so make this meeting fun and social to ensure members show up.

7. *Determine meeting schedule.* The right frequency is a delicate balance: meeting too often feels like too much work, while too little reduces compliance. During the fast, try to meet weekly, in person, by phone, or even via group text to maximize support and compliance, and to problem solve as needs change. Following the fast, try to meet once a month and adjust as needed. If and when one or more members start to feel things are backsliding, meet more frequently and in person until everyone is back on track.

8. *Reinforce your vision.* At the beginning and end of each meeting, state your group's purpose: why you've all come together, and what changes you'd like to see. For example, "This Reset Club has been formed because we're concerned about the health implications of too much technology, and we want to optimize our children's brain, body, and character development."

9. *Schedule Reset "checkups."* As the host or leader, place an ongoing calendar reminder every six months to check in with the group. Invariably families will revert back to their old screen habits, so determine whether the Reset needs to be repeated. Alternatively, some members may have realized their child cannot tolerate any screen-time at all, in which case these parents may wish to work more closely with a smaller group (for example, with only parents of autistic children).

10. *Expect attrition and change.* As with any group, attrition will occur, although some members may return if they begin experiencing serious difficulties again. Needs and circumstances may change over time as well.

Generally, parents will be able to offer different resources. Some parents are good at brainstorming and organizing group games, others might be available to give rides or watch the children, and others may contribute by buying snacks or contributing monetarily. Single parents will likely need to depend on other parents more — but that's the beauty of "the village" mentality.

A valuable benefit of this method is that it can provide everyone regular, planned breaks. What mother wouldn't die for a day when she has a few solid hours to herself? Remember, since you're replacing "screen breaks" with organized activities and kid time, you need to replace those breaks more than ever. Overall, forming a Reset club requires more time and effort in the beginning, but it also affords a great deal of support.

Talk to Physicians and Mental Health Clinicians

Bring this book or relevant articles from my blog (perhaps on subjects that are relevant to your child) to your child's physician or therapist's office. Again, the aforementioned articles "Electronic Screen Syndrome: An Unrecognized Disorder" and "Gray Matters: Too Much Screen Time Damages the Brain" are good places to start a conversation. The latter article provides a review of brain scan studies that may be particularly intriguing to physicians. You can share the results you observed from the Reset, including specific benefits to mood, focus, behavior, and sleep. Even if these discussions are restricted to issues pertaining to your child, the information may be relevant to many other families as well as colleagues that the practitioner works with. As such, sharing with clinicians can have a potentially very large butterfly effect.

Invite a Teacher to Reset the Entire Class

Today, teachers sometimes conduct electronic or technology fasts for a few days at a time as an assignment, and schools across the country now participate in "National Screen-Free Week" in May of each year, which is organized by the Campaign for a Commercial-Free Childhood (CCFC, www.screen free.org). But why not suggest the entire class try a fast for three weeks? The teacher would need to be willing to not assign any computer-related homework. Even if parents don't fully participate, the effort still raises awareness.

Share Info at a PTA Meeting

Ask if you can give a five-minute presentation at the end of a PTA meeting about ESS and the fast. Start a sign-up sheet for parents and teachers who want to hear more and provide the downloadable fact sheet from the book's website. This is also a great way to recruit parents for a community Reset.

Present to the School Board

As more schools require students to use school-issued iPads or laptops, more parents are feeling the need to intervene. I've received dozens of emails from parents about their plans to complain to the school board. Some are concerned about the effects of EMFs from WiFi (see appendix B), and others do not want to add more screen-time impacts on their children. This is a hot topic that will likely grow in scope. Check this book's website regularly for advice, presentation materials, and resources, including information about opting out; as parents send me more feedback, I will pass along what they've learned.

In the meantime, be sure to read "Fool's Gold: A Critical Look at Computers in Childhood," an eye-opening report produced by the Alliance for Childhood, which summarizes studies and issues regarding children, technology, and education (www.allianceforchildhood.org/fools_gold). And check out Dr. Aric Sigman's presentation on warnings about the impact of screen media on children to the European Parliament's Quality of Childhood Group; see endnotes for the link.[7]

Join Child Advocacy Groups

Dr. Richard Louv, author of *Last Child in the Woods: Saving Our Children from Nature Deficit Disorder*,[8] founded the Children and Nature Network, whose mission is to connect children, families, and communities to nature (www.childrenandnature.org). Campaign for a Commercial-Free Childhood (CCFC, www.screenfree.org) is concerned with not only screen-time but also the commercialization of childhood, including how most toys these days are heavily branded and how marketing to children often includes irresponsible messages that encourage poor nutrition, early sexualization, and dependency on screen activities.

Ask Corporations to Donate Funds

To support accessibility to safe outdoor play areas — which are particularly critical for children in urban areas — ask tech corporations to donate funds for building, repairing, and creating parks, playgrounds, community gardens, and nature walks. If tech companies are profiting from doing business with public entities, and wish us to believe they have good intentions, challenge them to donate funds that support healthy and safe outdoor play.

Network with Moms' Groups

As I say, mothers are often the ones who initiate a Reset, and they are also more likely to be a part of organized parenting communities. "Mommy and Me" groups can be found everywhere and encompass a wide range of ages and interests (visit www.mommy-me.meetup.com to find meetings in your area). Often these groups have a focus on healthy play, parenting, and bonding, so introducing the Reset might be met with welcoming arms. Another interesting group of proactive mothers is Moms Rising (www.momsrising .org), whose tagline is "Where moms and people who love them go to change our world." Finally, there are both grassroots groups of parents and formal organizations concerned about WiFi in schools; these groups are a natural fit for embracing the concept of ESS and the electronic fast. Visit www.wifiin schools.com for news items and research information, and check the book's website for updated information regarding groups dedicated to the safe use of technology in schools.

Share via Social Media, Blogs, and Listservs

Perhaps ironically, online communities have made the goal of global awareness of ESS and screen-time management much easier to achieve. When pediatric occupational therapist Cris Rowan blogged about ten reasons to ban handheld devices for children under twelve in the *Huffington Post*,[9] the article received more than a million views and hundreds of comments in a matter of days and was passed around on Facebook for months. The post obviously touched on a nerve!

There are also Listservs (such as Yahoo groups) and social media communities for parents and practitioners who want to discuss and share natural or integrative treatment information for complex psychiatric and neurological disorders. Members share links to articles or resources in addition to describing their experiences. Look for one that's associated with your child's particular struggles and share your experience with the Reset. (Of course, be careful about online communication becoming time or energy consuming.)

Never Stop Learning

You don't need to become a neuroscientist, but the better you understand the issues, the better you'll become at noticing when screen-time is affecting your own children, and the better equipped you'll be to help others. Pursue those topics that relate to your circumstances or concern you the most, and make yourself an expert in them.

Hopefully this book has provided you with a solid foundation, but it can also be used as a springboard. Make a note of which studies or references struck a chord with you; many of the articles in the endnotes can be downloaded and read in full, and of course they have their own references, too. Another good resource is Cris Rowan's blog (www.movingtolearn.ca). Rowan provides razor sharp insights on the impact of technology through a developmental lens, and the site provides toolkits, games, and a list of hundreds of research articles on screen-time's effects on learning, development, and attachment. The Campaign for a Commercial-Free Childhood (www .screenfree.org) also has a blog and a list of research articles with links.

Use the Media

If you identify a technology issue that affects the general public, particularly if it involves safety, unethical activity, or human rights, consider approaching journalists and media outlets.

Often, issues involving schools generate interest, since they affect many in the community and the public at large. Some themes that have regularly appeared in the media recently are the fallout from "teaching to the test" and issues related to the Common Core, investigations into staff members receiving kickbacks or "gifts" surrounding district-wide purchases of electronic devices or software, and parents and teachers objecting to WiFi in the classroom. There have also been stories that raise awareness or that point out small victories; for example, the aforementioned articles about tech execs limiting screen-time with their own children.

Media stories can sometimes force change when questionable actions are made public and can help spread the word when schools or communities make positive changes.

Looking Back, Looking Ahead

The medical school I attended happens to be one of the oldest in the nation. In one of the lecture halls, old black-and-white photographs line the walls, depicting a history of the hospital and its physicians since the mid-1800s. One of them shows several physicians standing outside a patient's room smoking cigarettes during what is presumably the doctors' morning rounds. Everyone got a kick out of this photo — how ironic it was! My hope is that eventually we'll have this same kind of feeling about present-day screen-time practices. We'll see how ironic it is to teach children with methods that impair concentration and creativity, to exercise them with mediums linked to obesity, or to parent them with devices that induce temper tantrums. It simply doesn't make sense.

And yet we cannot expect a parent to forgo reliance on a device if he or she cannot rely upon community. Parents and their children need easy access to safe, outdoor play areas, to greenery and nature indoors and out, and they need school environments that promote movement and creativity rather than easy access to yet more screens. We need to be conscious of how technology is being used and of how *mis*use is further deepening the divide between the more and less fortunate. Quality of life and success will always be optimized by a healthy brain, solid self-esteem, and a sense of true connectedness with others — *especially* for children struggling with other issues. Thus, to best raise our children, we must restore our trust in Mother Nature, choose truth and reality over technology's razzle-dazzle, and return to living in the manner in which individuals and society function best — as a village.

Ultimately, everything worthwhile in life takes work. In the quest to make this book happen, when I got so tired of writing that I wanted to cry (and often did), I'd turn to William Zinsser's classic *On Writing Well*[10] to inspire me, keep me on track, and remind me why I was writing in the first place — to help you help your child. You and I share the same goal. I'll leave you with his words, which will hopefully linger in your head as they did mine:

"Decide what you want to do. Then decide to do it. Then do it."

Chapter 12 Take-Home Points

- Parenting, education, and medicine all need to be conducted with mindful awareness of screen-time's impact on mental and physical health, learning, and overall development.
- The history of Big Tobacco teaches valuable lessons about how industries exploit biology and emotion in marketing products and in making products more addicting or compelling.
- Once screen management changes have been made in your own home, awareness can be expanded by sharing information at the local, institutional, and global levels, making it easier for other parents to implement changes for their own children.
- Locally, information can be shared via community Reset efforts with friends, neighbors, your child's playmate's parents, coaches, and teachers.
- Sharing information at the institutional level, such as with your child's school, can leverage efforts by reaching many parents and educators at once.
- Globally, the Internet allows for rapid dissemination of information via emails, Listservs, blogs, social media, and online communities — though of course online endeavors should be kept short and focused.
- Despite the ubiquitous nature of screens and the growth of handheld devices, individuals can make powerful contributions toward the growing screen-awareness movement by consciously choosing green-time over screen-time, practicing face-to-face over face-to-screen, and relying on one another so that no parent is forced to rely on a device.

APPENDIX A

TABLE OF PHYSIOLOGICAL MECHANISMS AND EFFECTS OF INTERACTIVE SCREEN-TIME

Multiple aspects of electronic screen device use trigger fight-or-flight reactions and compound chronic stress via changes in brain chemistry, hormones, blood flow, sensory processing, circadian rhythms, and the biofield. The following table outlines the pathways, mechanisms, and repercussions of electronic screen media use — all of which contribute to ESS. As such, it summarizes much of the information from chapter 2 and some from chapter 3, and it serves as a succinct reference for sharing information with others.

PATHWAY	MECHANISM	REPERCUSSIONS
Eyes	Visual stimulation	Sensory overload, overactive visual attention
	Electrical excitability	Erratic nerve firing, seizures, migraines, tics
	Blue light/intense light	Body clock disruption, melatonin suppression, sleep and hormone alterations, inflammation, dysregulation of serotonin, inflammation of retina
Brain	Dopamine dysregulation	Cravings, anxiety, withdrawal, mood swings, poor focus, disorganization, irritability, depression, activated reward/addiction pathways
	Blood flow shifts	Stunted frontal lobe development, poor executive functioning, mood dysregulation, poor impulse control
	Intense psychological engagement	intimacy issues, poor eye contact, addiction, suppressed creativity
	Orienting response and fight-or-flight	Hyperarousal, overstimulation, non-restorative sleep, body clock disruption, altered brain chemistry and hormones, inflammation
Body	Stagnation of blood flow despite fight-or-flight reaction	Weight gain, reduced nutrient absorption, toxin accumulation, muscle ache, repressed energy
	Fight-or-flight activation	Increased blood pressure and heart rate, hormonal imbalance, reduced heart rate variability (HRV), reduced blood flow to gut and other organs, suppressed immune system
	EMF interference with biofield	Stress response, nervous system electrical excitability, inflammation, cellular stress, DNA breaks, altered brain waves, disrupted blood-brain barrier?
	Prolonged sitting and repetitive movements	Musculoskeletal inflammation, muscle atrophy, repetitive stress injuries, blood clots, neck/back strain, weak "core" muscles

Table 5. Pathways, mechanisms, and repercussions of interactive screen-time

ELECTROMAGNETIC FIELDS (EMFs) AND HEALTH

A "Charged" Issue

Like electricity itself, the question of whether radiation from electronics causes harm is a polarizing force. People tend to believe either that EMFs are perfectly safe or that electronic-related radiation is the primary (or even only) reason that electronic screen devices produce dysfunction. But in fact the answer is not black or white, because the relationship between biology and manmade electromagnetic fields (EMFs) is nuanced and complex. At the same time, much of the science is not yet conclusive. That said, the following three points are abundantly clear: children absorb more radiation than adults; developing children are more sensitive to environmental exposures of all kinds; and impacts from environmental exposures can take decades to manifest.[1] Therefore, risk regarding EMFs need only be *plausible* to justify a precautionary approach — particularly in regard to children. The information presented here is far from comprehensive, but the better the general public understands what our youngest citizens face — who after all have no voice and no choice regarding what environmental impacts they're exposed to — the more likely it is that safe and ethical public policy will follow.

The term *radiation* itself contributes to the controversy surrounding EMFs because it's typically associated with the potency of nuclear power plants, cancer treatments, and X-rays. But radiation simply refers to the energy that's produced or sent out by electromagnetic fields in the form of waves, which vary in strength and wavelength (frequency), among other characteristics. In fact, natural things emit radiation, too, including the sun, the earth, and all forms of life. The problem is that radiation from manmade EMFs produced by electronic devices and wireless communications is multiplying rapidly, and it's unclear how the natural environment is handling such massive change.

The Biofield: The Body Electric

Along with the eyes, brain, and body, there exists another interface between electronic screen devices and your child: the *biofield*. The National Institute of Health now recognizes the term *biofield*[2] to describe the complex matrix of biological electromagnetic fields that emanate within, through, and around the human body. These include fields that are easily measured, such as those produced by the brain, heart, muscles, nerves, skin, and cell membranes, as well as extremely weak or "subtle" fields, which may serve to instantly transmit information in a non-linear fashion.[3] For example, coherent heart rhythm patterns induce coherent brain wave patterns within the same person, but they can also induce similar changes in those standing nearby, suggesting an energetic transfer of information.[4] Likewise, "clock" cells located in the brain can synchronize or desynchronize rhythms throughout the body instantaneously, by a kind of secret cell-to-cell communication. All these different fields have varying frequencies and intensities, and they also produce a field as a whole.

By definition, electromagnetic fields are physical fields produced by moving electrically charged objects that affect the behavior of other charged objects in their vicinity. In other words, fields influence one another if they're close enough to one another. Indeed, studies have demonstrated that EMFs from wireless communications can alter electromagnetic fields produced by the brain (as detected by EEG) and the heart (as detected by EKG).[5] It's much more difficult, however, to measure and understand the complex interactions between manmade fields and frequencies of individual brain cells or groups of brain cells, and how those interactions in turn impact the subtle fields.

Although the dynamics between electronics and the biofield are poorly understood, it is impossible to ignore this interface as a pathway contributing to electronic-related stress. Various electronic components, including screens, monitors, batteries, hard drives, and wiring, emit different types of radiation that can potentially disrupt the biofield. However, wireless communications produce microwave radiation* that may be particularly harmful, and our exposure to it has grown exponentially in recent years. Thus, hand-held devices with screens — whereby the user's hands are close to the battery and the eyes are close to the screen — that *also* use wireless signals may be particularly disruptive.

All Revved Up: Biological Effects from Manmade EMFs

Biophysicists who study radiation emitted from everyday electronic devices think that the radiation produced by unnatural EMFs perturbs the body's own energy fields. One theory is that when natural biological fields are disrupted by strong manmade fields, the biofield becomes disorganized or incoherent at the quantum (or the most fundamental) level, causing stress and interrupting information transmission.[6] This incoherence is an instantaneous response that gets transmitted to the *entire* biofield — not just at the point of contact. Others think that extremely weak manmade fields might be capable of desynchronizing cells or tissue via resonance or entrainment effects.[7]

Whatever the mechanism, tangible evidence of the EMF-stress relationship exists for both systemic (whole body) stress reactions and cellular stress reactions. Exposure studies have demonstrated systemic stress reactions in the form of high blood sugar, low heart-rate variability, altered circadian rhythms, disrupted sleep patterns, and impaired cognition.[8] Cellular stress has been evidenced by increased levels of heat shock proteins (HSPs, whose

---

* Microwaves (used by wireless communications) are a form of high-frequency radiation in the radiofrequency (RF) band of the electromagnetic spectrum. Thus, EMFs from wireless communication are referred to as "microwave," "RF," or "high frequency" (the latter of which differentiates them from extremely low frequency, or ELF, waves).

function is to stabilize other proteins when the cell is exposed to stress), oxidative stress (free radicals), breaks in DNA strands, and excessive unbound calcium inside the cell.[9]

In addition to these reactions, some animal studies suggest that manmade EMFs — including the frequencies produced by cell phones and WiFi — may disrupt the blood-brain barrier, leaving the brain vulnerable to substances it would otherwise be protected from.[10] This is a controversial area, and findings have not been consistent. Nevertheless, acute stress itself has been shown to trigger leakage of the blood-brain barrier via the activation of particular immune cells called mast cells.[11] Mast cells, in turn, have been shown to be activated by EMFs in some sensitive individuals,[12] so the link between EMFs and leakage of the blood-brain barrier is plausible. Another possible mechanism is related to the aforementioned heat shock proteins, which when overproduced can bind up the cell and make it more rigid. If the cell becomes too rigid or proteins in the membrane get pulled on, the membrane can ripple and/or the entire cell can shrink. When rippling or shrinkage occurs in rows of cells that are meant to provide a barrier from the outside world, gaps are created in between these cells, and the barrier becomes compromised. (Normally, barrier cells seal off areas by connecting with their next-door neighbors via "tight junctions," so they can closely control what goes in or out.) Similarly, HSPs and/or excess calcium can cause individual cell membranes to become more fragile, whereby the cell membrane itself (rather than the junctions between cells) leaks or becomes dysfunctional.

Most likely these processes proceed at different speeds depending on what other stressors the cells are being subjected to, such that leakiness doesn't occur until a tipping point is reached. This may explain why blood-brain barrier studies aren't always consistent. As with all cellular damage, this kind of effect is more likely to happen in vulnerable individuals whose nervous systems are less resilient to begin with.

Sensitive and Vulnerable: The Eyes, Brain, and Reproductive Organs

Generally speaking, sensitivity to radiation varies with tissue type and whether there is any "remodeling" going on within that tissue. Tissues that are actively growing or changing are more likely to absorb radiation, which is one reason why children are more sensitive to electromagnetic radiation. Children are also more vulnerable because their bodies contain more water, and their brains are more vulnerable because their skulls are thinner. [13] Indeed, imaging studies clearly demonstrate that a child's brain and eyes absorb more radiation when exposed to mobile devices than an adult's.

In regard to types of tissues, the eyes, brain, and sex organs are the organs most sensitive to electromagnetic radiation. In addition to the blood-brain barrier findings, studies have linked EMFs to retinal cell damage (tissue at the back of the eye involved with vision), loss of hippocampal cells (an area involved in memory), altered brain chemistry (such as from reduced amounts of GABA, the "calming" brain chemical), reduced antioxidant levels in the brain's cortex (suggesting inflammation), and aberrant firing of brain cells or networks. [14]

Other well-documented effects include lowered sperm count and sperm damage in males, which have been found with both mobile phone and WiFi exposure; animal studies suggest that EMFs may be detrimental to female fertility (and the embryo) as well. [15] The impact on fertility is compounded when mobile devices are placed on the lap because both thermal (heating) and non-thermal effects are stronger. [16] As an aside, the reason sperm cells are so vulnerable is because they are actively growing and dividing, and thus they are more vulnerable to oxidative stress and heat. It's much harder to analyze the effect of electronics on young girls' eggs — which are also actively developing, albeit more slowly. Nor is it easy to determine whether laptop use affects other organs, all of which are more sensitive in children.

Lastly, some research suggests that the offspring of mothers exposed to higher levels of mobile phone radiation are more likely to have behavioral issues. [17]

Figure 9 on the next page summarizes the mechanisms and possible effects related to radiation from electronics and wireless communications, roughly in descending order according to scale (from systemic to cellular).

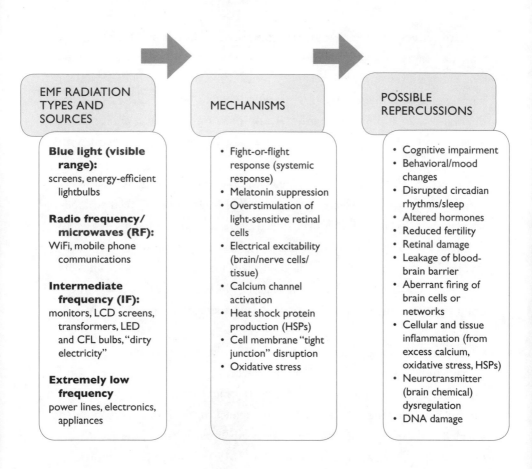

Figure 9. Potential mechanisms and repercussions from various types of radiation produced by electronics

It's Complicated...

Numerous experts who study the health effects of manmade EMFs maintain that they are causing a great deal more harm than regulatory agencies in the United States currently recognize. The discrepancy has arisen in part because US agencies primarily acknowledge only *thermal* (heating) effects from radiofrequency EMFs as damaging while virtually ignoring the growing body of research that has found damage from *non-thermal* effects. Already, however, nearly two thousand studies have documented non-thermal effects.[18]

The physics of non-thermal effects is complex and not altogether intuitive, contributing to the confusion. For example, a group of researchers at Lund

University Hospital in Sweden found delayed effects characterized by two discrete peaks in the days and weeks following exposure, and other research suggests there may be narrow "windows" of specific frequencies that cause harm.[19] These "non-linear" responses may explain why findings aren't always replicable, and they make findings difficult to understand. Meanwhile, non-thermal effects depend on a mind-boggling array of variables, including field frequency or wavelength, strength, nature (pulsed, intermittent, continuous, modulated), orientation, duration, and interaction with other fields. There are also variables involving individual differences in the person being exposed, such as age, gender, health, nutritional status, genetics, tissues involved, previous exposures, and so on. The more variables there are, the harder it is to replicate and compare studies. Most likely, non-thermal effects from manmade EMFs cause subtle and cumulative damage over time that is relatively hard to measure and difficult to prove. Considering all the difficulty in controlling variables and the oddly behaving physics, it's no wonder that the research is conflicting!

Other countries and governing agencies outside the United States, such as France, Israel, Germany, Switzerland, Russia, and the European Council, have been much more concerned about potential EMF effects, particularly in relation to children.[20] Medical organizations across Europe and in Canada and Australia have made objections to exposing children to wireless technology unnecessarily,[21] and the Parliamentary Assembly Council of Europe (PACE) considers WiFi use in schools to be a serious public health matter. PACE has warned: "Given the context of growing exposure of the population, in particular that of vulnerable groups, such as young people and children, there could be extremely high human and economic costs if early warnings are neglected."[22] In recent years, US medical organizations have also begun petitioning for a precautionary approach, including the American Academy of Environmental Medicine, which recommends children use wired-only Internet access,[23] and the American Academy of Pediatrics, which has written to the FCC and FDA recommending radiation limits be updated to reflect current use patterns and warning that children and pregnant women have unique vulnerabilities.[24] For more specifics regarding the growing use of WiFi in schools — which exposes children to daily and continuous amounts of radiofrequency radiation — see chapter 11 ("Exposure to EMFs from WiFi," page 268).

Autism: A Special Case?

Some experts feel the explosion of wireless communications has contributed to the growing rates of autism and ADHD, perhaps because of a breakdown of the gut and brain barriers.[25] Autism in particular is rising at an alarming rate; one recent study showed that even when diagnoses of milder cases and at younger ages were taken into account, autism increased more than five-fold from 1990 to 2006.[26]

Dr. Martha Herbert, a pediatric neurologist and autism expert at Harvard Medical School and Boston's Massachusetts General Hospital, published an extensive report in 2012 arguing that many of the pathological processes associated with autism parallel the effects observed in radiofrequency and other EMF research, and that it is therefore likely that use of electronic devices compounds autistic processes.[27] Dr. Herbert feels these effects should be considered a public health threat, not only because of the recent dramatic rise in autism and other mental disorders, but because WiFi is increasingly incorporated into our schools without regard for safety studies and without taking precautionary measures — such as simply using desktop computers with wired connections.

Effects gleaned from research on manmade EMFs that could theoretically trigger or worsen autism include: leakage of the blood-brain barrier, increased inflammation from oxidative stress, DNA damage and impaired repair mechanisms, abnormal calcium channel signaling in cells, an overly sensitized stress response, brain blood flow changes, excessive activation of mast cells, melatonin suppression, and electrical excitability.[28] Note that many of the effects thought to be produced by EMFs are the same as those discussed in chapter 2 from interactive screen-time — suggesting synergistic mechanisms may take place. These processes are likely occurring in all of us to some degree, but in a vulnerable autistic brain the consequences can be catastrophic.

Electrosensitivity vs. Electronic Screen Syndrome

Some people feel they are particularly sensitive to manmade EMFs. These *electrosensitive* or *electrohypersensitive* (EHS) individuals report that EMFs give them headaches, anxiety, depression, insomnia, and other stress-related symptoms. Although it's difficult to prove cause-and-effect with symptoms such as these that are subjective in nature, research indicates that some self-proclaimed sensitive individuals show objective skin inflammation markers when exposed to EMFs compared to controls.[29] There may be a connection to other sensitivities, too; children who have chemical, seasonal, or food allergies or sensitivities, including sensory issues, may be more affected by EMFs than others. In fact, the blood-brain barrier issues discussed above might explain why: that is, the same "tight junctions" between cells designed to protect the brain are also found in the barriers meant to protect the gut, eyes, skin, and lungs. These are tissues associated with modern-day conditions that are increasing in children and young adults — such as irritable bowel, autism, eczema, allergies, autoimmune disorders, and asthma. Interestingly, individuals who are electrosensitive may have lower electrical resistance (higher conductance).[30] Electrical changes in turn may cause calcium to flow into the cell, or cause the tight junctions to become leaky in various tissues, resulting in a wide variety of damage and symptoms.

Are ESS and EHS part of the same disorder? I contend that they are different entities that have synergistic mechanisms (such as altered circadian rhythms, melatonin suppression, and hyperarousal), as well as similar presentations — including issues with sleep, behavior, mood, and cognition. The clinical picture can look very similar. However, I started recognizing ESS phenomenon around the turn of the millennium, when children were playing a lot of video games but didn't own cell phones and wireless Internet wasn't widely available. So while these children had exposure to EMFs from electronic screen devices, they weren't exposed to the same level of wireless communications that they are today, and they weren't using handheld devices with screens held to their faces. Moreover, many parents today routinely implement the Reset successfully without turning off the WiFi in their home (although I wonder if they'd get even more dramatic results if they did). This suggests that much or most of the dysregulation in ESS is due to interacting with a screen device plus exposure to the bright screen itself. Likewise, many EHS sufferers "feel" WiFi or mobile phone signals without any screen devices visibly present, suggesting a mechanism independent of screen-time.

At present, an estimated 3 percent of adults suffer from EHS.[31] This number likely represents a smaller proportion of individuals compared to those affected by ESS, which I roughly estimate to be in the range of 15 to 20 percent of children. It is my feeling that because electrosensitive individuals have reactive systems, they are likely to be sensitive to ESS phenomenon *in addition* to EMFs. ESS sufferers, in contrast, may or may not suffer from EMF sensitivity. Children with environmentally sensitive disorders such as autism and allergies may be more prone to suffer from both, as may children with seizure disorders, tics, and ADHD.

Steps to Protect Your Child

Because of the nature of environmental exposures on physiology and development, it will take decades before some of the effects reveal themselves. In fact, some scientists speculate that it may be our *children's children* who show the full effects of the *present* level of exposure if DNA mutations are passed down to future generations. It's simply good medicine to take a conservative stance.

Although we can't hide from EMFs completely, here are some steps you can take that can dramatically reduce exposure:

1. *Turn off the wireless Internet access in your home.* Yes, I know this may seem extremely inconvenient, but try using hard-wired connections for a month and see if it makes a difference in your child (and in everyone else in the family, for that matter). EMF experts say you can see a difference in a sensitive individual in as little as three days. Wireless devices and routers emit electromagnetic radiation at all times, not just when the Internet is being used — but downloading increases the radiation many times over.[32] If you can't commit to giving up WiFi altogether, turn off the router each night manually or with a timer.

2. *Replace all compact fluorescent lightbulbs (CFLs).* Replace all CFL bulbs with incandescent (which is best), halogen (second best), or LEDs. All energy-efficient bulbs emit various kinds of radiation, but CFLs emit UV radiation as well. CFL and LED bulbs and LCD screens also emit blue-toned light that suppresses melatonin, and looking directly at screens is potentially damaging to the retina.[33] (See also chapter 7, "Unhealthy Lighting," page 197.)

3. *Reduce sources of EMFs where your child sleeps.* Move the clock radio from the nightstand to a dresser, move bedside lamps at least two feet from your child's head, and move any cords as far away from the bed as possible. If there is heavy wiring behind the wall

where your child's head lies, move the bed. Remove televisions and all other electronics from the room, and do not let your child keep a phone in the bedroom or use it in the evenings. The bed should be a sanctuary for rest.

4. *Use a landline for phone calls.* Make this a lifestyle choice for everyone in the house. Even better, use a corded phone. Pretend it's 1985.

5. *Use a wired headset.* If you must use your cell phone or a cordless phone for a call, use a wired headset or talk by speakerphone. Place the phone on a table as far away as you can. If you're downloading large files onto your smartphone, don't hold it in your hand; put it down and ideally far away from you.

6. *Put cell phones away when not in use.* When charging cell phones, overnight, and during "tech-free" times or in tech-free zones, put cell phones in another room. Even better, turn them off completely.

7. *Keep laptops and tablets off of the lap and mobile phones out of pockets.* This advice is especially important for children. As discussed above, EMFs affect sperm health in boys, may possibly damage girls' eggs, and they may affect other organs, too.

8. *Use a desktop computer whenever possible.* Desktops emit far less radiation than laptops or tablets; mobile devices emit stronger fields as well as more EMFs of varying frequencies, in part because their various electronic components are packaged into one device. Several types of radiation are emitted by laptop screens and touchscreens, and batteries, hard drives, wiring, and wireless signals contribute, too.[34] Furthermore, fingertips and the palms of the hands are highly conductive, which may magnify certain aspects of electropollution. Desktops also make it easier to maintain a distance of about two feet from your child's eyes and keep other components away from the body. If you only have mobile devices and don't have access to a desktop in your home, buy a separate (wired) keyboard and treat the mobile device as if it were a desktop. Note that WiFi capability needs to be actively *disabled* in laptops and tablets to eliminate the device from "searching."

9. *Opt your child out of school-based iPad or tablet programs.* Ask that your child be opted out of school programs that require the use of

wireless communication. In addition, if your child's school has WiFi powered on at all times, find out where the routers are and ask if your child can be placed in a WiFi-free classroom. If not, ask that the routers be turned on only when the class is using them. In 2014, a Los Angeles Unified teacher successfully petitioned to teach from a Wi-Fi-free classroom after she and several of her students experienced symptoms and illness following a school-wide WiFi installation.[35] (For more about WiFi in schools, see chapter 11.)

Public Policy and the Precautionary Principle

The essence of the precautionary principle is this: whenever research regarding a new technology suggests there is plausible risk for serious harm, we should take precautions to protect human and environmental health and use reasonable alternatives when we can, even if the science regarding such risk is not yet fully conclusive. Although the precautionary principle should be considered in regard to EMF hazards in general, it is especially applicable to the exposure of children to WiFi in schools. Aside from the fact that the World Health Organization recently classified radiofrequency fields as "possibly carcinogenic,"[36] there is enough evidence to suspect such fields stress the brain and other developing organs, and reasonable alternatives to wireless communications do exist.

For more information on the science, research, and policy regarding health effects of EMFs, visit the Environmental Health Trust (www.ehtrust.org) and the National Association for Children and Safe Technology (www.nacst.org). For more detailed research information and scientific summaries, visit BioInitiative 2012 (www.bioinitiative.org).

PARENTS' MOST
FREQUENTLY ASKED QUESTIONS

1. Is "an electronic fast" forever? Will moderation ever be okay?

How long you fast and the amount of use you allow after an electronic fast depend on several factors. The more risk factors your child has for developing ESS, and the more he or she is already struggling with ESS, the smaller the "dose" of screen exposure that can be tolerated. This means that following the Reset, some children will be able to reintroduce interactive screen-time in small amounts, while others won't be able to function well with any screen use at all. Regardless, parents who reintroduce devices afterward will have to learn by trial and error how much tech exposure, if any, their child can tolerate. How to mindfully manage screen-time after a Reset is the subject of chapter 9.

Notably, tolerability may increase with time and brain maturity, and some children can tolerate moderate amounts after being abstinent for longer periods (from months to years). For many children, teens, and young adults, continued elimination of all video games and banning all electronics from the bedroom is sufficient to prevent ESS from recurring.

2. Won't screen restrictions negatively affect my child's peer relationships — if they feel "out of the loop" regarding the latest computer programs, apps, Internet sites, and video games?

I have never seen a child's social life suffer as a result of screen limitations. Instead, one or more of the following occurs: One, the child complains that he or she can't talk about video games with certain friends, but in reality, relationships aren't "suffering" per se. If the child can't find other common ground with these friends, he or she migrates to other friends. Two, the child's peer relationships improve because the child now has improved frustration tolerance and mood, better eye contact, and an increased ability to converse. Three, the child starts to notice how much time his or her friends spend with devices, and so prompts friends to do other activities instead. And four, the child doesn't notice or care much about others' screen activities because his or her mind has naturally expanded and prefers healthier activities regardless.

In fact, if a child continues to excessively complain and beg to game or get a device back in the name of socializing throughout the fast, it may be a sign of addiction, which is all the more reason to continue restrictions. For more detail regarding technology's impact on social skills and relationships, as well as its impact on addiction pathways in the brain, see chapter 3.

3. How do I tell my other children they can't play video games when it doesn't seem to affect them the same way?

When it comes to treating Electronic Screen Syndrome (ESS), the analogy I use is that an electronic fast needs to be approached in the same way as food restrictions for a child with diabetes: if one child needs to be on a particular diet for serious health reasons, the entire family needs to share that diet. This is the best (and sometimes only) way to ensure compliance, and it conveys to the child that his or her needs are supported and respected. What I find is that if siblings aren't highly invested in screens themselves, they aren't bothered much by a fast, and siblings who *are* invested in screens, and who *are* bothered by a fast, will benefit from being screen-free by definition.

When the Reset is approached as a family, no one is singled out as if he or she is being "punished," and a sense of shared effort emerges instead. Further, when parents are mindful of their own screen-time and follow the "house rules" themselves, the Reset and screen-time in general become easier to manage, and healthier habits and interactions are reinforced. Chapter 4 describes the impact of healthy screen-management on family dynamics, chapter 5 covers how to prepare and involve the family for the fast itself, and chapter 10 outlines "house rules" to practice on an everyday basis.

4. How do video games affect my child's physical health? Is a more active video game system like the Wii any better for them?

All screen-time — including passive (television) and interactive (including gaming and Internet use) — has negative effects on physical health over time. Some of the impact is due to its sedentary nature, and some is due to various psychological and physiological stress reactions, including sleep disruption. Many of these mechanisms are described in chapters 2 and 3, particularly with regard to interactive screen-time.

In general, screen-time is associated with weight gain, high blood pressure, blood sugar dysregulation, and high cholesterol. Further, studies suggest screen-time increases risk for cardiovascular disease, diabetes, and metabolic syndrome — conditions that were essentially unheard of in children even one generation ago. These disorders may be more common now because of chronic stress reactions that occur with too much screen-time, and they are the same reactions that lead to dysregulation of the nervous system, or ESS. In addition, studies suggest that screen-time slows metabolism and impairs hunger and fullness cues, leading to overeating and weight gain. In fact, screen-time is associated with obesity regardless of physical activity, suggesting it has effects outside of simply displacing more physically active play.

Children who engage in too much screen-time may also develop repetitive stress injuries (such as carpal tunnel syndrome), posture problems from the tendency to move the head toward the screen, and neck and back pain. Because developing children have softer bones and more flexible ligaments and tendons, these habits can lead to irreversible changes, which may in turn become physically disabling. Increasing numbers of children complain of headaches and eyestrain every year as well, for similar reasons.

Active video games such as the Wii, also called exergames, are only marginally better than other video games in terms of energy expenditure. They don't burn anywhere near as many calories as the same sport played in real life, and they won't bring on a "nice and relaxed" state afterward like natural play will. Of the different kinds, dancing games are perhaps the most rigorous. Aside from that, an additional consideration is that the Wii may be more likely than other types of games to precipitate certain phenomenon, such as OCD and tics, as noted in chapter 3. Thus, there is no inherently "better" type of video game. Moreover, if your child is overweight, you'll be much better off drastically reducing screen-time than trying to incorporate exergames while attempting to control food intake because of the stress reactions and impaired hunger cues mentioned above. For more on the physiological changes that occur from electronic stress, see chapters 2 and 3.

5. How can I get my child's school to cooperate with this program?

The short answer is to simply ask, respectfully but firmly. School cultures vary widely, as do teachers' personalities and their attitudes toward and reliance on technology in the classroom. Who you approach and how really depends on your particular situation, but in general, do all you can to make it easy for teachers to comply with your requests. Whether or not you *need* to include school depends on what goes on at school as well as how severe your child's symptoms are. This is discussed in chapter 5 ("Reset Planning and School," page 158), as well as in chapter 7 as a troubleshooting issue.

If a discussion with the teacher or the school doesn't work, consider asking your child's doctor (or perhaps therapist) to write a letter (for a letter template, see page 159). While the Reset can often be done successfully without changing the amount of screen-time at school, this isn't always the case, and schools represent what can be a damaging constellation of screen-time issues and effects. For more on this, see chapter 11.

You may need to approach school personnel and state your request several times before you get cooperation. Framing what you want as an experiment or a temporary trial can help. Naturally, if your child already displays disruptive or otherwise problematic behaviors at school, then present your request as a means to accomplish the shared goal of reducing these behaviors, making it a win-win if successful.

6. My child's dream is to work on computers. How can she learn these skills without suffering from ESS?

It is important to distinguish learning a technology trade as a mature adult from the risks of too much screen-time as a still-developing child. This book is devoted to the proposal that too much screen-time at too young an age hinders brain development, and it can also spark a variety of negative symptoms, problematic behaviors, and even various other medical conditions. If a child is suffering from ESS, it is critical that it be taken seriously and addressed with strict screen management. Attention, mood, cognitive, and behavioral disorders will become a barrier to any future career, computer-related or not.

That doesn't necessarily mean that a child who is prone to ESS could never work with computers once he or she is older. Young adults, whose brains have developed more fully, are typically better able to tolerate screen-time than children. And nothing about the Reset Program will hamper any adult, young or old, from learning computer skills. In fact, a person's skills and mental abilities will be immeasurably improved by early screen-time limits, as I outline in chapter 4.

In the end, if a child suffers from ESS, worrying about his or her future computer skills is like worrying about watering the garden when the house is on fire — tend to what's critical to health first, and the future will take care of itself.

7. How do I reconcile the future of technology with my child's health?

As with your child's future career, don't let worries about the future of technology and society change what you do with your own child: *Always put health first.* Do whatever you need to do right now to protect and nurture your child, regardless of whether it goes against the flow of our current society, or against the culture of your child's peers. I discuss coping with personal doubts in more detail in chapter 8.

What does the future hold for technology? I'd like to hope that technology will become part of the solution to the problem it has created. The first step is for society to agree that technology *is* a problem, and I discuss some of these issues in chapter 12. It's quite possible that innovation will lead to ways we can protect ourselves from the dysregulating effects of interactive screen-time and electromagnetic stress. In the meantime, keep your child's mental health and brain development as your primary objective. You can't control the future, but you can control what happens in your family. No matter what technology brings, it is highly unlikely that it can beat simply aligning with nature. When considering the latest screen-based technological "advance" that promises the moon, you'll do well to remember this: *First, do no harm.*

8. Will my child get "left behind" because he or she's not as computer literate as other children?

Aside from the fact that research suggests that screen-time is detrimental to learning and academic success in general, studies suggest that computer skills are overemphasized in school, often to the detriment of other types of learning. For more on these findings, see chapter 11.

Further, in regard to earning potential, studies show that basic computer skills are easily learned and don't predict pay or job advancement, while math and reading skills do. Moreover, in the real world, an inability to focus, plan, get along with others, or tolerate frustration is much more likely to hold someone back; these are the traits that cause children or adults to get left behind in the game of life, not what he or she "knows" about technology. Lastly, consider that most kids today are plenty computer savvy already, and that much of to-day's technology may be obsolete by the time your child reaches adulthood.

9. What will happen as my child gets older and I can no longer protect him or her?

This question speaks to a dilemma facing all parents about any issue. Eventually, children grow up and become adults and must take personal re-sponsibility for themselves. As with other aspects of learning to successfully navigate life as an adult, your children may need to fall down a few times before figuring out what needs to be done to keep electronics use in check and to prevent screen-related symptoms from recurring. Certainly, technology has complicated life in ways previous generations haven't had to deal with. However, by following and teaching good screen management at home while your children are young and under your roof, you'll get them off to a good start — more so than you might think.

Also, it may be reassuring to keep the following in mind: First, adult brains are less sensitive to screen-time effects and are therefore less vulnera-ble to ESS, although ESS symptoms can and do occur in adults (see question 10 below). In fact, the brain is still actively developing until the mid-twenties, so it may be able to tolerate screen-time better once this stage has passed. Second, by protecting a child's brain as it develops, you'll help protect the child for the rest of their life. This is in part because children and adolescents who do not grow up closely attached to technology tend not to be as drawn to electronics as adults, and in part it's because strictly limiting screen-time pro-tects and strengthens the very parts of the brain that determine self-discipline and resiliency. In other words, protecting the brain now makes the brain less vulnerable later, and it raises the odds that children will use technology in a productive way rather than in a compulsive or coping way. For more on benefits and adjusting screen management over time, see chapters 4 and 9.

10. Does screen-time affect adults as well?

The short answer is a resounding *yes!* As an adult, you need to be able to do two things regarding screens: tolerate and moderate. We all have a screen-time "dose" we can tolerate without experiencing any negative side effects, though determining when this threshold has been crossed in adults may be more difficult than it is in children. Part of the reason I'm so in tune with what happens to children with ESS is that I'm sensitive to screen-time myself, and I know that if I'm using the Internet or my smartphone too much, I'll become disorganized and irritable, and I'll have trouble sleeping. Needless to say, writing and researching this book made me acutely aware of what dose I can tolerate. In a way, sensitivity as an adult provides built-in protection because it forces one to practice good screen habits. Many adults don't notice immediate effects, making it harder to appreciate a link between screen habits and health or functioning. Some red flags that electronics may be impacting you may include an inability to relax or feel rested in spite of getting enough sleep, an inability to follow through on commitments, and feeling as though you can't get anything done.

Adults with mental health issues should appreciate the effects of electronics use and light-at-night on depression, social isolation, attention, intimacy, motivation, and organization. Screen-time also impacts one's in-the-moment awareness and ability to problem-solve. Adults with addiction tendencies, social deficits, or psychiatric or neurological disorders are more likely to develop pathological screen-time habits. In regard to physical health, as mentioned earlier, screen-time and light-at-night are underestimated culprits in the development of weight gain, high cholesterol, heart disease, and diabetes — conditions that are common by the time we reach middle age and that become more difficult to reverse the longer they go on.

If you question whether you should moderate your own use, ask yourself: If asked to give up using your devices each evening — as it is suggested you do during the Reset — would you resist? If so, consider doing the electronic fast along with your child to break the cycle of compulsive use and to allow you time to self-reflect. To learn more on how doing so can benefit you, see "Six Reasons to Reduce Your Own Screen-Time During the Reset" (page 149).

ACKNOWLEDGMENTS

I'd first like to thank Lauralyn Kearney, whose spiritual guidance and words of wisdom regarding the book being part of my journey as a healer helped anchor me when I felt lost and free me when I felt stuck. I will always be grateful for my book coach, Lisa Tener, who came into my life at just the right time and always knew just the right thing to say. She helped focus the book's message, made me believe in its "bigness," and cheered me on tirelessly. She also encouraged me to go to the Harvard Medical School publishing course for health professionals, an event that became a turning point for me; it was also there that I met my agent Deirdre Mullane, with whom I instantly connected. I thank Deirdre for taking a chance on me as a first-time author and for all the advice, hand-holding, and encouragement she provided throughout this arduous process.

All the folks at New World Library have been wonderfully supportive and kind; I feel blessed to be working with a publisher with such dedication and integrity. I'm especially thankful for my editor, Jason Gardner, who was in tune with the book's message from the very beginning and who has been an absolute gem to work with — even when I drove him crazy with numerous revisions. Writing a book can be grueling and isolating, so working with people you like is life-saving. Many thanks to my copyeditor, Jeff Campbell, for pushing me to develop my ideas more fully and clearly and for his uncanny knack for keeping track of all the various elements. These two editors took the book far beyond my expectations.

I'm also indebted to kindred spirits Christopher Mulligan and Cris Rowan, who broadened and deepened my understanding of technology's impact on development and autism, respectively, and to Hilarie Cash, for all her organizational and administrative efforts in bringing like-minded clinicians and researchers together in one forum. I also want to acknowledge the open-access movement in academic publishing as well as ResearchGate, both of which provided me access to hundreds of journal articles from dozens of fields that would have been prohibitively expensive to consult otherwise.

Many thanks to all the friends and family who have listened to me talk about the subject of screen-time for over a decade now. I thank my parents and mother-in-law for their love and support — especially my mother, who wrote me notes of encouragement and took on much of the social media work so I wouldn't have to face more screen-time myself. Also big thanks to my sisters, who read my work and gave feedback at the drop of a hat. My biggest debt of gratitude goes to my husband, Ben; among other things, he tolerated my ESS-related meltdowns, made sure I ate, and helped me rehash too many sentences to count.

I also want to thank all the parents, grandparents, teachers, and health clinicians who've written to me with their insights. And finally, I thank all my patients and their families for working with me and for sharing what they've learned. They have truly paid it forward.

ENDNOTES

Introduction: Something Wicked This Way Comes

1 Carmen Moreno et al., "National Trends in the Outpatient Diagnosis and Treatment of Bipolar Disorder in Youth," *Archives of General Psychiatry* 64, no. 9 (September 2007): 1032–39, doi:10.1001/archpsyc.64.9.1032.

2 Hjördís Osk Atladóttir et al., "Time Trends in Reported Diagnoses of Childhood Neuropsychiatric Disorders: A Danish Cohort Study," *Archives of Pediatrics & Adolescent Medicine* 161, no. 2 (February 2007): 193–98, doi:10.1001/archpedi.161.2.193.

3 Emily R. Cox et al., "Trends in the Prevalence of Chronic Medication Use in Children: 2002–2005," *Pediatrics* 122, no. 5 (November 1, 2008): e1053–e1061, doi:10.1542/peds.2008-0214.

4 *SSI Annual Statistical Report, 2012* (Washington, DC: Social Security Administration, July 2013), http://www.ssa.gov/policy/docs/statcomps/ssi_asr/2012/ssi_asr12.pdf.

5 Victoria J. Rideout, Elizabeth A. Vandewater, and Ellen A. Wartella, "Zero to Six: Electronic Media in the Lives of Infants, Toddlers and Preschoolers," 2003, http://eric.ed.gov/?id=ED482302; D. A. Christakis et al., "Television, Video, and Computer Game Usage in Children under 11 Years of Age," *Journal of Pediatrics* 145, no. 5 (2004): 652–56.

6   "Facing the Screen Dilemma: Young Children, Technology and Early Education," *Campaign for a Commercial Free Childhood*, October 2012, http://www.commercial freechildhood.org/screendilemma.

7   Victoria J. Rideout, Ulla G. Foehr, and Donald F. Roberts, "Generation M2: Media in the Lives of 8- to 18-Year Olds," *Kaiser Family Foundation Study*, 2010, http://kff.org/other/poll-finding/report-generation-m2-media-in-the-lives/.

8   "Kids' Cell Phone Ownership Has Dramatically Increased in Past Five Years" (Mediamark Research & Intelligence, January 2010), http://www.gfkmri.com /PDF/MRIPR_010410_KidsAndCellPhones.pdf.

9   Rideout, Foehr, and Roberts, "Generation M2: Media in the Lives of 8- to 18-Year Olds," 2.

10 *U.S. Teen Mobile Report Calling Yesterday, Texting Today, Using Apps Tomorrow*, Nielsen Report, October 14, 2010, www.nielsen.com/us/en/insights /news/2010/u-s-teen-mobile-report-calling-yesterday-texting-today-using -apps-tomorrow.html.

11 John M. Grohol, "What Is Disruptive Mood Dysregulation Disorder?" *Psych Central*, May 16, 2012, psychcentral.com/blog/archives/2012/05/16/what-is -disruptive-mood-dysregulation-disorder/.

Chapter 1: Electronic Screen Syndrome

1   Simerpreet Ahuja and Santha Kumari, "The Impact of Extended Video Viewing on Cognitive, Affective and Behavioral Processes in Preadolescents" (doctoral thesis, School of Management and Social Sciences, Thapar University, Patiala-147001, 2009); A. E. Mark and I. Janssen, "Relationship Between Screen Time and Metabolic Syndrome in Adolescents," *Journal of Public Health* 30, no. 2 (April 2, 2008): 153–60, doi:10.1093/pubmed/fdn022.

2   David R. Fortin and Ruby Roy Dholakia, "Interactivity and Vividness Effects on Social Presence and Involvement with a Web-Based Advertisement," *Journal of Business Research* 58, no. 3 (March 2005): 387–96, doi:10.1016/S0148-2963(03)00106-1.

3   David N. Greenfield, "Psychological Characteristics of Compulsive Internet Use: A Preliminary Analysis," *CyberPsychology & Behavior* 2, no. 5 (October 1, 1999): 403–12, doi:10.1089/cpb.1999.2.403; Fortin and Dholakia, "Interactivity and Vividness Effects on Social Presence and Involvement with a Web-Based Advertisement."

4   Yusuke Kondo et al., "Association between Feeling upon Awakening and Use of Information Technology Devices in Japanese Children," *Journal of Epidemiology /Japan Epidemiological Association* 22, no. 1 (2012): 12–20.

5   Markus Dworak et al., "Impact of Singular Excessive Computer Game and Television Exposure on Sleep Patterns and Memory Performance of School-Aged Children," *Pediatrics* 120, no. 5 (November 2007): 978–85, doi:10.1542/peds.2007-0476.

6   Michael Gradisar et al., "The Sleep and Technology Use of Americans: Findings from the National Sleep Foundation's 2011 Sleep in America Poll," *Journal of Clinical Sleep Medicine: JCSM: Official Publication of the American Academy of Sleep Medicine* 9, no. 12 (2013): 1291–99, doi:10.5664/jcsm.3272.

7   Chuan-Bo Weng et al., "Gray Matter and White Matter Abnormalities in Online Game Addiction," *European Journal of Radiology* 82, no. 8 (August 2013): 1308–12, doi:10.1016/j.ejrad.2013.01.031.

8   Council on Communications and Media, "Children, Adolescents, and the Media," *Pediatrics* (October 28, 2013), doi:10.1542/peds.2013-2656.

9   Stephen Heyman, "Reading Literature on Screen: A Price for Convenience?" *New York Times*, August 13, 2014, http://www.nytimes.com/2014/08/14/arts /reading-literature-on-screen-a-price-for-convenience.html?_r=0; Anne Mangen, Bente R. Walgermo, and Kolbjørn Brønnick, "Reading Linear Texts on Paper versus Computer Screen: Effects on Reading Comprehension," *International Journal of Educational Research* 58 (January 2013): 61–68, doi:10.1016 /j.ijer.2012.12.002.

10   Angeline S. Lillard and Jennifer Peterson, "The Immediate Impact of Different Types of Television on Young Children's Executive Function," *Pediatrics* 128, no. 4 (October 2011): 644–49, doi:10.1542/peds.2010-1919.

11   Martin Blank and Reba Goodman, "Electromagnetic Fields Stress Living Cells," *Pathophysiology: The Official Journal of the International Society for Pathophysiology / ISP* 16, no. 2–3 (August 2009): 71–78, doi:10.1016/j.pathophys.2009.01.006. Tamir S. Aldad et al., "Fetal Radiofrequency Radiation Exposure From 800-1900 Mhz-Rated Cellular Telephones Affects Neurodevelopment and Behavior in Mice," *Scientific Reports* 2 (March 15, 2012), doi:10.1038/srep00312; Martha R. Herbert and Cindy Sage, "Autism and EMF? Plausibility of a Pathophysiological Link — Part I," *Pathophysiology: The Official Journal of the International Society for Pathophysiology / ISP* 20, no. 3 (June 2013): 191–209, doi:10.

12   "Media and Children," *American Academy of Pediatrics*, accessed July 20, 2014, http://www.aap.org/en-us/advocacy-and-policy/aap-health-initiatives/Pages /Media-and-Children.aspx; A. Sigman, "Time for a View on Screen Time," *Archives of Disease in Childhood* 97, no. 11 (October 8, 2012): 935–42, doi:10.1136 /archdischild-2012-302196.

13   Douglas A. Gentile et al., "Well-Child Visits in the Video Age: Pediatricians and the American Academy of Pediatrics' Guidelines for Children's Media Use," *Pediatrics* 114, no. 5 (November 2004): 1235–41, doi:10.1542/peds.2003-1121-L.

14   Colleen Cordes and Edward Miller, "Fool's Gold: A Critical Look at Computers in Childhood" (2000), 28–39; Tara Ehrcke, "21st Century Learning Inc.," *Our Schools/Our Selves* (Winter 2013), accessed October 30, 2014, http://www.nl1630 .policyalternatives.ca/sites/default/files/uploads/publications/National%20 Office/2013/02/osos110_21stCenturyLearning_0.pdf.

Chapter 2: All Revved Up and Nowhere to Go

1   Jun Kohyama, "A Newly Proposed Disease Condition Produced by Light Exposure during Night: Asynchronization," *Brain and Development* 31, no. 4 (April 2009): 255–73, doi:10.1016/j.braindev.2008.07.006.

2   Cris Rowan, "Unplug — Don't Drug: A Critical Look at the Influence of Technology on Child Behavior with an Alternative Way of Responding Other than Evaluation and Drugging," *Ethical Human Psychology and Psychiatry* 12, no. 1 (April 1, 2010): 60–68, doi:10.1891/1559-4343.12.1.60.

3   N. Kozeis, "Impact of Computer Use on Children's Vision," *Hippokratia* 13, no. 4 (October 2009): 230–31.

4   Eva Chamorro et al., "Effects of Light-Emitting Diode Radiations on Human Retinal Pigment Epithelial Cells in Vitro," *Photochemistry and Photobiology* 89, no. 2 (April 2013): 468–73, doi:10.1111/j.1751-1097.2012.01237.x; Toshio Narimatsu et al., "Disruption of Cell-Cell Junctions and Induction of Pathological Cytokines in the Retinal Pigment Epithelium of Light-Exposed Mice," *Investigative Ophthalmology & Visual Science* 54, no. 7 (July 2013): 4555–62, doi:10.1167/iovs.12-11572.

5   B. Gopinath et al., "Influence of Physical Activity and Screen Time on the Retinal Microvasculature in Young Children," *Arteriosclerosis, Thrombosis, and Vascular Biology* 31, no. 5 (April 20, 2011): 1233–39, doi:10.1161/ATVBAHA.110.219451.

6   Emmanuel Stamatakis, Mark Hamer, and David W. Dunstan, "Screen-Based Entertainment Time, All-Cause Mortality, and Cardiovascular Events: Population-Based Study with Ongoing Mortality and Hospital Events Follow-Up," *Journal of the American College of Cardiology* 57, no. 3 (January 18, 2011): 292–99, doi:10.1016/j.jacc.2010.05.065; A. E. Mark and I. Janssen, "Relationship Between Screen Time and Metabolic Syndrome in Adolescents," *Journal of Public Health* 30, no. 2 (April 2, 2008): 153–60, doi:10.1093/pubmed/fdn022; Valerie Carson and Ian Janssen, "Neighborhood Disorder and Screen Time among 10-16 Year Old Canadian Youth: A Cross-Sectional Study," *The International Journal of Behavioral Nutrition and Physical Activity* 9 (2012): 66, doi:10.1186/1479-5868-9-66; B. Gopinath et al., "Influence of Physical Activity and Screen Time on the Retinal Microvasculature in Young Children," *Arteriosclerosis, Thrombosis, and Vascular Biology* 31, no. 5 (April 20, 2011): 1233–39, doi:10.1161/ATVBAHA.110.219451; B. Gopinath et al., "Relationship between a Range of Sedentary Behaviours and Blood Pressure during Early Adolescence," *Journal of Human Hypertension* 26, no. 6 (June 2012): 350–56, doi:10.1038/jhh.2011.40.

7   Mark and Janssen, "Relationship Between Screen Time and Metabolic Syndrome in Adolescents."

8   Rowan, "Unplug — Don't Drug."

9   James D. Ivory and Sriram Kalyanaraman, "The Effects of Technological Advancement and Violent Content in Video Games on Players' Feelings of Presence, Involvement, Physiological Arousal, and Aggression," *Journal of Communication* 57, no. 3 (September 2007): 532–55, doi:10.1111/j.1460-2466.2007.00356.x; B. H. Detenbur, R. F. Simons, and G. G. Bennett Jr., "The Effects of Picture Motion

on Emotional Responses.," *Journal of Broadcasting and Electronic Media*, no. 42 (1998): 113–27; Robert F. Simons et al., "Emotion Processing in Three Systems: The Medium and the Message," *Psychophysiology* 36, no. 5 (1999): 619–27; Ko-hyama, "A Newly Proposed Disease Condition Produced by Light Exposure during Night: Asynchronization."

10   Jessica Solodar, "Commentary: ILAE Definition of Epilepsy," *Epilepsia* 55, no. 4 (2014): 491, doi:10.1111/epi.12594; Center for Neurosciences, "Headache /Migraine," accessed July 5, 2014, http://www.neurotucson.com/medical -specialties/pediatric-neurology/headache-migraine/; American Nutrition Asso-ciation, "Tics and Tourette's — Tracing the True Triggers," accessed November 4, 2013, http://americannutritionassociation.org/newsletter/tics-tourettes -tracing-true-triggers.

11   *CNN World News*, "Cartoon-Based Illness Mystifies Japan," December 17, 1997, http://www.cnn.com/world/9712/17/japan.cartoon/.

12   Angelica B. Ortiz de Gortari and Mark D. Griffiths, "Altered Visual Perception in Game Transfer Phenomena: An Empirical Self-Report Study," *International Jour-nal of Human-Computer Interaction* 30, no. 2 (September 25, 2013): 95–105, doi:10.10 80/10447318.2013.839900.

13   Cris Rowan, "The Impact of Technology on Child Sensory and Motor Develop-ment," 2010, http://www.sensoryprocessinginfo/CrisRowan.pdf.

14   John Hopson, "Behavioral Game Design," *Gamasutra*, April 27, 2001, http://www.gamasutra.com/view/feature/3085/behavioral_game_design .php?page=1.

15   Ivory and Kalyanaraman, "The Effects of Technological Advancement and Violent Content in Video Games on Players' Feelings"; D. A. Gentile and W. Stone, "Vio-lent Video Game Effects on Children and Adolescents: A Review of the Literature," *Minerva Pediatrica* 57, no. 6 (December 2005): 337–58; Aric Sigman, "Visual Voo-doo: The Biological Impact of Watching TV," *Biologist* 54, no. 1 (2007): 12–17.

16   Brian D. Ng and Peter Wiemer-Hastings, "Addiction to the Internet and Online Gaming," *Cyberpsychology & Behavior: The Impact of the Internet, Multimedia and Virtual Reality on Behavior and Society* 8, no. 2 (April 2005): 110–13, doi:10.1089 /cpb.2005.8.110.

17   Shang Hwa Hsu, Ming-Hui Wen, and Muh-Cherng Wu, "Exploring User Expe-riences as Predictors of MMORPG Addiction," *Computers & Education* 53, no. 3 (November 2009): 990–99, doi:10.1016/j.compedu.2009.05.016.

18   Mark Ward, "Why Minecraft Is More than Just Another Video Game," *BBC News*, September 6, 2013, http://www.bbc.com/news/magazine-23572742.

19   Mary Lee Barron, "Light Exposure, Melatonin Secretion, and Menstrual Cycle Parameters: An Integrative Review," *Biological Research for Nursing* 9, no. 1 (July 2007): 49–69, doi:10.1177/1099800407303337; E. Kasuya et al., "Light Exposure during Night Suppresses Nocturnal Increase in Growth Hormone Secretion in Holstein Steers," *Journal of Animal Science* 86, no. 8 (August 2008): 1799–1807, doi:10.2527/jas.2008-0877.

20   Shigekazu Higuchi et al., "Effects of Vdt Tasks with a Bright Display at Night on
      Melatonin, Core Temperature, Heart Rate, and Sleepiness," *Journal of Applied
      Physiology* 94, no. 5 (May 2003): 1773–76, doi:10.1152/japplphysiol.00616.2002;
      Kohyama, "A Newly Proposed Disease Condition Produced by Light Exposure
      during Night: Asynchronization."

21   R. Luboshitzky and P. Lavie, "Melatonin and Sex Hormone Interrelationships — a
      Review," *Journal of Pediatric Endocrinology & Metabolism* 12, no. 3 (June 1999):
      355–62; Daniel A. Rossignol and Richard E. Frye, "Melatonin in Autism Spectrum
      Disorders: A Systematic Review and Meta-Analysis," *Developmental Medicine and
      Child Neurology* 53, no. 9 (September 2011): 783–92, doi:10.1111/j.1469
      -8749.2011.03980.x; L. Wetterberg et al., "Age, Alcoholism and Depression Are
      Associated with Low Levels of Urinary Melatonin," *Journal of Psychiatry & Neuro-
      science* 17, no. 5 (November 1992): 215–24.

22   Kasuya et al., "Light Exposure during Night Suppresses Nocturnal Increase in
      Growth Hormone Secretion in Holstein Steers."

23   Christian Cajochen et al., "Evening Exposure to a Light-Emitting Diodes
      (led)-Backlit Computer Screen Affects Circadian Physiology and Cognitive Perfor-
      mance," *Journal of Applied Physiology* 110, no. 5 (May 2011): 1432–38, doi:10.1152
      /japplphysiol.00165.2011; Higuchi et al., "Effects of Vdt Tasks with a Bright Dis-
      play at Night on Melatonin, Core Temperature, Heart Rate, and Sleepiness."

24   *Harvard Health Publications*, "Blue Light Has a Dark Side," May 2012,
      http://www.health.harvard.edu/newsletters/Harvard_Health_Letter/2012
      /May/blue-light-has-a-dark-side?utm_source=health&utm_medium=press
      release&utm_campaign=health0512.

25   Suchinda Jarupat et al., "Effects of the 1900MHz Electromagnetic Field Emitted
      from Cellular Phone on Nocturnal Melatonin Secretion," *Journal of Physiological
      Anthropology and Applied Human Science* 22, no. 1 (2003): 61–63.

26   Mary A. Carskadon, "Sleep's Effects on Cognition and Learning in Adolescence,"
      Progress in Brain Research 190 (2011): 137–43, doi:10.1016/B978-0-444-53817
      -8.00008-6.

27   Catharine Paddock, "Bedtime Texting, Internet Use, Disturbs Sleep and Mood in
      Teens," *Medical News Today*, November 3, 2010, http://www.medicalnewstoday
      .com/articles/206546.php.

28   Norihito Oshima et al., "The Suicidal Feelings, Self-Injury, and Mobile Phone Use
      After Lights Out in Adolescents," *Journal of Pediatric Psychology* 37, no. 9 (Octo-
      ber 1, 2012): 1023–30, doi:10.1093/jpepsy/jss072; Yuan-Sheng Yang et al., "The
      Association between Problematic Cellular Phone Use and Risky Behaviors and
      Low Self-Esteem among Taiwanese Adolescents," *BMC Public Health* 10 (2010):
      217, doi:10.1186/1471-2458-10-217; Paddock, "Bedtime Texting, Internet Use,
      Disturbs Sleep and Mood in Teens."

29   Jun Kohyama, "Neurochemical and Neuropharmacological Aspects of Circadian
      Disruptions: An Introduction to Asynchronization," *Current Neuropharmacology* 9,
      no. 2 (2011): 330.

30 Jan Van den Bulck, "Adolescent Use of Mobile Phones for Calling and for Sending Text Messages after Lights Out: Results from a Prospective Cohort Study with a One-Year Follow-Up," *Sleep* 30, no. 9 (September 2007): 1220–23.

31 Yueji Sun et al., "Brain fMRI Study of Crave Induced by Cue Pictures in Online Game Addicts (Male Adolescents)," *Behavioural Brain Research* 233, no. 2 (August 1, 2012): 563–76, doi:10.1016/j.bbr.2012.05.005; Doug Hyun Han et al., "Brain Activity and Desire for Internet Video Game Play," *Comprehensive Psychiatry* 52, no. 1 (January 2011): 88–95, doi:10.1016/j.comppsych.2010.04.004.

32 Doug Hyun Han et al., "Changes in Cue-Induced, Prefrontal Cortex Activity with Video-Game Play," *Cyberpsychology, Behavior and Social Networking* 13, no. 6 (December 2010): 655–61, doi:10.1089/cyber.2009.0327.

33 Yan Zhou et al., "Gray Matter Abnormalities in Internet Addiction: A Voxel-Based Morphometry Study," *European Journal of Radiology* 79, no. 1 (July 2011): 92–95, doi:10.1016/j.ejrad.2009.10.025; Chuan-Bo Weng et al., "Gray Matter and White Matter Abnormalities in Online Game Addiction," *European Journal of Radiology* 82, no. 8 (August 2013): 1308–12, doi:10.1016/j.ejrad.2013.01.031; Chuan-Bo Weng et al., "[A voxel-based morphometric analysis of brain gray matter in online game addicts]," *Zhonghua yi xue za zhi* 92, no. 45 (December 4, 2012): 3221–23; Kai Yuan et al., "Microstructure Abnormalities in Adolescents with Internet Addiction Disorder," ed. Shaolin Yang, *PLoS ONE* 6, no. 6 (June 3, 2011): e20708, doi:10.1371/journal.pone.0020708; Soon-Beom Hong et al., "Reduced Orbitofrontal Cortical Thickness in Male Adolescents with Internet Addiction," *Behavioral and Brain Functions* 9, no. 1 (2013): 11, doi:10.1186/1744-9081-9-11; Kai Yuan et al., "Cortical Thickness Abnormalities in Late Adolescence with Online Gaming Addiction," ed. Bogdan Draganski, *PLoS ONE* 8, no. 1 (January 9, 2013): e53055, doi:10.1371/journal.pone.0053055.

34 M. J. Koepp et al., "Evidence for Striatal Dopamine Release during a Video Game," *Nature* 393, no. 6682 (May 21, 1998): 266–68, doi:10.1038/30498.

35 George Koob and Mary Jeanne Kreek, "Stress, Dysregulation of Drug Reward Pathways, and the Transition to Drug Dependence," *American Journal of Psychiatry* 164, no. 8 (August 1, 2007): 1149, doi:10.1176/appi.ajp.2007.05030503.

36 Joseph Hilgard, Christopher R. Engelhardt, and Bruce D. Bartholow, "Individual Differences in Motives, Preferences, and Pathology in Video Games: The Gaming Attitudes, Motives, and Experiences Scales (GAMES)," *Frontiers in Psychology* 4 (2013): 608, doi:10.3389/fpsyg.2013.00608.

37 Geoffrey L. Ream, Luther C. Elliott, and Eloise Dunlap, "Playing Video Games While Using or Feeling the Effects of Substances: Associations with Substance Use Problems," *International Journal of Environmental Research and Public Health* 8, no. 12 (October 18, 2011): 3979–98, doi:10.3390/ijerph8103979.

38 Detenbur, Simons, and Bennett, "The Effects of Picture Motion on Emotional Responses"; Sigman, "Visual Voodoo."

39 Byron Reeves et al., "The Effects of Screen Size and Message Content on Attention and Arousal," *Media Psychology* 1, no. 1 (March 1, 1999): 49–67, doi:10.1207/s1532785xmep0101_4.

40 S. Shyam Sundar and Carson B. Wagner, "The World Wide Wait: Exploring Physiological and Behavioral Effects of Download Speed," *Media Psychology* 4, no. 2 (May 1, 2002): 173–206, doi:10.1207/S1532785XMEP0402_04; Detenbur, Simons, and Bennett, "The Effects of Picture Motion on Emotional Responses."

41 Ivory and Kalyanaraman, "The Effects of Technological Advancement and Violent Content in Video Games on Players' Feelings."

42 Gloria Mark, Yiran Wang, and Melissa Niiya, "Stress and Multitasking in Everyday College Life: An Empirical Study of Online Activity," *CHI '14: Proceedings of the SIGCHI Conference on Human Factors in Computing Systems* (ACM Press, 2014): 41–50, doi:10.1145/2556288.2557361; Mark W. Becker, Reem Alzahabi, and Christopher J. Hopwood, "Media Multitasking Is Associated with Symptoms of Depression and Social Anxiety," *Cyberpsychology, Behavior and Social Networking* 16, no. 2 (February 2013): 132–35, doi:10.1089/cyber.2012.0291; Stuart Wolpert, "Russell Poldrack: Multi-Tasking Adversely Affects the Brain's Learning Systems," UCLA Department of Psychology, July 25, 2006, http://www.psych.ucla.edu/news /russell-poldrack-multi-tasking-adversely-affects-the-brains-learning-systems.

43 Marjut Wallenius, "Salivary Cortisol in Relation to the Use of Information and Communication Technology (ICT) in School-Aged Children," *Psychology* 01, no. 02 (2010): 88–95, doi:10.4236/psych.2010.12012; T. A. Bedrosian et al., "Light at Night Alters Daily Patterns of Cortisol and Clock Proteins in Female Siberian Hamsters," *Journal of Neuroendocrinology* 25, no. 6 (June 2013): 590–96, doi:10.1111/jne.12036.

44 Panagiota Pervanidou and George P. Chrousos, "Stress and Obesity/Metabolic Syndrome in Childhood and Adolescence," *International Journal of Pediatric Obesity: IJPO: An Official Journal of the International Association for the Study of Obesity* 6, Suppl 1 (September 2011): 21–28, doi:10.3109/17477166.2011.615996.

45 Pablo A. Nepomnaschy et al., "Stress and Female Reproductive Function: A Study of Daily Variations in Cortisol, Gonadotrophins, and Gonadal Steroids in a Rural Mayan Population," *American Journal of Human Biology: The Official Journal of the Human Biology Council* 16, no. 5 (October 2004): 523–32, doi:10.1002/ajhb.20057; Andrea C. Gore, Barbara Attardi, and Donald B. DeFranco, "Glucocorticoid Repression of the Reproductive Axis: Effects on GnRH and Gonadotropin Subunit mRNA Levels," *Molecular and Cellular Endocrinology* 256, no. 1–2 (August 15, 2006): 40–48, doi:10.1016/j.mce.2006.06.002; Panagiota Pervanidou and George P. Chrousos, "Metabolic Consequences of Stress during Childhood and Adolescence," *Metabolism: Clinical and Experimental* 61, no. 5 (May 2012): 611–19, doi:10.1016/j.metabol.2011.10.005.

46 Narimatsu et al., "Disruption of Cell-Cell Junctions and Induction of Pathological Cytokines in the Retinal Pigment Epithelium of Light-Exposed Mice."

47 Paddock, "Bedtime Texting, Internet Use, Disturbs Sleep and Mood in Teens"; P. M. Maras et al., "Preferential Loss of Dorsal-Hippocampus Synapses Underlies Memory Impairments Provoked by Short, Multimodal Stress," *Molecular Psychiatry* 19, no. 7 (July 2014): 811–22.

48 Pei-Luen Patrick Rau, Shu-Yun Peng, and Chin-Chow Yang, "Time Distortion for Expert and Novice Online Game Players," *Cyberpsychology & Behavior: The Impact of the Internet, Multimedia and Virtual Reality on Behavior and Society* 9, no. 4 (August 2006): 396–403, doi:10.1089/cpb.2006.9.396.

49 R. Kraut et al., "Internet Paradox. A Social Technology That Reduces Social Involvement and Psychological Well-Being?" *The American Psychologist* 53, no. 9 (September 1998): 1017–31.

Chapter 3: Insidious Shape-Shifter

1 E. F. Schumacher, *Small Is Beautiful: Economics as If People Mattered* (New York: Harper Perennial, 2010).

2 A. R. Pachner, "Borrelia Burgdorferi in the Nervous System: The New 'Great Imitator,'" *Annals of the New York Academy of Sciences* 539 (1988): 56–64.

3 Haifeng Hou et al., "Reduced Striatal Dopamine Transporters in People with Internet Addiction Disorder," *Journal of Biomedicine & Biotechnology* (2012): 854524, doi:10.1155/2012/854524; Sang Hee Kim et al., "Reduced Striatal Dopamine D2 Receptors in People with Internet Addiction," *Neuroreport* 22, no. 8 (June 11, 2011): 407–11, doi:10.1097/WNR.0b013e328346e16e.

4 Erick Messias et al., "Sadness, Suicide, and Their Association with Video Game and Internet Overuse Among Teens: Results from the Youth Risk Behavior Survey 2007 and 2009," *Suicide & Life-Threatening Behavior* 41, no. 3 (June 2011): 307–15, doi:10.1111/j.1943-278X.2011.00030.x; Yotaro Katsumata et al., "Electronic Media Use and Suicidal Ideation in Japanese Adolescents," *Psychiatry and Clinical Neurosciences* 62, no. 6 (December 2008): 744–46, doi:10.1111/j.1440 -1819.2008.01880.x; Catriona M. Morrison and Helen Gore, "The Relationship Between Excessive Internet Use and Depression: A Questionnaire-Based Study of 1,319 Young People and Adults," *Psychopathology* 43, no. 2 (2010): 121–26, doi:10.1159/000277001.

5 Rosalina Richards et al., "Adolescent Screen Time and Attachment to Parents and Peers," *Archives of Pediatrics & Adolescent Medicine* 164, no. 3 (March 2010): 258–62, doi:10.1001/archpediatrics.2009.280; Adriano Schimmenti et al., "Attachment Disorganization and Dissociation in Virtual Worlds: A Study on Problematic Internet Use among Players of Online Role Playing Games," *Clinical Neuropsychiatry* 9, no. 5 (2012): 195–202; R. Kraut et al., "Internet Paradox. A Social Technology that Reduces Social Involvement and Psychological Well-Being?" *The American Psychologist* 53, no. 9 (September 1998): 1017–31.

6 Ethan Kross et al., "Facebook Use Predicts Declines in Subjective Well-Being in Young Adults," ed. Cédric Sueur, *PLoS ONE* 8, no. 8 (August 14, 2013): e69841, doi:10.1371/journal.pone.0069841; Hui-Tzu Grace Chou and Nicholas Edge, "'They Are Happier and Having Better Lives than I Am': The Impact of Using Facebook on Perceptions of Others' Lives," *Cyberpsychology, Behavior and Social Networking* 15, no. 2 (February 2012): 117–21, doi:10.1089/cyber.2011.0324.

7   Victoria Dunckley, "The Link Between Light-at-Night, Depression & Suicidal-
     ity," *Psychology Today,* "Mental Wealth" (March 30, 2014), http://www
     .psychologytoday.com/blog/mental-wealth/201403/the-link-between
     -light-night-depression-suicidality; Norihito Oshima et al., "The Suicidal Feel-
     ings, Self-Injury, and Mobile Phone Use After Lights Out in Adolescents," *Journal
     of Pediatric Psychology* 37, no. 9 (October 1, 2012): 1023–30, doi:10.1093/jpepsy
     /jss072; Katsumata et al., "Electronic Media Use and Suicidal Ideation in Japanese
     Adolescents."

8   Mark W. Becker, Reem Alzahabi, and Christopher J. Hopwood, "Media Multitask-
     ing Is Associated with Symptoms of Depression and Social Anxiety," *Cyberpsychol-
     ogy, Behavior and Social Networking* 16, no. 2 (February 2013): 132–35, doi:10.1089
     /cyber.2012.0291; J. Lee, K. Lee, and T. Choi, "The Effects of Smartphone and
     Internet/Computer Addiction on Adolescent Psychopathology" (poster presented
     at the 166th Annual Meeting of the American Psychiatric Association, San Fran-
     cisco, CA, 2013; NR6-41).

9   Rune Aune Mentzoni et al., "Problematic Video Game Use: Estimated Prevalence
     and Associations with Mental and Physical Health," *Cyberpsychology, Behavior and
     Social Networking* 14, no. 10 (October 2011): 591–96, doi:10.1089/cyber.2010.0260;
     Messias et al., "Sadness, Suicide, and Their Association with Video Game and In-
     ternet Overuse among Teens"; Rani A. Desai et al., "Video-Gaming Among High
     School Students: Health Correlates, Gender Differences, and Problematic Gam-
     ing," *Pediatrics* 126, no. 6 (December 1, 2010): e1414–e1424, doi:10.1542
     /peds.2009-2706.

10   D. A. Gentile et al., "Pathological Video Game Use Among Youths: A Two-
     Year Longitudinal Study," *Pediatrics,* 127, no. 2 (January 17, 2011): e319–e329,
     doi:10.1542/peds.2010-1353.

11   Ibid.

12   Jun Kohyama, "Neurochemical and Neuropharmacological Aspects of Circadian
     Disruptions: An Introduction to Asynchronization," *Current Neuropharmacology* 9,
     no. 2 (2011): 330.

13   Victoria Dunckley, "Misdiagnosed? Bipolar Disorder Is All the Rage!," *Psychology
     Today*, "Mental Wealth" (June 7, 2011), http://www.psychologytoday.com/blog
     /mental-wealth/201106/misdiagnosed-bipolar-disorder-is-all-the-rage.

14   Christina J. Calamaro, Thornton B. A. Mason, and Sarah J. Ratcliffe, "Adolescents
     Living the 24/7 Lifestyle: Effects of Caffeine and Technology on Sleep Duration
     and Daytime Functioning," *Pediatrics* 123, no. 6 (June 1, 2009): e1005–e1010,
     doi:10.1542/peds.2008-3641; Paddock, "Bedtime Texting, Internet Use, Disturbs
     Sleep and Mood in Teens"; Peter G. Polos et al., "The Effect of Sleep Time Re-
     lated Information and Communication Technology (STRICT) on Sleep Patterns
     and Daytime Functioning in Children and Young Adults: A Pilot Study," *CHEST
     Journal* 138, no. 4 (October 1, 2010): 911A, doi:10.1378/chest.9771.

15   Douglas A. Gentile et al., "Video Game Playing, Attention Problems, and Impul-
     siveness: Evidence of Bidirectional Causality," *Psychology of Popular Media Culture*
     1, no. 1 (2012): 62–70, doi:10.1037/a0026969.

16   Doug Hyun Han et al., "The Effect of Methylphenidate on Internet Video Game Play in Children with Attention-Deficit/Hyperactivity Disorder," *Comprehensive Psychiatry* 50, no. 3 (June 2009): 251–56, doi:10.1016/j.comppsych.2008.08.011; Doug Hyun Han, Jun Won Hwang, and Perry F. Renshaw, "Bupropion Sustained Release Treatment Decreases Craving for Video Games and Cue-Induced Brain Activity in Patients with Internet Video Game Addiction," *Experimental and Clinical Psychopharmacology* 18, no. 4 (August 2010): 297–304, doi:10.1037/a0020023.

17   C. Shawn Green and Daphne Bavelier, "Action Video Game Modifies Visual Selective Attention," *Nature* 423, no. 6939 (May 29, 2003): 534–37.

18   Kathleen Beullens, Keith Roe, and Jan Van den Bulck, "Excellent Gamer, Excellent Driver? The Impact of Adolescents' Video Game Playing on Driving Behavior: A Two-Wave Panel Study," *Accident; Analysis and Prevention* 43, no. 1 (January 2011): 58–65, doi:10.1016/j.aap.2010.07.011.

19   D. A. Christakis et al., "Early Television Exposure and Subsequent Attentional Problems in Children," *Pediatrics* 113, no. 4 (2004): 708–13; C. E. Landhuis et al., "Does Childhood Television Viewing Lead to Attention Problems in Adolescence? Results From a Prospective Longitudinal Study," *Pediatrics* 120, no. 3 (August 31, 2007): 532–37, doi:10.1542/peds.2007-0978; Ignacio David Acevedo-Polakovich et al., "Disentangling the Relation Between Television Viewing and Cognitive Processes in Children with Attention-Deficit/Hyperactivity Disorder and Comparison Children," *Archives of Pediatrics & Adolescent Medicine* 160, no. 4 (April 1, 2006): 354, doi:10.1001/archpedi.160.4.354; Jeffrey G. Johnson et al., "Extensive Television Viewing and the Development of Attention and Learning Difficulties during Adolescence," *Archives of Pediatrics & Adolescent Medicine* 161, no. 5 (May 2007): 480–86, doi:10.1001/archpedi.161.5.480.

20   Stéphanie Bioulac, Lisa Arfi, and Manuel P. Bouvard, "Attention Deficit/Hyperactivity Disorder and Video Games: A Comparative Study of Hyperactive and Control Children," *European Psychiatry: The Journal of the Association of European Psychiatrists* 23, no. 2 (March 2008): 134–41, doi:10.1016/j.eurpsy.2007.11.002; Philip Chan and Terry Rabinowitz, "A Cross-Sectional Analysis of Video Games and Attention Deficit Hyperactivity Disorder Symptoms in Adolescents," *Annals of General Psychiatry* 5, no. 1 (2006): 16; Edward L. Swing et al., "Television and Video Game Exposure and the Development of Attention Problems," *Pediatrics* 126, no. 2 (August 2010): 214–21, doi:10.1542/peds.2009-1508; Ju-Yu Yen et al., "The Comorbid Psychiatric Symptoms of Internet Addiction: Attention Deficit and Hyperactivity Disorder (ADHD), Depression, Social Phobia, and Hostility," *The Journal of Adolescent Health: Official Publication of the Society for Adolescent Medicine* 41, no. 1 (July 2007): 93–98, doi:10.1016/j.jadohealth.2007.02.002; H. J. Yoo et al., "Attention Deficit Hyperactivity Symptoms and Internet Addiction," *Psychiatry and Cliical Neuroscience* 58, no. 5 (2004): 487–94.

21   Markus Dworak et al., "Impact of Singular Excessive Computer Game and Television Exposure on Sleep Patterns and Memory Performance of School-Aged Children," *Pediatrics* 120, no. 5 (November 2007): 978–85, doi:10.1542/peds.2007-0476.

22 Swing et al., "Television and Video Game Exposure and the Development of Attention Problems."

23 Gentile et al., "Video Game Playing, Attention Problems, and Impulsiveness."

24 Swing et al., "Television and Video Game Exposure and the Development of Attention Problems."

25 Angeline S. Lillard and Jennifer Peterson, "The Immediate Impact of Different Types of Television on Young Children's Executive Function," *Pediatrics* 128, no. 4 (October 2011): 644–49, doi:10.1542/peds.2010-1919.

26 Aysegul Yolga Tahiroglu et al., "Short-Term Effects of Playing Computer Games on Attention," *Journal of Attention Disorders* 13, no. 6 (May 2010): 668–76, doi:10.1177/1087054709347205.

27 Pei-Luen Patrick Rau, Shu-Yun Peng, and Chin-Chow Yang, "Time Distortion for Expert and Novice Online Game Players," *Cyberpsychology & Behavior: The Impact of the Internet, Multimedia and Virtual Reality on Behavior and Society* 9, no. 4 (August 2006): 396–403, doi:10.1089/cpb.2006.9.396.

28 Peter Fischer et al., "The Racing-Game Effect: Why Do Video Racing Games Increase Risk-Taking Inclinations?," *Personality and Social Psychology Bulletin* 35, no. 10 (October 1, 2009): 1395–1409, doi:10.1177/0146167209339628.

29 Christian Cajochen et al., "Evening Exposure to a Light-Emitting Diodes (led)-Backlit Computer Screen Affects Circadian Physiology and Cognitive Performance," *Journal of Applied Physiology* 110, no. 5 (May 2011): 1432–38, doi:10.1152/japplphysiol.00165.2011; Calamaro, Mason, and Ratcliffe, "Adolescents Living the 24/7 Lifestyle: Effects of Caffeine and Technology on Sleep Duration and Daytime Functioning"; Seog Ju Kim et al., "Relationship between Weekend Catch-up Sleep and Poor Performance on Attention Tasks in Korean Adolescents," *Archives of Pediatrics & Adolescent Medicine* 165, no. 9 (September 2011): 806–12, doi:10.1001/archpediatrics.2011.128; Polos et al., "The Effect of Sleep Time Related Information and Communication Technology (STRICT) on Sleep Patterns and Daytime Functioning in Children and Young Adults."

30 Shigekazu Higuchi et al., "Effects of Vdt Tasks with a Bright Display at Night on Melatonin, Core Temperature, Heart Rate, and Sleepiness," *Journal of Applied Physiology* 94, no. 5 (May 2003): 1773–76, doi:10.1152/japplphysiol.00616.2002.

31 Stuart Wolpert, "Russell Poldrack: Multi-Tasking Adversely Affects the Brain's Learning Systems," *UCLA Department of Psychology*, July 25, 2006, http://www.psych.ucla.edu/news/russell-poldrack-multi-tasking-adversely -affects-the-brains-learning-systems; David Meyer, *Multitasking and Task Switching* (Brain, Cognition and Action Laboratory: University of Michigan, 2006), http://www.umich.edu/~bcalab/multitasking.html.

32 Larry D. Rosen, L. Mark Carrier, and Nancy A. Cheever, "Facebook and Texting Made Me Do It: Media-Induced Task-Switching While Studying," *Computers in Human Behavior* 29, no. 3 (May 2013): 948–58, doi:10.1016/j.chb.2012.12.001.

33 Robert Weis and Brittany C. Cerankosky, "Effects of Video-Game Ownership on Young Boys' Academic and Behavioral Functioning: A Randomized,

Controlled Study," *Psychological Science* 21, no. 4 (April 2010): 463–70, doi:10.1177/0956797610362670.

34 Jacob Vigdor and Helen Ladd, *Scaling the Digital Divide: Home Computer Technology and Student Achievement*, National Center for Analysis of Longitudinal Data in Education Reseach (CALDER, The Urban Institute, June 2010), http://www.caldercenter.org/publications/scaling-digital-divide-home -computer-technology-and-student-achievement.

35 Ofer Malamud and Cristian Pop-Eleches, *Home Computer Use and the Development of Human Capital* (National Bureau of Economic Research, 2010), http://www.nber.org/papers/w15814.

36 Leonard Sax, *Boys Adrift: The Five Factors Driving the Growing Epidemic of Unmotivated Boys and Underachieving Young Men* (New York: Basic Books, 2009).

37 Nicholas Carr, "Is Google Making Us Stupid?" *The Atlantic*, July/August 2008, accessed July 18, 2014, http://www.theatlantic.com/magazine/archive/2008/07 /is-google-making-us-stupid/306868/.

38 Salvatore Mannuzza et al., "Significance of Childhood Conduct Problems to Later Development of Conduct Disorder among Children with ADHD: A Prospective Follow-up Study," *Journal of Abnormal Child Psychology* 32, no. 5 (October 2004): 565–73.

39 Stephen Kaplan and Janet Frey Talbot, "Psychological Benefits of a Wilderness Experience," in *Behavior and the Natural Environment*, ed. Irwin Altman and Joachim F. Wohlwill (New York: Springer, 1983), 163–203, http://dx.doi .org/10.1007/978-1-4613-3539-9_6.

40 Frances E. Kuo and William C. Sullivan, "Aggression and Violence in the Inner City: Effects of Environment via Mental Fatigue," *Environment and Behavior* 33, no. 4 (July 1, 2001): 543–71, doi:10.1177/00139160121973124; Andrea Faber Taylor, Frances E. Kuo, and William C. Sullivan, "Coping with ADD: The Surprising Connection to Green Play Settings," *Environment and Behavior* 33, no. 1 (2001): 54–77; Andrea Faber Taylor and Frances E. Kuo, "Children With Attention Deficits Concentrate Better After Walk in the Park," *Journal of Attention Disorders* 12, no. 5 (March 1, 2009): 402–9, doi:10.1177/1087054708323000; Nancy M. Wells, "At Home with Nature: Effects of 'Greenness' on Children's Cognitive Functioning," *Environment and Behavior* 32, no. 6 (November 1, 2000): 775–95, doi:10.1177/00139160021972793.

41 Victoria Dunckley, "Computer, Video Games & Psychosis: Cause for Concern," *Psychology Today*, "Mental Wealth" (June 30, 2012), http://www.psychology today.com/blog/mental-wealth/201206/computer-video-games-psychosis -cause-concern.

42 Sean A. Spence, "Nintendo Hallucinations: A New Phenomenological Entity," *Irish Journal of Psychological Medicine* 10, no. 2, (June 1993): 98–99; R. Forsyth, R. Harland, and T. Edwards, "Computer Game Delusions," *Journal of the Royal Society of Medicine* 94, no. 4 (April 2001): 184–85; Konstantinos S. Bonotis, "Manifestations of Psychotic Symptomatology during Excessive Internet Use," *Psychology*

and Behavioral Sciences 2, no. 2 (2013): 28, doi:10.11648/j.pbs.20130202.12; Uri Nitzan et al., "Internet-Related Psychosis — A Sign of the Times," *The Israel Journal of Psychiatry and Related Sciences* 48, no. 3 (2011): 207–11.

43   Angelica B. Ortiz de Gortari and Mark D. Griffiths, "Altered Visual Perception in Game Transfer Phenomena: An Empirical Self-Report Study," *International Journal of Human-Computer Interaction* 30, no. 2 (September 25, 2013): 95–105, doi:10.10 80/10447318.2013.839900.

44   Margaret D. Weiss et al., "The Screens Culture: Impact on ADHD," *ADHD Attention Deficit and Hyperactivity Disorders* 3, no. 4 (September 24, 2011): 327–34, doi:10.1007/s12402-011-0065-z.

45   Marny R. Hauge and Douglas A. Gentile, "Video Game Addiction among Adolescents: Associations with Academic Performance and Aggression," Society for Research in Child Development Conference, 2003.

46   Michael A. Irvine et al., "Impaired Decisional Impulsivity in Pathological Videogamers," ed. Leonardo Fontenelle, *PLoS ONE* 8, no. 10 (October 16, 2013): e75914, doi:10.1371/journal.pone.0075914; Yen et al., "The Comorbid Psychiatric Symptoms of Internet Addiction."

47   Gentile et al., "Video Game Playing, Attention Problems, and Impulsiveness."

48   Craig A. Anderson et al., "Violent Video Game Effects on Aggression, Empathy, and Prosocial Behavior in Eastern and Western Countries: A Meta-Analytic Review," *Psychological Bulletin* 136, no. 2 (2010): 151–73, doi:10.1037/a0018251.

49   Lee, Lee, and Choi, "The Effects of Smartphone and Internet/Computer Addiction on Adolescent Psychopathology"; Valerie Carson, William Pickett, and Ian Janssen, "Screen Time and Risk Behaviors in 10- to 16-Year-Old Canadian Youth," *Preventive Medicine* 52, no. 2 (February 2011): 99–103, doi:10.1016/j .ypmed.2010.07.005.

50   Cheng-Fang Yen, Bryan H. King, and Tze-Chun Tang, "The Association between Short and Long Nocturnal Sleep Durations and Risky Behaviours and the Moderating Factors in Taiwanese Adolescents," *Psychiatry Research* 179, no. 1 (August 30, 2010): 69–74, doi:10.1016/j.psychres.2009.02.016.

51   Christopher P. Barlett, Richard J. Harris, and Ross Baldassaro, "Longer You Play, the More Hostile You Feel: Examination of First Person Shooter Video Games and Aggression during Video Game Play," *Aggressive Behavior* 33, no. 6 (December 2007): 486–97, doi:10.1002/ab.20227.

52   David R. Ewoldsen et al., "Effect of Playing Violent Video Games Cooperatively or Competitively on Subsequent Cooperative Behavior," *Cyberpsychology, Behavior, and Social Networking* 15, no. 5 (May 2012): 277–80, doi:10.1089 /cyber.2011.0308; Mike Schmierbach, "'Killing Spree': Exploring the Connection Between Competitive Game Play and Aggressive Cognition," *Communication Research* 37, no. 2 (April 1, 2010): 256–74, doi:10.1177/0093650209356394; Brad E. Sheese and William G. Graziano, "Deciding to Defect: The Effects of Video-Game Violence on Cooperative Behavior," *Psychological Science* 16, no. 5 (May 2005): 354–57, doi:10.1111/j.0956-7976.2005.01539.x; Tobias Greitemeyer, "Effects

of Prosocial Media on Social Behavior: When and Why Does Media Exposure Affect Helping and Aggression?," *Current Directions in Psychological Science* 20, no. 4 (August 1, 2011): 251–55, doi:10.1177/0963721411415229.

53   Schmierbach, "'Killing Spree': Exploring the Connection Between Competitive Game Play and Aggressive Cognition."

54   Council on Communications and Media, "Media Violence," *Pediatrics* 124, no. 5 (November 1, 2009): 1495–1503, doi:10.1542/peds.2009-2146.

55   L. Rowell Huesmann et al., "Longitudinal Relations between Children's Exposure to TV Violence and Their Aggressive and Violent Behavior in Young Adulthood: 1977–1992," *Developmental Psychology* 39, no. 2 (March 2003): 201–21; Daniel R. Anderson, "A Neuroscience of Children and Media?," *Journal of Children and Media* 1, no. 1 (February 1, 2007): 77–85, doi:10.1080/17482790601005215.

56   D. A. Gentile and W. Stone, "Violent Video Game Effects on Children and Adolescents: A Review of the Literature," *Minerva Pediatrica* 57, no. 6 (December 2005): 337–58.

57   Anderson et al., "Violent Video Game Effects on Aggression, Empathy, and Prosocial Behavior in Eastern and Western Countries"; Bruce D. Bartholow, Marc A. Sestir, and Edward B. Davis, "Correlates and Consequences of Exposure to Video Game Violence: Hostile Personality, Empathy, and Aggressive Behavior," *Personality and Social Psychology Bulletin* 31, no. 11 (November 1, 2005): 1573–86, doi:10.1177/0146167205277205; Douglas A. Gentile and Craig A. Anderson, "Violent Video Games: Effects on Youth and Public Policy Implications," in *Handbook of Children, Culture, and Violence,* eds. Nancy E. Dowd, Dorothy G. Singer, Robin F. Wilson (Thousand Oaks, CA: Sage, 2006), 225–46.

58   Christopher R. Engelhardt et al., "This Is Your Brain on Violent Video Games: Neural Desensitization to Violence Predicts Increased Aggression Following Violent Video Game Exposure," *Journal of Experimental Social Psychology* 47, no. 5 (September 2011): 1033–36, doi:10.1016/j.jesp.2011.03.027; Bruce D. Bartholow, Brad J. Bushman, and Marc A. Sestir, "Chronic Violent Video Game Exposure and Desensitization to Violence: Behavioral and Event-Related Brain Potential Data," *Journal of Experimental Social Psychology* 42, no. 4 (July 2006): 532–39, doi:10.1016/j.jesp.2005.08.006.

59   Nicholas L. Carnagey, Craig A. Anderson, and Brad J. Bushman, "The Effect of Video Game Violence on Physiological Desensitization to Real-Life Violence," *Journal of Experimental Social Psychology* 43, no. 3 (May 2007): 489–96, doi:10.1016/j.jesp.2006.05.003.

60   Patrick M. Markey and Charlotte N. Markey, "Vulnerability to Violent Video Games: A Review and Integration of Personality Research," *Review of General Psychology* 14, no. 2 (2010): 82–91, doi:10.1037/a0019000; Jan Frölich, Gerd Lehmkuhl, and Manfred Döpfner, [Computer games in childhood and adolescence: relations to addictive behavior, ADHD, and aggression], *Zeitschrift für Kinder- und Jugendpsychiatrie und Psychotherapie* 37, no. 5 (September 2009): 393–402; quiz 403–404, doi:10.1024/1422-4917.37.5.393.

61   J. L. Sherry, "The Effects of Violent Video Games on Aggression," *Human Com-munication Research* 27, no. 3 (2001): 409–31, doi:10.1111/j.1468-2958.2001 .tb00787.x; James D. Ivory and Sriram Kalyanaraman, "The Effects of Techno-logical Advancement and Violent Content in Video Games on Players' Feelings of Presence, Involvement, Physiological Arousal, and Aggression," *Journal of Com-munication* 57, no. 3 (September 2007): 532–55, doi:10.1111/j.1460-2466.2007 .00356.x; Christopher P. Barlett and Christopher Rodeheffer, "Effects of Realism on Extended Violent and Nonviolent Video Game Play on Aggressive Thoughts, Feelings, and Physiological Arousal," *Aggressive Behavior* 35, no. 3 (June 2009): 213–24, doi:10.1002/ab.20279.

62   Carson, Pickett, and Janssen, "Screen Time and Risk Behaviors in 10- to 16-Year-Old Canadian Youth"; Yuan-Sheng Yang et al., "The Association between Prob-lematic Cellular Phone Use and Risky Behaviors and Low Self-Esteem among Taiwanese Adolescents," *BMC Public Health* 10 (2010): 217, doi:10.1186/1471 -2458-10-217.

63   Carson, Pickett, and Janssen, "Screen Time and Risk Behaviors in 10- to 16-Year-Old Canadian Youth."

64   Yen, King, and Tang, "The Association between Short and Long Nocturnal Sleep Durations and Risky Behaviours and the Moderating Factors in Taiwanese Ado-lescents."

65   Chih-Hung Ko et al., "Predictive Values of Psychiatric Symptoms for Internet Addiction in Adolescents: A 2-Year Prospective Study," *Archives of Pediatrics & Adolescent Medicine* 163, no. 10 (October 2009): 937 –43, doi:10.1001/arch pediatrics.2009.159; Gentile et al., "Pathological Video Game Use Among Youths"; Randy A. Sansone and Lori A. Sansone, "Cell Phones: The Psychosocial Risks," *Innovations in Clinical Neuroscience* 10, no. 1 (January 2013): 33–37.

66   Richards et al., "Adolescent Screen Time and Attachment to Parents and Peers."

67   Chuan-bo Weng et al., "[A voxel-based morphometric analysis of brain gray mat-ter in online game addicts]," *Zhonghua yi xue za zhi* 92, no. 45 (December 4, 2012): 3221–23; Atsunobu Suzuki, "[Emotional functions of the insula]," *Brain and Nerve = Shinkei Kenkyo No Shinpo* 64, no. 10 (October 2012): 1103–12.

68   Sara H. Konrath, Edward H. O'Brien, and Courtney Hsing, "Changes in Disposi-tional Empathy in American College Students Over Time: A Meta-Analysis," *Personality and Social Psychology Review* 15, no. 2 (May 1, 2011): 180–98, doi:10.1177/1088868310377395.

69   Roy Pea et al., "Media Use, Face-to-Face Communication, Media Multitasking, and Social Well-Being among 8- to 12-Year-Old Girls," *Developmental Psychology* 48, no. 2 (March 2012): 327–36, doi:10.1037/a0027030.

70   Yalda T. Uhls et al., "Five Days at Outdoor Education Camp without Screens Im-proves Preteen Skills with Nonverbal Emotion Cues," *Computers in Human Behav-ior* 39 (October 2014): 387–92, doi:10.1016/j.chb.2014.05.036.

71   Rideout, Foehr, and Roberts, "Generation M2: Media in the Lives of 8- to 18-Year-Olds."

72 Dimitri Christakis, "Internet Addiction: A 21st Century Epidemic?," *BMC Medicine* 8, no. 1 (2010): 61; Gentile et al., "Pathological Video Game Use Among Youths."

73 Ivory and Kalyanaraman, "The Effects of Technological Advancement and Violent Content in Video Games on Players' Feelings of Presence, Involvement, Physiological Arousal, and Aggression."

74 Chuan-Bo Weng et al., "Gray Matter and White Matter Abnormalities in Online Game Addiction," *European Journal of Radiology* 82, no. 8 (August 2013): 1308–12, doi:10.1016/j.ejrad.2013.01.031; Kai Yuan et al., "Internet Addiction: Neuroimaging Findings," *Communicative & Integrative Biology* 4, no. 6 (2011): 637–39.

75 Fuchun Lin et al., "Abnormal White Matter Integrity in Adolescents with Internet Addiction Disorder: A Tract-Based Spatial Statistics Study," *PloS One* 7, no. 1 (2012): e30253, doi:10.1371/journal.pone.0030253.

76 Gentile et al., "Pathological Video Game Use Among Youths."

77 Aviv Weinstein and Abraham Weizman, "Emerging Association between Addictive Gaming and Attention-Deficit/hyperactivity Disorder," *Current Psychiatry Reports* 14, no. 5 (October 2012): 590–97, doi:10.1007/s11920-012-0311-x; Ko et al., "Predictive Values of Psychiatric Symptoms for Internet Addiction in Adolescents."

78 Paddock, "Bedtime Texting, Internet Use, Disturbs Sleep and Mood in Teens."

79 Lee, Lee, and Choi, "The Effects of Smartphone and Internet/Computer Addiction on Adolescent Psychopathology"; Kiyoko Kamibeppu and Hitomi Sugiura, "Impact of the Mobile Phone on Junior High-School Students' Friendships in the Tokyo Metropolitan Area," *Cyberpsychology & Behavior: The Impact of the Internet, Multimedia and Virtual Reality on Behavior and Society* 8, no. 2 (April 2005): 121–30, doi:10.1089/cpb.2005.8.121; Norihito Oshima et al., "The Suicidal Feelings, Self-Injury, and Mobile Phone Use After Lights Out in Adolescents," *Journal of Pediatric Psychology* 37, no. 9 (October 1, 2012): 1023–30, doi:10.1093/jpepsy/jss072.

80 "The Effect of Drugs on the Adolescent Brain," *SAMA Foundation, Science and Management of Addiction*, accessed July 19, 2014, http://samafoundation.org/youth-substance-addiction/effects-of-drugs-on-adolescent-brain/.

81 Geoffrey L. Ream, Luther C. Elliott, and Eloise Dunlap, "Playing Video Games While Using or Feeling the Effects of Substances: Associations with Substance Use Problems," *International Journal of Environmental Research and Public Health* 8, no. 12 (October 18, 2011): 3979–98, doi:10.3390/ijerph8103979.

82 Victoria Dunckley, "Case: OCD Precipitated by Wii Video Game," *Psychology Today*, "Mental Wealth" (September 16, 2012), http://www.psychologytoday.com/blog/mental-wealth/201209/case-ocd-precipitated-wii-video-game.

83 Michelle M. Garrison, Kimberly Liekweg, and Dimitri A Christakis, "Media Use and Child Sleep: The Impact of Content, Timing, and Environment," *Pediatrics* 128, no. 1 (July 2011): 29–35, doi:10.1542/peds.2010-3304.

84 Hjördís Osk Atladóttir et al., "Time Trends in Reported Diagnoses of Childhood Neuropsychiatric Disorders: A Danish Cohort Study," *Archives of Pediatrics*

& *Adolescent Medicine* 161, no. 2 (February 2007): 193–98, doi:10.1001 /archpedi.161.2.193.

85 "Tics and Tourette's — Tracing the True Triggers," *American Nutrition Association*, accessed November 4, 2013, http://americannutritionassociation.org /newsletter/tics-tourettes-tracing-true-triggers.

86 Christopher Mulligan, "The Toxic Relationship: Technology and Autism," 2012, http://www.teenvideogameaddiction.com/The_toxicrelationshipautismand technology.pdf.

87 Micah O. Mazurek and Christopher R. Engelhardt, "Video Game Use and Problem Behaviors in Boys with Autism Spectrum Disorders," *Research in Autism Spectrum Disorders* 7, no. 2 (February 2013): 316–24, doi:10.1016/j.rasd.2012.09.008; Micah O. Mazurek and Colleen Wenstrup, "Television, Video Game and Social Media Use Among Children with ASD and Typically Developing Siblings," *Journal of Autism and Developmental Disorders* 43, no. 6 (June 2013): 1258–71, doi:10.1007/s10803-012-1659-9.

88 Martha Herbert and Cindy Sage, "Findings in Autism (ASD) Consistent with Electromagnetic Fields (EMF) and Radiofrequency Radiation (RFR)," 2012, http://www.bioinitiative.org/report/wp-content/uploads/pdfs/sec20_2012 _Findings_in_Autism.pdf.

89 Brenda Nally, Bob Houlton, and Sue Ralph, "Researches in Brief: The Management of Television and Video by Parents of Children with Autism," *Autism* 4, no. 3 (September 1, 2000): 331–37, doi:10.1177/1362361300004003008.

90 Mazurek and Wenstrup, "Television, Video Game and Social Media Use Among Children with ASD and Typically Developing Siblings."

91 Micah O. Mazurek and Christopher R. Engelhardt, "Video Game Use in Boys with Autism Spectrum Disorder, ADHD, or Typical Development," *Pediatrics* 132, no. 2 (August 2013): 260–66, doi:10.1542/peds.2012-3956.

92 J. Melke et al., "Abnormal Melatonin Synthesis in Autism Spectrum Disorders," *Molecular Psychiatry* 13, no. 1 (May 15, 2007): 90–98.

93 Scott D. Tomchek and Winnie Dunn, "Sensory Processing in Children with and without Autism: A Comparative Study Using the Short Sensory Profile," *American Journal of Occupational Therapy* 61, no. 2 (2007): 190–200.

94 Michael Waldman, Sean Nicholson, and Nodir Adilov, *Does Television Cause Autism?* (National Bureau of Economic Research, 2006), http://www.nber.org /papers/w12632.

95 Herbert and Sage, "Findings in Autism (ASD) Consistent with Electromagnetic Fields (EMF) and Radiofrequency Radiation (RFR)."

96 Cris Rowan, "Unplug — Don't Drug: A Critical Look at the Influence of Technology on Child Behavior with an Alternative Way of Responding Other than Evaluation and Drugging," *Ethical Human Psychology and Psychiatry* 12, no. 1 (April 1, 2010): 60–68, doi:10.1891/1559-4343.12.1.60.

97 L. Strathearn, "Maternal Neglect: Oxytocin, Dopamine and the Neurobiology of Attachment," *Journal of Neuroendocrinology* 23, no. 11 (November 2011): 1054–65, doi:10.1111/j.1365-2826.2011.02228.x.

98 Thomas R. Insel, "Is Social Attachment an Addictive Disorder?," *Physiology &
    Behavior* 79, no. 3 (August 2003): 351–57, doi:10.1016/S0031-9384(03)00148-3.

99 Rowan, "Unplug — Don't Drug."

100 "Cartoon-Based Illness Mystifies Japan," *CNN World News*, December 17, 1997,
    http://www.cnn.com/WORLD/9712/17/japan.cartoon/.

101 John R. Hughes, "The Photoparoxysmal Response: The Probable Cause of
    Attacks during Video Games," *Clinical EEG and Neuroscience* 39, no. 1 (January
    2008): 1–7.

102 Jessica Solodar, "Commentary: ILAE Definition of Epilepsy," *Epilepsia* 55, no. 4
    (2014): 491, doi:10.1111/epi.12594.

Chapter 4: The Brain Liberated

1   Michael Shayer, Denise Ginsburg, and Robert Coe, "Thirty Years on — a Large
    Anti-Flynn Effect? The Piagetian Test Volume & Heaviness Norms 1975–
    2003," *British Journal of Educational Psychology* 77, no. 1 (March 2007): 25–41,
    doi:10.1348/000709906X96987.

2   Suzy Welch, *10-10-10: A Life Transforming Idea* (London: Simon & Schuster, 2009).

3   Carmi Schooler, "Environmental Complexity and the Flynn Effect," in *The Rising
    Curve: Long-Term Gains in IQ and Related Measures*, ed. Ulric Neisser (Washing-
    ton, DC: American Psychological Association, 1998), 67–79, http://content.apa
    .org/books/10270-002.

4   Shayer, Ginsburg, and Coe, "Thirty Years on — a Large Anti-Flynn Effect?"

5   Thomas W. Teasdale and David R. Owen, "Secular Declines in Cognitive Test
    Scores: A Reversal of the Flynn Effect," *Intelligence* 36, no. 2 (March 2008):
    121–26, doi:10.1016/j.intell.2007.01.007.

6   Dan J. Siegel, "An Interpersonal Neurobiology Approach to Psychotherapy,"
    Psychiatric Annals 36, no. 4 (April 1, 2006).

7   Christopher Mulligan, "The Toxic Relationship: Technology and Autism," 2012,
    http://www.tecnvideogameaddiction.com/The_toxicrelationshipautismand
    technology.pdf.

8   Heather L. Kirkorian et al., "The Impact of Background Television on Parent-
    Child Interaction," *Child Development* 80, no. 5 (October 2009): 1350–59,
    doi:10.1111/j.1467-8624.2009.01337.x; Rosalina Richards et al., "Adolescent Screen
    Time and Attachment to Parents and Peers," *Archives of Pediatrics & Adolescent
    Medicine* 164, no. 3 (March 2010): 258–62, doi:10.1001/archpediatrics.2009.280.

9   Adriano Schimmenti et al., "Attachment Disorganization and Dissociation in Vir-
    tual Worlds: A Study on Problematic Internet Use among Players of Online Role
    Playing Games," *Clinical Neuropsychiatry* 9, no. 5 (2012): 195–202.

10 Anne Fishel, *The Family Dinner Project*, FAQ page, accessed July 20, 2014,
    http://thefamilydinnerproject.org/resources/faq/.

11 Douglas A. Gentile et al., "Protective Effects of Parental Monitoring of Children's
    Media Use: A Prospective Study," *JAMA Pediatrics* 168, no. 5 (May 2014): 479–84,
    doi:10.1001/jamapediatrics.2014.146.

12 Dan J. Siegel, "An Interpersonal Neurobiology Approach to Psychotherapy."

Chapter 5: Week 1: Getting Ready

1   Warren Farrell, *Father and Child Reunion: How to Bring the Dads We Need to the Children We Love* (New York: Tarcher, 2001), 29–36.
2   R. Koestner, C. Franz, and J. Weinberger, "The Family Origins of Empathic Concern: A 26-Year Longitudinal Study," *Journal of Personality and Social Psychology* 58, no. 4 (April 1990): 709–17.
3   Farrell, *Father and Child Reunion*, 31, 55–56.
4   Jeffrey Masson, *The Emperor's Embrace: Reflections on Animal Families and Fatherhood* (New York: Atria Books, 2014), 38–44.
5   Aric Sigman, "The Impact of Screen Media on Children: A Eurovision for Parliament," *Improving the Quality of Childhood in Europe* 3 (2012): 88–121; Douglas A. Gentile et al., "Video Game Playing, Attention Problems, and Impulsiveness: Evidence of Bidirectional Causality," *Psychology of Popular Media Culture* 1, no. 1 (2012): 62–70, doi:10.1037/a0026969; Victoria Dunckley, "Gray Matters: Too Much Screen Time Damages the Brain," *Psychology Today*, "Mental Wealth" (February 27, 2014), http://www.psychologytoday.com/blog/mental -wealth/201402/gray-matters-too-much-screen-time-damages-the-brain.

Chapter 6: Weeks 2–4: The Electronic Fast

1   F. Waldhauser et al., "Serum Melatonin in Central Precocious Puberty Is Lower than in Age-Matched Prepubertal Children," *The Journal of Clinical Endocrinology and Metabolism* 73, no. 4 (October 1991): 793–96, doi:10.1210/jcem-73-4-793.
2   Rollin McCraty, Mike Atkinson, and William Tiller, "The Role of Physiological Coherence in the Detection and Measurement of Cardiac Energy Exchange Between People," in *Proceedings of the Tenth International Montreux Congress on Stress* (Montreux, Switzerland, 1999).

Chapter 7: Tracking and Troubleshooting

1   T. Morita and H. Tokura, "Effects of Lights of Different Color Temperature on the Nocturnal Changes in Core Temperature and Melatonin in Humans," *Applied Human Science: Journal of Physiological Anthropology* 15, no. 5 (September 1996): 243–46; M. R. Basso, "Neurobiological Relationships Between Ambient Lighting and the Startle Response to Acoustic Stress in Humans," *International Journal of Neuroscience* 110, no. 3–4 (January 1, 2001): 147–57, doi:10.3109/00207450108986542; Tomoaki Kozaki et al., "Effect of Color Temperature of Light Sources on Slow-Wave Sleep," *Journal of Physiological Anthropology and Applied Human Science* 24, no. 2 (March 2005): 183–86.
2   Mariana G. Figueiro and Mark S. Rea, "The Effects of Red and Blue Lights on Circadian Variations in Cortisol, Alpha Amylase, and Melatonin," *International Journal of Endocrinology* 2010 (2010): 1–9, doi:10.1155/2010/829351; Eva Chamorro et al., "Effects of Light-Emitting Diode Radiations on Human Retinal

Pigment Epithelial Cells in Vitro," *Photochemistry and Photobiology* 89, no. 2 (April 2013): 468–73, doi:10.1111/j.1751-1097.2012.01237.x.

3   Magda Havas, *Health Concerns Associated with Energy Efficient Lighting and Their Electromagnetic Emissions*, Scientific Committee on Emerging and Newly Indentified Health Risks (SCENIHR), (June 2008); Tatsiana Mironava et al., "The Effects of UV Emission from Compact Fluorescent Light Exposure on Human Dermal Fibroblasts and Keratinocytes *In Vitro*," *Photochemistry and Photobiology* 88, no. 6 (November 2012): 1497–1506, doi:10.1111/j.1751-1097.2012.01192.x; A. J. Wilkins et al., "Fluorescent Lighting, Headaches and Eyestrain," *Lighting Research and Technology* 21, no. 1 (March 1, 1989): 11–18, doi:10.1177/096032718902100102.

Chapter 9: Elimination vs. Moderation

1   Robert M. Pressman et al., "Examining the Interface of Family and Personal Traits, Media, and Academic Imperatives Using the Learning Habit Study," *The American Journal of Family Therapy* 42, no. 5 (October 20, 2014): 347–63, doi:10.10 80/01926187.2014.935684.

2   Douglas A. Gentile et al., "Protective Effects of Parental Monitoring of Children's Media Use: A Prospective Study," *JAMA Pediatrics* 168, no. 5 (May 2014): 479–84, doi:10.1001/jamapediatrics.2014.146.

3   "Media and Children," *American Academy of Pediatrics*, accessed July 20, 2014, http://www.aap.org/en-us/advocacy-and-policy/aap-health-initiatives/Pages/Media-and-Children.aspx.

Chapter 10: Everyday House Rules and Protective Practices

1   "Blue Light Has a Dark Side," *Harvard Health Publications*, May 2012, http://www.health.harvard.edu/staying-healthy/blue-light-has-a-dark-side; Sarah L. Chellappa et al., "Acute Exposure to Evening Blue-Enriched Light Impacts on Human Sleep," *Journal of Sleep Research* 22, no. 5 (October 2013): 573–80, doi:10.1111/jsr.12050.

2   "Blue Light Has a Dark Side."

3   Stéphanie van der Lely et al., "Blue Blocker Glasses as a Countermeasure for Alerting Effects of Evening Light-Emitting Diode Screen Exposure in Male Teenagers," *Journal of Adolescent Health* (January 2015), doi:10.1016/j.jadohealth .2014.08.002.

4   Dan J. Siegel, "An Interpersonal Neurobiology Approach to Psychotherapy," *Psychiatric Annals* 36, no. 4 (April 1, 2006).

5   David Meyer, *Multitasking and Task Switching* (Brain, Cognition, and Action Laboratory, University of Michigan, 2006), http://www.umich.edu/~bcalab/multitasking.html; Donald T. Stuss et al., "Dissociation within the Anterior Attentional System: Effects of Task Complexity and Irrelevant Information on Reaction Time Speed and Accuracy," *Neuropsychology* 16, no. 4 (2002): 500–13,

doi:10.1037//0894-4105.16.4.500; E. Ophir, C. Nass, and A. D. Wagner, "Cognitive Control in Media Multitaskers," *Proceedings of the National Academy of Sciences* 106, no. 37 (September 15, 2009): 15583–87, doi:10.1073/pnas.0903620106.

6   Stephen Kaplan, "The Restorative Benefits of Nature: Toward an Integrative Framework," *Journal of Environmental Psychology* 15, no. 3 (1995): 169–82; Andrea Faber Taylor and Frances E. Kuo, "Children With Attention Deficits Concentrate Better After Walk in the Park," *Journal of Attention Disorders* 12, no. 5 (March 1, 2009): 402–9, doi:10.1177/1087054708323000; Frances E. Kuo and William C. Sullivan, "Aggression and Violence in the Inner City: Effects of Environment via Mental Fatigue," *Environment and Behavior* 33, no. 4 (July 1, 2001): 543–71, doi:10.1177/00139160121973124; Nancy M. Wells, "At Home with Nature: Effects of 'Greenness' on Children's Cognitive Functioning," *Environment and Behavior* 32, no. 6 (November 1, 2000): 775–95, doi:10.1177/00139160021972793.

7   Kaplan, "The Restorative Benefits of Nature."

8   Wells, "At Home with Nature: Effects of 'Greenness' on Children's Cognitive Functioning"; Kuo and Sullivan, "Aggression and Violence in the Inner City: Effects of Environment via Mental Fatigue."

9   Rick Nauert, "Does Sunlight & Climate Influence Prevalence of ADHD?" *Psych Central*, October 22, 2013, http://psychcentral.com/news/2013/10/22/does-sunlight-climate-influence-prevalence-of-adhd/61026.html.

10 A. J. Lewy, R. L. Sack, and C. M. Singer, "Melatonin, Light and Chronobiological Disorders," *Ciba Foundation Symposium* 117 (1985): 231–52; Palmiero Monteleone, Vassilis Martiadis, and Mario Maj, "Circadian Rhythms and Treatment Implications in Depression," *Progress in Neuro-Psychopharmacology & Biological Psychiatry* 35, no. 7 (August 15, 2011): 1569–74, doi:10.1016/j.pnpbp.2010.07.028.

11 John J. Ratey and Eric Hagerman, *Spark: The Revolutionary New Science of Exercise and the Brain* (New York, NY: Little, Brown and Co., 2013), 3–5.

12 Stefanie L. Wells, "Moving Through the Curriculum: The Effect of Movement on Student Learning, Behavior, and Attitude," *Rising Tide* 5 (Summer 2012): 1–17.

13 Michelle A. Short et al., "Time for Bed: Parent-Set Bedtimes Associated with Improved Sleep and Daytime Functioning in Adolescents," *Sleep* 34, no. 6 (June 2011): 797–800, doi:10.5665/SLEEP.1052.

14 Peter Suedfeld, Janet Metcalfe, and Susan Bluck, "Enhancement of Scientific Creativity by Flotation REST (restricted Environmental Stimulation Technique)," *Journal of Environmental Psychology* 7, no. 3 (1987): 219–31.

15 Simerpreet Ahuja and Santha Kumari, "The Impact of Extended Video Viewing on Cognitive, Affective and Behavioral Processes in Preadolescents" (Ph.D. diss., School of Management and Social Sciences, Thapar University, Patiala, Punjab, India, 2009), 21–23.

16 Do-Hyung Kang et al., "The Effect of Meditation on Brain Structure: Cortical Thickness Mapping and Diffusion Tensor Imaging," *Social Cognitive and Affective Neuroscience* 8, no. 1 (January 2013): 27–33, doi:10.1093/scan/nss056.

17 Lisa Flook et al., "Effects of Mindful Awareness Practices on Executive Functions

in Elementary School Children," *Journal of Applied School Psychology* 26, no. 1 (February 9, 2010): 70–95, doi:10.1080/15377900903379125.

18 L. Strathearn, "Maternal Neglect: Oxytocin, Dopamine and the Neurobiology of Attachment," *Journal of Neuroendocrinology* 23, no. 11 (November 2011): 1054–65, doi:10.1111/j.1365-2826.2011.02228.x; Roy Pea et al., "Media Use, Face-to-Face Communication, Media Multitasking, and Social Well-Being among 8- to 12-Year-Old Girls," *Developmental Psychology* 48, no. 2 (March 2012): 327–36, doi:10.1037/a0027030.

19 Rosalina Richards et al., "Adolescent Screen Time and Attachment to Parents and Peers," *Archives of Pediatrics & Adolescent Medicine* 164, no. 3 (March 2010): 258–62, doi:10.1001/archpediatrics.2009.280; Adriano Schimmenti et al., "Attachment Disorganization and Dissociation in Virtual Worlds: A Study on Problematic Internet Use among Players of Online Role Playing Games," *Clinical Neuropsychiatry* 9, no. 5 (2012): 195–202; Douglas Gentile, "Pathological Video-Game Use among Youth Ages 8 to 18: A National Study," *Psychological Science* 20, no. 5 (May 2009): 594–602, doi:10.1111/j.1467-9280.2009.02340.x; Valerie Carson and Ian Janssen, "Neighborhood Disorder and Screen Time among 10–16 Year Old Canadian Youth: A Cross-Sectional Study," *The International Journal of Behavioral Nutrition and Physical Activity* 9 (2012): 66, doi:10.1186/1479-5868-9-66.

20 Helen Y. Weng et al., "Compassion Training Alters Altruism and Neural Responses to Suffering," *Psychological Science* 24, no. 7 (July 1, 2013): 1171–80, doi:10.1177/0956797612469537.

21 Barry Sanders, *A Is for Ox: The Collapse of Literacy and the Rise of Violence in an Electronic Age* (New York: Vintage Books, 1995).

22 Robert J. Rossi and Samuel C. Stringfield, "What We Must Do for Students Placed at Risk," *Phi Delta Kappan* 77, no. 1 (1995): 173–77; Colleen Cordes and Edward Miller, "Fool's Gold: A Critical Look at Computers in Childhood.," 2000, 28–39.

Chapter 11: School Daze

1 Aric Sigman, "Does Not Compute, Revisited: Screen Technology in Early Years Education," in *Too Much, Too Soon?*, ed. Richard House (Gloucestershire, England: Hawthorn Press, 2011), 265–89.

2 "How Smart Are Monkeys?" *The Tulane National Primate Research Center*, 2006, http://tulane.edu/tnprc/outreach/public-faq/#q20; Lindsay Nemelka, "Apps for Animals: iPads Used in Communicating with Apes, Dolphins," *Deseret News*, May 10, 2012, http://www.deseretnews.com/article/765575082/Apps-for-animals-iPads-used-in-communicating-with-apes-dolphins.html?pg=all.

3 Lex Borghans and Bas ter Weel, "Are Computer Skills the New Basic Skills? The Returns to Computer, Writing and Math Skills in Britain," *Labour Economics* 11, no. 1 (February 2004): 85–98, doi:10.1016/S0927-5371(03)00054-X.

4 Julia Parish-Morris et al., "Once Upon a Time: Parent-Child Dialogue and Storybook Reading in the Electronic Era: Preschool Reading in the Electronic Era,"

Mind, Brain, and Education 7, no. 3 (September 2013): 200–11, doi:10.1111 /mbe.12028; Weerasak Chonchaiya and Chandhita Pruksananonda, "Television Viewing Associates with Delayed Language Development," *Acta Pædiatrica* 97, no. 7 (2008): 977–82, doi:10.1111/j.1651-2227.2008.00831.x.

5   Association of Waldorf Schools of North America, "Why Waldorf Works — Frequently Asked Questions," accessed July 4, 2014, http://www.whywaldorfworks .org/02_W_Education/faq_about.asp.

6   Matt Richtel, "A Silicon Valley School That Doesn't Compute," *New York Times*, October 22, 2011, http://www.nytimes.com/2011/10/23/technology/at-waldorf -school-in-silicon-valley-technology-can-wait.html.

7   Nick Bilton, "Steve Jobs Was a Low-Tech Parent," *New York Times*, September 10, 2014, http://www.nytimes.com/2014/09/11/fashion/steve-jobs-apple-was -a-low-tech-parent.html.

8   Alicia Senauer Loge and Cheryl Charles, "Children's Contact with the Outdoors and Nature: A Focus on Educators and Educational Settings," Children and Nature Network (2012), http://www.childrenandnature.org/downloads/C&NN EducationBenefits2012.pdf; Nancy M. Wells, "At Home with Nature: Effects of 'Greenness' on Children's Cognitive Functioning," *Environment and Behavior* 32, no. 6 (November 1, 2000): 775–95, doi:10.1177/00139160021972793; Olga Jarrett, "A Researched-Based Case for Recess," US Play Coalition (November 2013), http://usplaycoalition.clemson.edu/resources/articles/13.11.5_Recess_final _online.pdf.

9   American Academy of Pediatrics, "Media and Children," accessed July 20, 2014, http://www.aap.org/en-us/advocacy-and-policy/aap-health-initiatives/Pages /Media-and-Children.aspx.

10 Adrian M. Owen et al., "Putting Brain Training to the Test," *Nature* 465, no. 7299 (June 10, 2010): 775–78, doi:10.1038/nature09042; Tamar Lewin, "No Einstein in Your Crib? Get a Refund," *New York Times*, October 23, 2009, http://www .nytimes.com/2009/10/24/education/24baby.html; Colleen Cordes and Edward Miller, "Fool's Gold: A Critical Look at Computers in Childhood," Alliance for Childhood, 2000, 28–39.

11 Cellular Phone Task Force, "Governments and Organizations That Ban or Warn against Wireless Technology," accessed July 20, 2014, http://www.cellphonetask force.org/?page_id=128; Lloyd Burrell, "WiFi Banned from Pre-School Childcare Facilities in a Bold Move by French Government," *Natural News*, January 29, 2014, http://www.naturalnews.com/043695_electrosensitivity_WiFi_French _government.html.

12 American Academy of Environmental Medicine, "Statement on WiFi in Schools," October 3, 2012, http://aaemonline.org/WiFischool.html.

13 Bonnie Rochman, "Pediatricians Say Cell Phone Radiation Standards Need Another Look," *Time*, July 20, 2012, http://healthland.time.com/2012/07/20 /pediatricians-call-on-the-fcc-to-reconsider-cell-phone-radiation-standards/.

14 Howard Blume, "Former L.A. Schools Chief Calls iPad Program Illegal," *LA*

Times, February 27, 2014, http://www.latimes.com/local/lanow/la-me-ln-former
-schools-chief-ipad-illegal-20140227-story.html.

15   Cornell University Ergonomics Web, "5 Tips for Using a Laptop Computer,"
accessed July 21, 2014, http://ergo.human.cornell.edu/culaptoptips.html; J.
Wahlstrom, "Ergonomics, Musculoskeletal Disorders and Computer Work," *Occupational Medicine* 55, no. 3 (March 9, 2005): 168–76, doi:10.1093/occmed/kqi083.

16   Diana DeStefano and Jo-Anne LeFevre, "Cognitive Load in Hypertext Reading: A Review," *Computers in Human Behavior* 23, no. 3 (May 2007): 1616–41,
doi:10.1016/j.chb.2005.08.012.

17   Sara Rimer, "A Campus Fad That's Being Copied: Internet Plagiarism Seems on
the Rise," *New York Times*, September 3, 2003, http://www.nytimes.com
/2003/09/03/nyregion/a-campus-fad-that-s-being-copied-internet-plagiarism
-seems-on-the-rise.html.

18   Thomas Fuchs and Ludger Woessman, "Computers and Student Learning: Bivariate and Multivariate Evidence on the Availability and Use of Computers at Home
and at School" (CESifo working papers, November 2004), http://www.econstor
.eu/handle/10419/18686.

19   Gemma Moss, Great Britain, and Department for Education and Skills, *The Interactive Whiteboards, Pedagogy and Pupil Performance Evaluation: An Evaluation of
the Schools Whiteboard Expansion (SWE) Project: London Challenge* (Nottingham:
DfES Publications, 2007).

20   BioInitiative 2012, "BioInitiative Report: A Rationale for a Biologically-Based
Public Exposure Standard for Electromagnetic Fields (ELF and RF),"2012,
http://www.bioinitiative.org/.

21   WiFi in Schools, "LAUSD Testimony," accessed July 21, 2014, http://www.wifi
inschools.com/lausd-testimony.html.

22   *Safe Schools 2012: Medical and Scientific Experts Call for Safe Technologies in
Schools*, Wifiinschools.org.uk, 2012, http://www.wifiinschools.org.uk/resources
/safeschools2012.pdf.

23   Ibid.

24   Parliamentary Assembly, Council of Europe, "Resolution 1815 (2011): The Potential Dangers of Electromagnetic Fields and Their Effect on the Environment"
(2011), http://www.assembly.coe.int/Mainf.asp?link=/Documents/Adopted
Text/ta11/ERES1815.htm.

25   D. M. Fenton and R. Penney, "The Effects of Fluorescent and Incandescent
Lighting on the Repetitive Behaviours of Autistic and Intellectually Handicapped
Children," *Journal of Intellectual and Developmental Disability* 11, no. 3 (January 1,
1985): 137–41, doi:10.3109/13668258508998632.

26   Lindsey Gruson, "Color Has a Powerful Effect on Behavior," *New York Times*,
October 19, 1982, http://www.nytimes.com/1982/10/19/science/color-has-a
-powerful-effect-on-behavior-researchers-assert.html.

27   Aaron E. Carroll et al., "Household Computer and Internet Access: The Digital
Divide in a Pediatric Clinic Population," *AMIA Annual Symposium Proceedings
Archive*, 2005, 111–15.

28   Larry Cuban, quoted in Valerie Strauss, "Magical Thinking about Technology in
      Education," *Washington Post*, March 21, 2013, http://www.washingtonpost.com
      /blogs/answer-sheet/wp/2013/03/21/magical-thinking-about-technology
      -in-education/.

29   Larry Cuban, quoted in Valerie Strauss, "The Problem with Evidenced-Based Ed-
      ucation Policy: The Evidence," *Washington Post*, April 10, 2014, http://www
      .washingtonpost.com/blogs/answer-sheet/wp/2014/04/10/the-problem
      -with-evidence-based-education-policy-the-evidence/; Larry Cuban, quoted in
      Stephanie McCrummen, "Some Educators Question if Whiteboards, other High-
      Tech Tools Raise Achievement," *Washington Post*, June 11, 2010, http://www
      .washingtonpost.com/wp-dyn/content/article/2010/06/10/AR2010061005522
      .html.

30   Learning Matters, "First to Worst," PBS, April 30, 2004, 14–15. Transcript ac-
      cessed at http://learningmatters.tv/images/blog/First.pdf.

31   Tara Ehrcke, "21st Century Learning Inc.," *Our Schools/Our Selves*, Winter 2013,
      accessed October 30, 2014, https://www.policyalternatives.ca/sites/default
      /files/uploads/publications/National%20Office/2013/02/0sos110_21st
      CenturyLearning_0.pdf.

32   Jacob Vigdor and Helen Ladd, *Scaling the Digital Divide: Home Computer Technol-
      ogy and Student Achievement*, National Center for Analysis of Longitudinal Data in
      Education Reseach (CALDER, The Urban Institute, June 2010), http://www
      .caldercenter.org/sites/default/files/CALDERWorkingPaper_48.pdf.

33   Fuchs and Woessman, "Computers and Student Learning: Bivariate and Multivar-
      iate Evidence."

34   Ofer Malamud and Cristian Pop-Eleches, "Home Computer Use and the Develop-
      ment of Human Capital" (National Bureau of Economic Research, March 2010),
      http://www.nber.org/papers/w15814.

35   Borghans and ter Weel, "Are Computer Skills the New Basic Skills?"

36   Frederick J. Zimmerman and Dimitri A. Christakis, "Children's Television View-
      ing and Cognitive Outcomes: A Longitudinal Analysis of National Data," *Archives
      of Pediatrics & Adolescent Medicine* 159, no. 7 (July 2005): 619–25, doi:10.1001/
      archpedi.159.7.619; Robert Weis and Brittany C. Cerankosky, "Effects of Video-
      Game Ownership on Young Boys' Academic and Behavioral Functioning: A Ran-
      domized, Controlled Study," *Psychological Science* 21, no. 4 (April 2010): 463–70,
      doi:10.1177/0956797610362670.

37   Dana Gioia, *To Read or Not to Read: A Question of National Consequence*, National
      Endowment for the Arts (DIANE Publishing, November 2007), http://arts.gov
      /sites/default/files/ToRead_ExecSum.pdf

38   Leonard Sax, *Boys Adrift the Five Factors Driving the Growing Epidemic of Unmo-
      tivated Boys and Underachieving Young Men* (New York: Basic Books, 2009), 8–9,
      53–57.

39   Laura E. Levine, Bradley M. Waite, and Laura L. Bowman, "Electronic Media
      Use, Reading, and Academic Distractibility in College Youth," *CyberPsychology &
      Behavior* 10, no. 4 (August 2007): 560–66, doi:10.1089/cpb.2007.9990.

40   Bernice E. Cullinan, "Independent Reading and School Achievement," *School Library Media Research* 3, no. 3 (2000).

41   Maria T. de Jong and Adriana G. Bus, "Quality of Book-Reading Matters for Emergent Readers: An Experiment with the Same Book in a Regular or Electronic Format," *Journal of Educational Psychology* 94, no. 1 (2002): 145–55, doi:10.1037/0022-0663.94.1.145.

42   Alison Garton, *Learning to Be Literate: The Development of Spoken and Written Language*, 2nd ed (Malden, MA: Blackwell, 1998).

43   Daniel R. Anderson and Tiffany A. Pempek, "Television and Very Young Children," *American Behavioral Scientist* 48, no. 5 (January 1, 2005): 505–22, doi:10.1177/0002764204271506; Gretchen Geng and Leigh Disney, "A Case Study: Exploring Video Deficit Effect in 2-Year-Old Children's Playing and Learning with an iPad," *Proceedings of the 21st International Conference on Computers in Education 2013* (Bali, Indonesia), http://espace.cdu.edu.au/view/cdu :40222.

44   Marie Evans Schmidt et al., "The Effects of Background Television on the Toy Play Behavior of Very Young Children," *Child Development* 79, no. 4 (August 2008): 1137–51, doi:10.1111/j.1467-8624.2008.01180.x; D. A. Christakis et al., "Early Television Exposure and Subsequent Attentional Problems in Children," *Pediatrics* 113, no. 4 (2004): 708–13.

45   Cris Rowan, "Ten Reasons to NOT Use Technology in Schools for Children under the Age of 12 Years," *Moving to Learn*, January 1, 2014, http://moving tolearn.ca/2014/ten-reasons-to-not-use-technology-in-schools-for-children -under-the-age-of-12-years.

46   William Klemm, "Biological and Psychology Benefits of Learning Cursive," *Psychology Today*, "Memory Medic" (August 5, 2013), http://www.psychologytoday .com/blog/memory-medic/201308/biological-and-psychology-benefits-learn ing-cursive.

47   Carrie B. Fried, "In-Class Laptop Use and Its Effects on Student Learning," *Computers & Education* 50, no. 3 (April 2008): 906–14, doi:10.1016/j.compedu.2006 .09.006.

48   Pam A. Mueller and Daniel M. Oppenheimer, "The Pen Is Mightier Than the Keyboard: Advantages of Longhand Over Laptop Note Taking," *Psychological Science*, April 23, 2014, doi:10.1177/0956797614524581.

49   Kevin Yamamoto, "Banning Laptops in the Classroom: Is It Worth the Hassles?" *Journal of Legal Education* 57 (2007): 477.

50   Cris Rowan, "The Impact of Technology on the Developing Child," *Huffington Post*, May 29, 2013, http://www.huffingtonpost.com/cris-rowan/technology -children-negative-impact_b_3343245.html.

51   Robert M. Pressman et al., "Examining the Interface of Family and Personal Traits, Media, and Academic Imperatives Using the Learning Habit Study," *The American Journal of Family Therapy* 42, no. 5 (October 20, 2014): 347–63, doi:10.10 80/01926187.2014.935684.

Chapter 12: From Grassroots to Global Awareness

1   Al Gore et al., *An Inconvenient Truth* (Hollywood, CA: Paramount, 2006).
2   Martin Fischer, *Fischerisms*, ed. Howard Fabing and Ray Marr (Springfield, IL: Charles C. Thomas, 1944).
3   Naomi Oreskes and Erik M. Conway, *Merchants of Doubt: How a Handful of Scientists Obscured the Truth on Issues from Tobacco Smoke to Global Warming* (New York: Bloomsbury Press, 2010).
4   Kelly D. Brownell and Kenneth E. Warner, "The Perils of Ignoring History: Big Tobacco Played Dirty and Millions Died. How Similar Is Big Food?" *Milbank Quarterly* 87, no. 1 (March 2009): 259–94, doi:10.1111/j.1468-0009.2009.00555.x.
5   Tara Ehrcke, "21st Century Learning Inc.," *Our Schools/Our Selves* Winter 2013, accessed October 30, 2014, https://www.policyalternatives.ca/sites/default/files/uploads/publications/National%20Office/2013/02/osos110_21stCentury Learning_0.pdf.
6   Victoria Dunckley, "Electronic Screen Syndrome: An Unrecognized Disorder?," *Psychology Today*, "Mental Wealth" (July 23, 2012), http://www.psychology today.com/blog/mental-wealth/201207/electronic-screen-syndrome-unrecog nized-disorder; "Gray Matters: Too Much Screen Time Damages the Brain," *Psychology Today*, "Mental Wealth" (February 27, 2014), http://www.psychology today.com/blog/mental-wealth/201402/gray-matters-too-much-screen-time -damages-the-brain; "Wired and Tired: Electronics and Sleep Disturbance in Children," *Psychology Today*, "Mental Wealth" (March 12, 2011), http://www .psychologytoday.com/blog/mental-wealth/201103/wired-and-tired-electronics -and-sleep-disturbance-in-children.
7   Aric Sigman, "The Impact of Screen Media on Children: A Eurovision for Parliament," *Improving the Quality of Childhood in Europe* 3 (2012): 88–121, www.ecswe .com/downloads/publications/QOC-V3/Chapter-4.pdf.
8   Richard Louv, *Last Child in the Woods: Saving Our Children from Nature-Deficit Disorder* (Chapel Hill, NC: Algonquin Books of Chapel Hill, 2008).
9   Cris Rowan, "10 Reasons Why Handheld Devices Should Be Banned for Children Under the Age of 12," *Huffington Post*, March 6, 2014, http://www.huffington post.com/cris-rowan/10-reasons-why-handheld-devices-should-be-banned_b _4899218.html.
10 William Knowlton Zinsser, *On Writing Well: The Classic Guide to Writing Nonfiction*, 7th ed. (New York: HarperCollins, 2006) p. 280.

Appendix B: Electromagnetic Fields (EMFs) and Health

1   L. Lloyd Morgan, Santosh Kesari, and Devra Lee Davis, "Why Children Absorb More Microwave Radiation than Adults: The Consequences," *Journal of Microscopy and Ultrastructure*, no. 0 (n.d.), doi:10.1016/j.jmau.2014.06.005; Leeka Kheifets et al., "The Sensitivity of Children to Electromagnetic Fields," *Pediatrics* 116, no. 2 (August 1, 2005): e303–13, doi:10.1542/peds.2004-2541.

2   Beverly Rubik, "The Biofield Hypothesis: Its Biophysical Basis and Role in Medi-
    cine," *Journal of Alternative & Complementary Medicine* 8, no. 6 (2002): 703–17.

3   Rubik, "The Biofield Hypothesis," 703–17.

4   Rollin McCraty and Mike Atkinson, "Influence of Afferent Cardiovascular Input
    on Cognitive Performance and Alpha Activity," in *Proceedings of the Annual Meet-
    ing of the Pavlovian Society* (Tarrytown, NY, 1999); Rollin McCraty, Mike Atkin-
    son, and William Tiller, "The Role of Physiological Coherence in the Detection
    and Measurement of Cardiac Energy Exchange Between People," in *Proceedings of
    the Tenth International Montreux Congress on Stress* (Montreux, Switzerland, 1999).

5   Sabine J. Regel et al., "Pulsed Radio-Frequency Electromagnetic Fields: Dose-
    Dependent Effects on Sleep, the Sleep EEG and Cognitive Performance," *Journal
    of Sleep Research* 16, no. 3 (2007): 253–58, doi:10.1111/j.1365-2869.2007.00603.x;
    Magda Havas, "Radiation from Wireless Technology Affects the Blood, the Heart,
    and the Autonomic Nervous System," *Reviews on Environmental Health* 28, no. 2–3
    (January 1, 2013), doi:10.1515/reveh-2013-0004.

6   Beverly Rubik, "Sympathetic Resonance Technology: Scientific Foundation and
    Summary of Biologic and Clinical Studies," *Journal of Alternative and Complemen-
    tary Medicine* 8, no. 6 (December 2002): 823–56, doi:10.1089/10755530260511838.

7   "BioInitiative Report: A Rationale for a Biologically-Based Public Exposure Stan-
    dard for Electromagnetic Fields (ELF and RF)," *BioInitiative* 2012, http://www
    .bioinitiative.org/.

8   Magda Havas, "Dirty Electricity Elevates Blood Sugar among Electrically Sen-
    sitive Diabetics and May Explain Brittle Diabetes," *Electromagnetic Biology and
    Medicine* 27, no. 2 (2008): 135–46, doi:10.1080/15368370802072075; Bogdan
    Lewczuk et al., "Influence of Electric, Magnetic, and Electromagnetic Fields on
    the Circadian System: Current Stage of Knowledge," *BioMed Research Interna-
    tional* 2014 (2014), doi:10.1155/2014/169459. Havas, "Radiation from Wireless
    Technology"; Regel et al., "Pulsed Radio-Frequency Electromagnetic Fields."

9   Martin Blank and Reba Goodman, "Electromagnetic Fields Stress Living Cells,"
    Pathophysiology: The Official Journal of the International Society for Pathophysiology
    16, no. 2–3 (August 2009): 71–78, doi:10.1016/j.pathophys.2009.01.006; Myrtill
    Simkó, "Cell Type Specific Redox Status Is Responsible for Diverse Electromag-
    netic Field Effects," *Current Medicinal Chemistry* 14, no. 10 (2007): 1141–52; Martin
    L. Pall, "Electromagnetic Fields Act via Activation of Voltage-Gated Calcium
    Channels to Produce Beneficial or Adverse Effects," *Journal of Cellular and Molec-
    ular Medicine* 17, no. 8 (August 2013): 958–65, doi:10.1111/jcmm.12088.

10 Leif G. Salford et al., "Nerve Cell Damage in Mammalian Brain after Exposure to
    Microwaves from GSM Mobile Phones," *Environmental Health Perspectives* 111, no.
    7 (June 2003): 881–83; discussion A408; Jacob L. Eberhardt et al., "Blood-Brain
    Barrier Permeability and Nerve Cell Damage in Rat Brain 14 and 28 Days after
    Exposure to Microwaves from GSM Mobile Phones," *Electromagnetic Biology and
    Medicine* 27, no. 3 (2008): 215–29, doi:10.1080/15368370802344037.

11 P. Esposito et al., "Acute Stress Increases Permeability of the Blood-Brain-Barrier

through Activation of Brain Mast Cells," *Brain Research* 888, no. 1 (January 5, 2001): 117–27; Theoharis C. Theoharides and Robert Doyle, "Autism, Gut-Blood-Brain Barrier, and Mast Cells:," *Journal of Clinical Psychopharmacology* 28, no. 5 (October 2008): 479–83, doi:10.1097/JCP.0b013e3181845f48.

12 Olle Johansson, "Electrohypersensitivity: State-of-the-Art of a Functional Impairment," *Electromagnetic Biology and Medicine* 25, no. 4 (2006): 245–58, doi:10.1080/15368370601044150.

13 Morgan, Kesari, and Davis, "Why Children Absorb More Microwave Radiation than Adults."

14 Eva Chamorro et al., "Effects of Light-Emitting Diode Radiations on Human Retinal Pigment Epithelial Cells in Vitro," *Photochemistry and Photobiology* 89, no. 2 (April 2013): 468–73, doi:10.1111/j.1751-1097.2012.01237.x; A. L. Mausset et al., "Effects of Radiofrequency Exposure on the GABAergic System in the Rat Cerebellum: Clues from Semi-Quantitative Immunohistochemistry," *Brain Research* 912, no. 1 (August 31, 2001): 33–46; Salford et al., "Nerve Cell Damage in Mammalian Brain"; Pall, "Electromagnetic Fields Act via Activation of Voltage-Gated Calcium Channels."

15 Sandro La Vignera et al., "Effects of the Exposure to Mobile Phones on Male Reproduction: A Review of the Literature," *Journal of Andrology* 33, no. 3 (June 2012): 350–56, doi:10.2164/jandrol.111.014373; Myung Chan Gye and Chan Jin Park, "Effect of Electromagnetic Field Exposure on the Reproductive System," *Clinical and Experimental Reproductive Medicine* 39, no. 1 (2012): 1, doi:10.5653/cerm.2012.39.1.1.

16 Conrado Avendaño et al., "Use of Laptop Computers Connected to Internet through WiFi Decreases Human Sperm Motility and Increases Sperm DNA Fragmentation," *Fertility and Sterility* 97, no. 1 (n.d.): 39–45.e2, accessed July 21, 2014, doi:10.1016/j.fertnstert.2011.10.012; "Laptops Can Cause 'Toasted Skin Syndrome': Medical Reports," *Sydney Morning Herald*, October 4, 2010, http://www.smh.com.au/digital-life/computers/laptops-can-cause-toasted-skin-syndrome-medical-reports-20101004-163li.html.

17 Yoon-Hwan Byun et al., "Mobile Phone Use, Blood Lead Levels, and Attention Deficit Hyperactivity Symptoms in Children: A Longitudinal Study," *PloS One* 8, no. 3 (2013): e59742, doi:10.1371/journal.pone.0059742; Tamir S. Aldad et al., "Fetal Radiofrequency Radiation Exposure From 800-1900 Mhz-Rated Cellular Telephones Affects Neurodevelopment and Behavior in Mice," *Scientific Reports* 2 (March 15, 2012), doi:10.1038/srep00312.

18 "BioInitiative Report: A Rationale for a Biologically-Based Public Exposure Standard."

19 Rubik, "The Biofield Hypothesis"; Eberhardt et al., "Blood-Brain Barrier Permeability and Nerve Cell Damage"; G. Franceschetti and I. Pinto, "Cell Membrane Nonlinear Response to an Applied Electromagnetic Field," *IEEE Transactions on Microwave Theory and Techniques*, 32, no. 7 (July 1984): 653–58, doi:10.1109/TMTT.1984.1132749; V. S. Rao et al., "Nonthermal Effects of

Radiofrequency-Field Exposure on Calcium Dynamics in Stem Cell-Derived Neuronal Cells: Elucidation of Calcium Pathways," *Radiation Research* 169, no. 3 (March 2008): 319–29, doi:10.1667/RR1118.1.

20 Lloyd Burrell, "WiFi Banned from Pre-School Childcare Facilities in a Bold Move by French Government," *Natural News*, January 29, 2014, http://www .naturalnews.com/043695_electrosensitivity_wifi_French_government.html; *Safe Schools 2012: Medical and Scientific Experts Call for Safe Technologies in Schools*, 2012, http://www.wifiinschools.org.uk/resources/safeschools2012.pdf; "WiFi in Schools Australia: Worldwide," *WiFi in Schools Australia*, accessed November 5, 2014, http://www.wifi-in-schools-australia.org/p/worldwide.html.

21 *Safe Schools 2012: Medical and Scientific Experts Call for Safe Technologies in Schools*.

22 *Resolution 1815 (2011): The Potential Dangers of Electromagnetic Fields and Their Effect on the Environment*, Parliamentary Assembly of Council of Europe (2011), http://www.assembly.coe.int/Mainf.asp?link=/Documents/AdoptedText/ta11 /ERES1815.htm.

23 "Statement on WiFi in Schools," *American Academy of Environmental Medicine*, October 3, 2012, http://aaemonline.org/wifischool.html.

24 Bonnie Rochman, "Pediatricians Say Cell Phone Radiation Standards Need Another Look," *Time*, July 20, 2012, http://healthland.time.com/2012/07/20 /pediatricians-call-on-the-fcc-to-reconsider-cell-phone-radiation-standards/; The American Academy of Pediatrics to the Federal Communications Commission and the US Food and Drug Administration, on proposed reassessment of exposure to radiofrequency electromagnetic fields limits and policies, August 29, 2013, http://apps.fcc.gov/ecfs/document/view?id=7520941318.

25 Martha Herbert and Cindy Sage, "Findings in Autism (ASD) Consistent with Electromagnetic Fields (EMF) and Radiofrequency Radiation (RFR)," *BioInitiative 2012* (2012), http://www.bioinitiative.org/report/wp-content/uploads /pdfs/sec20_2012_Findings_in_Autism.pdf; Byun et al., "Mobile Phone Use, Blood Lead Levels, and Attention Deficit."

26 Irva Hertz-Picciotto and Lora Delwiche, "The Rise in Autism and the Role of Age at Diagnosis," *Epidemiology* 20, no. 1 (January 2009): 84–90, doi:10.1097 /EDE.0b013e3181902d15.

27 Herbert and Sage, "Findings in Autism (ASD) Consistent with Electromagnetic Fields (EMF)."

28 Mustafa Emre et al., "Oxidative Stress and Apoptosis in Relation to Exposure to Magnetic Field," *Cell Biochemistry and Biophysics* 59, no. 2 (March 2011): 71–77, doi:10.1007/s12013-010-9113-0; Suchinda Jarupat et al., "Effects of the 1900MHz Electromagnetic Field Emitted from Cellular Phone on Nocturnal Melatonin Secretion," *Journal of Physiological Anthropology and Applied Human Science* 22, no. 1 (2003): 61–63; Eberhardt et al., "Blood-Brain Barrier Permeability and Nerve Cell Damage"; Salford et al., "Nerve Cell Damage in Mammalian Brain"; Blank and Goodman, "Electromagnetic Fields Stress Living Cells"; Rao et al., "Nonthermal

Effects of Radiofrequency-Field Exposure"; Lewczuk et al., "Influence of Electric, Magnetic, and Electromagnetic Fields on the Circadian System."

29   Chiara De Luca et al., "Metabolic and Genetic Screening of Electromagnetic Hypersensitive Subjects as a Feasible Tool for Diagnostics and Intervention," *Mediators of Inflammation* 2014 (2014): 924184, doi:10.1155/2014/924184; Johansson, "Electrohypersensitivity."

30   Johansson, "Electrohypersensitivity."

31   Patrick Levallois et al., "Study of Self-Reported Hypersensitivity to Electromagnetic Fields in California," *Environmental Health Perspectives* 110, Suppl 4 (August 2002): 619–23; Joerg Schrottner and Norbert Leitgeb, "Sensitivity to Electricity — Temporal Changes in Austria," *BMC Public Health* 8, no. 1 (2008): 310.

32   Board of the American Academy of Environmental Medicine, "Wireless Radiofrequency Radiation in Schools," November 14, 2013, http://aaemonline.org/docs/WiredSchools.pdf.

33   "Blue Light Has a Dark Side," Harvard Health Publications (May 1, 2012), accessed July 6, 2014, http://www.health.harvard.edu/newsletters/Harvard_Health_Letter/2012/May/blue-light-has-a-dark-side/; Chamorro et al., "Effects of Light-Emitting Diode Radiations on Human."

34   "Safer Use of Computers," *Create Healthy Homes*, accessed November 4, 2014, http://www.createhealthyhomes.com/safercomputers.php.

35   "Los Angeles Unified School District Removes Wi-Fi Routers from Classroom After Teacher Experiences Adverse Health Effects," *Stop Smart Meters Irvine*, October 10, 2014, http://stopsmartmetersirvine.com/2014/10/10/los-angeles-unified-school-district-removes-wi-fi-routers-from-classroom-after-teacher-experiences-adverse-health-effects/.

36   World Health Organization, "IARC Classifies Radiofrequency Electromagnetic Fields as Possibly Carcinogenic to Humans," press release no. 208, (May 31, 2011), www.iarc.fr/en/media-centre/pr/2011/pdfs/pr208_E.pdf.

INDEX

ABOUT THE AUTHOR

Victoria L. Dunckley, MD, is an integrative child, adolescent, and adult psychiatrist with more than fifteen years of clinical experience in the private and public health sectors. A regular consultant to schools, interdisciplinary treatment teams, and the courts, she specializes in working with children and families who have failed to respond to previous treatments, by utilizing environmental and lifestyle interventions, natural medicines, and conventional treatment strategies. She is a frequent media commentator and has appeared as a mental health expert on such media outlets as the *TODAY* show, *NBC Nightly News*, and the Investigation Discovery network. Dr. Dunckley has won numerous patient care awards, including the Patient's Choice Award and Compassionate Doctor Award by Vitals.com, and was recently recognized as one of "America's Top Psychiatrists" by the Consumers' Research Council of America.

Dr. Dunckley received her medical degree from Albany Medical College in New York and completed her adult and child psychiatry training at University of California at Irvine's Neuropsychiatric Institute. She is board-certified by the American Board of Psychiatry and Neurology, the American Academy of Child and Adolescent Psychiatry, and the American Board of Integrative Holistic Medicine. She is an active board member of Doctors for Safer Schools and is currently in private practice at the Centre for Life in Los Angeles. She blogs for *Psychology Today*.

For more information, see her websites at www.DrDunckley.com and www.ResetYourChildsBrain.com.

NEW WORLD LIBRARY is dedicated to publishing books and other media that inspire and challenge us to improve the quality of our lives and the world.

We are a socially and environmentally aware company. We recognize that we have an ethical responsibility to our customers, our staff members, and our planet.

We serve our customers by creating the finest publications possible on personal growth, creativity, spirituality, wellness, and other areas of emerging importance. We serve New World Library employees with generous benefits, significant profit sharing, and constant encouragement to pursue their most expansive dreams.

As a member of the Green Press Initiative, we print an increasing number of books with soy-based ink on 100 percent postconsumer-waste recycled paper. Also, we power our offices with solar energy and contribute to non-profit organizations working to make the world a better place for us all.

Our products are available in bookstores everywhere.

www.newworldlibrary.com

At NewWorldLibrary.com you can download our catalog,
subscribe to our e-newsletter, read our blog,
and link to authors' websites, videos, and podcasts.

Find us on Facebook, follow us on Twitter, and watch us on YouTube.

Send your questions and comments our way!
You make it possible for us to do what we love to do.

Phone: 415-884-2100 or 800-972-6657
Catalog requests: Ext. 10 | Orders: Ext. 52 | Fax: 415-884-2199
escort@newworldlibrary.com

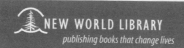
NEW WORLD LIBRARY
publishing books that change lives   14 Pamaron Way, Novato, CA 94949

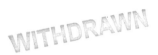

POWER & RIGHTS
IN US CONSTITUTIONAL LAW

Thomas Lundmark

OCEANA PUBLICATIONS, INC.
Dobbs Ferry, New York

Information contained in this work has been obtained by Oceana Publications from sources believed to be reliable. However, neither the Publisher nor its authors guarantee the accuracy or completeness of any information published herein, and neither Oceana nor its authors shall be responsible for any errors, omissions or damages arising from the use of this information. This work is published with the understanding that Oceana and its authors are supplying information, but are not attempting to render legal or other professional services. If such services are required, the assistance of an appropriate professional should be sought.

You may order this or any other Oceana publications by visiting Oceana's website at http://www.oceanalaw.com

Library of Congress Cataloging-in-Publication Data

Lundmark, Thomas.
    Power & rights in US constitutional law / by Thomas Lundmark.
        p. cm.
    Includes bibliographical references.
    ISBN 0-379-21439-3 (alk. paper)
    1. Constitutional law–United States. 2. Civil rights–United States.
    3. United States–Politics and government. I. Title: Power and rights
    in United States constitutional law. II. Title.

    KF4550.Z9 L86 2001
    342.73–dc21

                                                    2001034653

ISBN 0-379-21439-3 (alk. paper)